PUT PREVENTION INTO PRACTICE

Clinician's Handbook of Preventive Services

2nd Edition

U.S. DEPARTMENT OF HEALTH AND HUMAN SERVICES
PUBLIC HEALTH SERVICE
OFFICE OF PUBLIC HEALTH AND SCIENCE
OFFICE OF DISEASE PREVENTION AND HEALTH PROMOTION

1998

For sale by the U.S. Government Printing Office
Superintendent of Documents, Mail Stop: SSOP, Washington, DC 20402-9328
ISBN 0-16-049227-0

TABLE OF CONTENTS

INDEX

FOREWORD

It is my pleasure to present the second edition of the *Clinician's Handbook of Preventive Services*, an updated and expanded version of the original text. This handbook is the cornerstone of the Put Prevention Into Practice (PPIP) campaign. Since its introduction in 1994, PPIP has provided clinicians with helpful information and practical tools for adopting a non-categorical, systematic approach to the delivery of clinical preventive services. PPIP has been a welcome addition to many clinical practices, helping to improve the delivery of clinical preventive services.

Over the past 200 years, public health and preventive medicine efforts have dramatically improved health and well-being in the United States. Life expectancy has steadily increased, however, the vast majority of premature death and disability in our country results from preventable causes. Furthermore, unacceptable discrepancies in health and longevity between sub-populations still remain in our nation. Improved delivery of clinical preventive services can help resolve these descrepancies.

Unfortunately, barriers to the delivery of clinical preventive services continue to exist. Many missed opportunities for prevention can be attributed to the lack of a prevention plan and a reference resource for prevention. The *Clinicians's Handbook of Preventive Services* provides practical information for developing and implementing a prevention plan tailored to the needs of clinicians in a variety of settings. I hope this edition of the *Clinician's Handbook* will prove to be a useful tool for clinicians as they work to improve the health of all Americans.

Claude Earl Fox, M.D., M.P.H.
Deputy Assistant Secretary for Health
September 1997

Overview

i

INTRODUCTION

The *Clinician's Handbook of Preventive Services*, a practical and comprehensive guide to clinical preventive services, is the cornerstone of the Put Prevention Into Practice (PPIP) initiative. The goal of PPIP, which was developed by the US Public Health Service's Office of Disease Prevention and Health Promotion, is to enhance the delivery of clinical preventive services. This handbook discusses screening tests for early detection of disease, immunizations and prophylaxis to prevent disease, and counseling to modify risk factors that lead to disease.

The *Clinician's Handbook* is written for a wide variety of readers including health care providers, educators, students and health service administrators and planners. It can be used as a reference book for clinical preventive guidelines, or as a practical guide to delivering clinical preventive services and implementing a preventive care protocol. In addition, the *Clinician's Handbook* provides references for patient and provider educational materials and resources.

Organization

The *Clinician's Handbook* has been organized to facilitate quick reference. The main text is divided into two sections: preventive services for children/adolescents (up to age 18 years) and preventive services for adults/older adults. The overview chapters provide background information on topics such as: the basic epidemiologic principles of prevention, occupational and environmental considerations and the implementation of a preventive care protocol. In addition, several appendices provide supplementary information including timelines and risk factor tables (Appendix A); general information on immunizations, including information on reporting adverse effects (Appendix B); notifiable diseases (Appendix C); and a list of major authorities cited (Appendix D).

The Children and Adolescents and Adults and Older Adults sections are divided into three subsections: (1) screening guidelines, (2) immunization and prophylaxis recommendations, and (3) counseling information.

Chapters are broken down into six subsections. Each chapter is organized in the following format:

1. A brief introduction describing the burden of suffering of the disease, risk factors, and the effectiveness of the preventive intervention.

2. A summary of the recommendations of major authorities.

3. Technical information describing how to perform each preventive service.

4. A resource list for patients—pamphlets, books, videotapes, and other materials that can be provided to patients for reinforcement of health messages.

5. A resource list for providers—information for supplemental reading on each topic.

6. Selected (bibliographic) references—references used in the chapter.

Content

The criterion for inclusion of a preventive service in the *Clinician's Handbook* is a recommendation for its routine use in the care of asymptomatic persons by a major US authority such as: a Federal health agency (eg, Centers for Disease Control and Prevention, National Institutes of Health), a non-Federal expert panel (eg, US Preventive Services Task Force), a national professional organization (eg, American Academy of Family Physicians, American Academy of Pediatrics), or a national voluntary health organization (eg, American Cancer Society, American Heart Association). Recommendations of the Canadian Task Force on the Periodic Health Examination have also been included.

Because the *Clinician's Handbook* focuses on preventive care for the general population without special risk factors, the following types of preventive care have not been included: tertiary prevention (treatment to prevent progression of known disease), prenatal and perinatal care, and preventive care for certain high-risk groups. Preventive services not recommended by at least one major authority have been excluded. However, the exclusion of a medical procedure does not suggest that it is ineffective in diagnosing and treating disease. The clinician should exercise judgement on a case-by-case basis with respect to preventive services not addressed in the *Clinician's Handbook*.

Every effort has been made to ensure that recommendations of major authorities listed in each chapter accurately represent the current positions of these authorities. Recommendations are listed alphabetically by organization. Similar recommendations are often grouped together to facilitate comparisons by the reader. Appearance in the *Clinician's Handbook* does not imply that either the US Department of Health and Human Services or the Public Health Service endorses a specific authority or its recommendations; clinicians are encouraged to consult the references provided to evaluate the scientific basis for each organization's recommendations. Similarly, the citation of a group's recommendations does not imply that the group has endorsed the *Clinician's Handbook* or its contents.

The "Basics" of providing services sections were derived from a compilation of sources, including expert opinion. In many instances, the recommendations of major authorities, as well as expert researchers, were combined.

The items listed in the "Patient and Provider Resource" sections of the chapters have been selected after an extensive review of materials solicited from government agencies and professional and voluntary organizations. However, this list is not exhaustive and there are undoubtedly other, equally useful publications that have not been included. The materials listed provide a starting point for clinicians to build a library of high-quality literature and resources for themselves and their patients. The individual clinician must determine the appropriateness of each material in any specific case.

The publications listed in the "Selected References" sections were chosen because of their use in preparing the chapters and their potential usefulness to the clinician. These lists are not intended to be a comprehensive bibliography of the literature, but provide a core set of references for the reader.

No single set of preventive services is appropriate for all patients in all settings. The *Clinician's Hand book* is designed to facilitate the design and implementation of a preventive care program for practices of all sizes and types. Chapter ii discusses the principles of prevention, such as general principles of screening, immunizations, and counseling. This information, when combined with the more specific recommendations of authorities, relevant patient risk factors given in each chapter, and the summary risk-factor tables in Appendix A, should help clinicians select a set of preventive services appropriate for their patients and practice. Chapter iv provides practical information on establishing and implementing a preventive care protocol.

A goal of the *Clinician's Handbook* is to describe areas of consensus among the recommendations of major authorities regarding clinical preventive services. Important clinical differences in recommendations are reflected. However, the differences in the processes by which authorities arrived at their recommendations are not described. Some recommendations of major authorities are based strictly on expert opinion and others incorporate evidenced-based approaches. Names and addresses of all major authorities cited are listed in Appendix D and readers are encouraged to contact the organization to ascertain how guidelines were formulated.

Sources

The data for the *Clinician's Handbook* were obtained from scientific literature identified by searching computerized data bases and reference lists of primary sources; policy statements and position papers issued by government agencies, professional groups, and voluntary associations; educational brochures, booklets, and other materials from government agencies, professional groups, and voluntary associations; and consultation with experts.

The National Coordinating Committee on Clinical Preventive Services

Oversight of the Put Prevention Into Practice campaign is provided by the National Coordinating Committee on Clinical Preventive Services (NCCCPS). The NCCCPS was formed in 1989 to accelerate the integration of clinical preventive services into primary care delivery in the United States. Members of this group provided extensive review of the Put Prevention Into Practice materials during their development. NCCCPS member organizations include:

Ambulatory Pediatric Association
American Academy of Family Physicians
American Academy of Pediatrics
American Academy of Physician Assistants
American Association of Colleges of Nursing
American Association of Health Plans
American College of Obstetricians and Gynecologists
American College of Occupational and Environmental Medicine
American College of Physicians
American College of Preventive Medicine
American Hospital Association
American Medical Association
American Nurses Association
American Osteopathic Association
American Osteopathic College of Occupational and Preventive Medicine
American Public Health Association
Association of Academic Health Centers
Association of American Medical Colleges
Association of Health Services Research
Association of Schools of Public Health
Association of State and Territorial Health Officials
Association of Teachers of Preventive Medicine
Blue Cross Blue Shield Association
Institute of Medicine
National Alliance of Nurse Practitioners
National Association of Community Health Centers

National Association of County and City Health Officials
North American Primary Care Research Group
Society of General Internal Medicine
Society for Public Health Education
Society of Teachers of Family Medicine

Federal Liaisons to the National Coordinating Committee on Clinical Preventive Services

Department of Health and Human Services
   Agency for Health Care Policy and Research
   Centers for Disease Control and Prevention
   Food and Drug Administration
   Indian Health Service
   Health Resources and Services Administration
   Health Care Financing Administration
   National Institutes of Health
   Office of the Assistant Secretary for Planning and Evaluation
   Substance Abuse Mental Health Services Administration
Department of Defense
Department of Transportation
   US Coast Guard
Department of Veterans Affairs
Office of Personnel Management

Review

The chapters of this book have been reviewed for scientific accuracy by experts in the following divisions in the Department of Health and Human Services:

Administration for Children and Families
Agency for Health Care Policy and Research
Administration on Aging
Centers for Disease Control and Prevention
Food and Drug Administration
Health Care Financing Administration
Health Resources and Services Administration
Indian Health Service
National Institutes of Health
Office of HIV/AIDS Policy
Office of Minority Health
Office of Population Affairs
Office of the Surgeon General
Office on Women's Health
Substance Abuse and Mental Health Services Administration

Acknowledgments

Preparation of this *Clinician's Handbook of Preventive Services* was coordinated by staff in the Office of Disease Prevention and Health Promotion, Office of Public Health and Science, US Department of Health and Human Services, under the general supervision of Claude Earl Fox, III, MD, MPH, Deputy Assistant Secretary for Health (Disease Prevention and Health Promotion).

Principal staff responsible for the preparation of this edition were:

Rika Maeshiro, MD, MPH, Co-Editor
Lynn M. Soban, MPH, RN, Project Coordinator and Co-Editor

Other staff members of the Office of Disease Prevention and Health Promotion who contributed to the preparation of this edition were:

David R. Baker
Kate-Louise Gottfried, JD, MSPH
Kathryn McMurry, MS
Linda D. Meyers, PhD
Janice T. Radak
Mark Smolinski, MD, MPH

Valuable research and writing contributions were made by the following preventive medicine residents during rotations at the Office of Disease Prevention and Health Promotion:

Liz Ribadenyra, MD   University of Maryland
Annette Kussmaul, MD   State University of New York at Stony Brook
Tamera Coyne-Beasley, MD   University of North Carolina, Chapel Hill
Margaret Savage, MD   Johns Hopkins University
Ron Hale, MD   Johns Hopkins University
Allen Brinker, MD   University of Maryland
Renee Kanan, MD   University of Washington
Robert A. Gilchick, MD   San Diego State University/University of
                                     California, San Diego
Shelley Levesque, MD   University of Massachusetts Medical Center
Linda E. Hertz, MD   University of South Carolina

Special thanks to the following individuals and organizations for their contributions:

Larry L. Dickey, MD, MPH, Chief, Office of Clinical Preventive Medicine, California Department of Health Services, who updated the Recommendations of Major Authorities;

Bradley Evanoff, MD, MPH, Assistant Professor, Section of Occupational and Environmental Medicine, Department of Medicine, Washington University

School of Medicine, St. Louis, Missouri, who prepared the chapter on Occupational and Environmental Exposures;

Crystal Wilkinson, MSN, RN, CNS, Texas Department of Health, who prepared the chapter on Implementing a Preventive Care Protocol;

The American Society of Clinical Pathologists for their contributions to the chapter on Papanicolaou Smear Screening.

Other contributors included:

Jacqelyn B. Admire, MSPH
Patti Auer, RN, MSN
Susan Bradford
Cheri Hahn, MS, RN
Melissa Koenig

Tammy L. Lin, MD
Rosemarie Perrin
Kristine Samson
Yu Ning Wong

Acknowledgments for the First Edition of the Clinician's Handbook of Preventive Services

Preparation of the *Clinician's Handbook of Preventive Services* was coordinated by staff in the Office of Disease Prevention and Health Promotion, Public Health Services, US Department of Health and Human Services, under the general supervision J. Michael McGinnis, MD, Deputy Assistant Secretary for Health (Disease Prevention and Health Promotion). Principal staff responsible for the preparation of this book were:

Larry L. Dickey, MD, MPH, Luther Terry Senior Fellow
(Scientific editor and principal writer)

Hurdis M. Griffith, PhD, RN, Senior Policy Advisor
(review coordinator and writer)

Douglas B. Kamerow, MD, MPH, Director, Clinical Preventive Services Staff
(managing editor)

Other staff members of the Office of Disease Prevention and Health Promotion who contributed to preparation of this book were:

David R. Baker
Rachel Ballard-Barbash, MD, MPH.
Elena Carbone, MS, RD
Carolyn DiGuiseppi, MD, MPH
Walter H. Glinsman, MD

Linda D. Meyers, PhD
Janice T. Radak
Susan Simmons, RN, PhD
Marilyn G. Stephenson, MS, RD

Valuable research and writing contributions were made by the following preventive medicine residents from Johns Hopkins University and the University of Maryland during rotations at the Office of Disease Prevention and Health Promotion.

Robert Beardall, MD, MPH
Karen S. Collins, MD, MPH
Paul Denning, MD, MPH
Tina Farup, MD
Clarice Green, MD
Lana Jeng, MD, MPH

S. Patrick Kachur, MD, MPH
Cynthia Mobley, MD, MPH
Peter W. Pendergrass, MD, MPH
Donald Robinson, MD, MPH
William Schluter, MD
Suzanne Steinberg, MD

Material on preventive services for older adults was researched and prepared by fellows of the Multi campus Division of Geriatric Medicine and Gerontology at the University of California, Los Angeles (listed below). David B. Reuben, MD was supervising editor for this component of *Clinician's Handbook* preparation.

Nelson C. Apostol, MD
Christopher J. Bula, MD
Russel E. Hoxie, MD
David Kelley, MD
Michael E. Lim, MD
Matthew K. McNabney, MD
Alison A. Moore, MD
Michael Temporal, MD
Emil Yagudin, MD
Michael P. Zeitlin, MD

Assistance in researching and preparing the chapters on sexually transmitted diseases was provided by C. Patrick Chaulk, MD, MPH, Johns Hopkins School, of Hygiene and Public Health.

Copy editor was Barbara Ravage.

ii

CONCEPTS OF PREVENTION

"Clinicians should be selective in ordering tests and providing preventive services."[1]

This chapter introduces fundamental aspects of preventive services, including the epidemiologic principles that help influence decisions regarding the appropriateness of preventive services, the concepts that help determine the usefulness of screening tests, guidance for counseling patients, and an examination of prevention at the community or population level.

General Clinical Preventive Services

The primary and secondary clinical preventive services presented in the *Clinician's Handbook* target asymptomatic persons based on individual risk profiles. The basic epidemiologic principles used to develop preventive services guidelines also provide the context in which to consider these general recommendations and their relevance to particular populations, communities, and patients. The following questions have been adapted from Woolf (1996) for clinicians to consider when prioritizing their assessment of risk factors that can increase a patient's potential for future disease. These questions can be applied to all clinical preventive services:

- How important is the target condition?
- How important is the risk factor?
- Is the preventive service effective?
- How accurately can the risk factor or target condition be identified?

How important is the target condition?

The *target condition* is the health or disease outcome that the preventive care intervention avoids (primary prevention) or identifies early (secondary prevention). The *frequency* and the *severity* of target conditions help define their importance. The *frequency* of a target condition is usually measured by its *incidence rate* and *prevalence rate* (Key Concepts 1).

---

[1]A principal finding of the US Preventive Services Task Force from US Preventive Services Task Force. *Guide to Clinical Preventive Services. 2nd ed. Washington, DC: US Department of Health and Human Services; 1996: chap xxix-xxxii.*

Key Concepts 1

$$\text{\textit{Incidence Rate} during a given time period} = \frac{\text{number of new cases of a target condition during the given time period}}{\text{population at risk for developing the target condition during the given time period}}$$

The denominator, "population at risk for developing the target condition," does not refer to any specific high risk group, but includes all members of the population of interest whose probability of becoming a *new* case is greater than zero. Thus, if one is studying the annual incidence of HIV seropositivity among US adolescent males, then the population at risk for developing the target condition (HIV seropositivity) includes all adolescent males residing in the US, **with the exception of those who are already HIV positive prior to the beginning of the time period.** One cannot become a *new* case of HIV seropositivity if one is already HIV positive prior to the start of the time period.

EXAMPLE: In a year, there are an estimated 1,500,000 new or recurrent episodes of coronary attacks* among 101,570,000 Americans age 29 years and over. The annual incidence of new or recurrent coronary attacks* among Americans aged 29 years and over is

$$\frac{1,500,000}{101,570,000} = .015 = 1.5\%.$$

Each year, 15 of every 1000 Americans age 29 years and over (1.5%) has a new or recurrent episode of coronary attack.*

$$\text{\textit{Prevalence Rate} during a given time} = \frac{\text{total number of new cases (new and old) of a target condition at the given time}}{\text{total population at the given time}}$$

EXAMPLE: In 1994, approximately 13,670,000 out of 185,390,000 Americans age 20 years and over had a history of coronary heart disease.* The prevalence of coronary heart disease* among Americans age 20 years and over in 1994 is

$$\frac{13,670,000}{185,390,000} = .074 = 7.4\%.$$

In 1994, 74 of every 1000 Americans age 20 years and over (7.4%) had a history of coronary heart disease.*

---

*Both terms, "coronary attack" and "coronary heart disease," refer to a group of diagnoses under the general heading of ischemic heart disease, specifically ICD-9 410-414.

Source: American Heart Association. *1997 Heart and Stroke Statistical Update.* Dallas, Tex: American Heart Association; 1996.

The *severity* of a target condition can be described by several measures: mortality, morbidity, and survival rates. Target conditions with higher frequencies in specific populations, as well as conditions of greater severity, may merit greater preventive attention.

How important is the risk factor?

Risk factors are the attributes associated with target conditions. They can help predict outcomes but may not cause the target condition. Risk factors include demographic variables, such as gender, ethnicity, or age; behavioral risk factors, such as smoking or driving without seatbelts; and environmental factors, such as the area of residence. Ascertaining the presence or absence of risk factors (*risk assessment)* is accomplished through thorough patient histories, targeted examinations, and laboratory tests. Specific health risk appraisal tools have also been developed to ascertain risk status (chapter iv).

The *frequency* and *magnitude* of risks contribute to their importance. The *frequency* of risk factors are also described by their *incidence* and *prevalence* in the population of interest (Key Concepts 2).

Key Concepts 2

$$\text{\textit{Incidence Rate} during a given time period} = \frac{\text{number of new individuals exhibiting the risk factor during the given time period}}{\text{population at risk for developing the risk factor in the given time period}}$$

EXAMPLE: In 1995, approximately 4.5 million out of 22.2 million youths age 12-17 were current smokers. If approximately 1 million youths become smokers annually, the annual incidence rate of smoking among youths age 12-17 is

$$\frac{1,000,000 \text{ new smoking youths}}{17,700,000^* \text{ million non-smoking youths}} = .056 = 5.6\%$$

In 1995, 56 of every 1000 youths ages 12 to 17 (5.6%) who had not been smokers began to smoke.

*The 17.7 million nonsmoking youths are calculated by subtracting the already smoking youths from the total population of 12 to 17 year old youths (22.2 million − 4.5 million).

$$\text{Prevalence Rate at a given time period} = \frac{\text{total number of individuals exhibiting the risk factor at the given time}}{\text{total population at the given time}}$$

EXAMPLE: In 1995, approximately 56.4 million of the 189.3 million adults age ≥18 years were current cigarette smokers. The prevalence of current cigarette smoking in the United States among adults age ≥18 years is

$$\frac{56,400,000 \text{ million current adult smokers} \geq 18 \text{ years}}{189,300,000 \text{ million adults} \geq 18 \text{ years}} = 0.298 = 29.8\%$$

In 1995, 298 of every 1000 Americans age 18 years or older (29.8%) were current smokers.

Source: Substance Abuse and Mental Health Services Administration, US Department of Health and Human Services. *Preliminary Estimates from the 1995 National Household Survey on Drug Abuse.* Rockville, Md: Substance Abuse and Mental Health Services Administration, US Department of Health and Human Services; 1995.

The *magnitude* of risk helps to quantify the association between the risk factor and the target condition. Because a variety of risk measures exist, clinicians need to be aware that there are important differences between these risk measures and their implications for disease prevention. An understanding of basic risk measures may aid clinicians in interpreting risks for their patients (Key Concepts 3).

Key Concepts 3

The *absolute risk* is the incidence of the target condition in the population with the risk factor.

EXAMPLE: Out of 1000 men who smoke, 172 will develop lung cancer. The absolute risk for lung cancer in men who smoke is 172/1000 = .172 = 17.2%.

The *relative risk* ratio is the ratio of the incidence of disease among persons with the risk factor to the incidence of disease among those without the risk factor. Relative risk does not measure the probability that any given person with the risk factor will develop the condition.

EXAMPLE: The risk of death from lung cancer in men who smoke is 341.3 deaths per 100,000 person years. The risk of death from lung cancer in men who do not smoke is 14.7 deaths per 100,000 person years. The relative risk of death from lung cancer in men who smoke is

$$\frac{341.3 \text{ deaths from lung cancer per 100,000 person years}}{14.7 \text{ deaths from lung cancer per 100,000 person years}} = 23.2$$

Men who smoke have 23.2 times the risk of dying from lung cancer of men who do not smoke.

The *attributable risk* measures the amount of risk that can be attributed to one particular risk factor and is calculated by subtracting the incidence rate of the population without the factor from the incidence rate among the population with the factor. The *excess* amount experienced by the exposed group represents the attributable risk.

EXAMPLE: The attributable risk for death from lung cancer that is associated
with smoking is

$$\begin{array}{r} 341.3 \text{ deaths from lung cancer per } 100{,}000 \text{ person years} \\ -\ \underline{14.7 \text{ deaths from lung cancer per } 100{,}000 \text{ person years}} \\ 326.6 \end{array}$$

Of the 341.3 lung cancers occurring in smokers, 326.6 can be attributed to smoking.

Source: Office on Smoking and Health, National Center for Chronic Disease Prevention and Health Promotion, Centers for Disease Control and Prevention; US Department of Health and Human Services.

Is the preventive service effective?

The strongest quality of scientific evidence to evaluate the effects of preventive services comes from well designed intervention studies and observational studies that link risk modification with improved outcomes. Many major authorities rely on scientific evidence to guide their recommendations. The US Preventive Services Task Force (USPSTF), a body of preventive care experts convened by the US Public Health Service, has developed a system for rating the quality of scientific evidence used in its deliberations. The USPSTF rating system for grading scientific evidence is given in Table ii.1.

Table ii.1. US Preventive Services Task Force Rating System of Quality of Scientific Evidence

I:	Evidence obtained from at least one properly designed randomized controlled trial
II-1:	Evidence obtained from well-designed controlled trials without randomization
II-2:	Evidence obtained from well-designed cohort or case-control analytic studies, preferably from more than one center or research group
II-3:	Evidence obtained from multiple time series with or without the intervention, or dramatic results in uncontrolled experiments (such as the results of the introduction of penicillin treatment in the 1940s)
III:	Opinions of respected authorities, based on clinical experience, descriptive studies, or reports of expert committees

From: US Preventive Services Task Force. Task Force Ratings. *Guide to Clinical Preventive Services*. Washington, DC: US Department of Health and Human Services; 1996:862.

Even with good evidence that an intervention is *efficacious* (the intervention results in true effects under ideal conditions), the intervention may be less *effective* in a routine practice setting. Potential benefits of a preventive intervention must be weighed against potential harms, costs, and implementation considerations.

Recently, *outcome measures* have been developed incorporating quality-of-life measures that attempt to capture functional status and preference as outcomes of clinical interventions, including preventive services. *Quality-adjusted life-years* and *disability-adjusted life-years* are measures that attempt to standardize quantitative and qualitative information into summary measures that can be used to compare various conditions and outcomes for different prevention strategies.

Unfortunately, for most of medical practice, there is insufficient evidence that a service is or is not effective in improving process or outcome measures. Therefore, decision-makers at the policy and at the clinical level often need to consider factors other than scientific evidence in determining whether to offer a preventive service. Particularly for asymptomatic patients, thresholds for performing preventive services differ depending on their potential for harm in the absence of strong evidence of benefit. Frame and Carlson (1975) summarized the circumstances that must exist for screening tests to be useful:

- The condition must have a significant effect on the quality and quantity of life.

- Acceptable methods of treatment must be available.

- The condition must have an asymptomatic period during which detection and treatment significantly reduce morbidity or mortality.

- Treatment in the asymptomatic phase must yield a therapeutic result superior to that obtained by delaying treatment until symptoms appear.

- Tests that are acceptable to patients must be available, at a reasonable cost, to detect the condition in the asymptomatic period.

- The incidence of the condition must be sufficient to justify the cost of the screening.

"The clinician and patient should share decision-making."[2]

Clinicians are responsible for providing patients with the best available information about potential benefits and harms of the preventive service, translat-

---

[2]A principal finding of the US Preventive Services Task Force from US Preventive Services Task Force. *Guide to Clinical Preventive Services. 2nd ed. Washington, DC: US Department of Health and Human Services; 1996: chap xxix-xxxii.*

ing what is known and not known about the likelihood of various outcomes, and explaining the probable consequences of different decisions. Patient preferences, which are important in all clinical decisions, are paramount to consider when contemplating preventive services of uncertain benefit.

How accurately can the risk factor or target condition be detected?

Efforts to detect risk factors or target conditions by screening tests may be ineffective or harmful if the test is inaccurate. The *accuracy* of a screening test is measured by its *sensitivity* and *specificity* (Key Concepts 4).

Key Concepts 4

Sensitivity refers to the proportion of persons with a condition who correctly test positive when screened.

> A test with poor sensitivity will miss many cases and therefore produce a large proportion of *false-negative results.*

Specificity refers to the proportion of persons without the condition who correctly test negative when screened.

> A test with poor specificity incorrectly labels persons as having the condition. The incorrect labeling of true negative results produce *false-positive cases.* False positive results can produce a series of adverse consequences including psychological stress and the risks associated with further tests and procedures.

Relative risk reduction is the percent reduction in risk of disease morbidity or mortality achieved through active prevention compared to a control group.

Absolute risk reduction is the actual difference between the risk of a condition with and without the preventive service.

Number needed to treat (or screen) is the reciprocal of absolute risk reduction and represents the number of patients needed to treat in order to prevent one case.

Positive predictive value (PPV) is the proportion of positive test results that are correct (true positives). The predictive value of a test for a particular condition in an individual depends on the prevalence of that condition in the population. If the prevalence of the condition is low, the *positive predictive value* also will be very low regardless of the accuracy of the screening test. The higher the prevalence, the more likely the positive test result reflects a true positive.

This is the basis for utilizing a *"high-risk"* strategy for screening illustrated in Appendix A.

Counseling

"Interventions that address patients' personal health practices are vitally important."[3]

The most prominent identifiable contributors to premature death in the United States are tobacco, diet and physical activity patterns, alcohol, microbial agents, toxic agents, firearms, sexual behavior, motor vehicles, and illicit use of drugs (McGinnis 1993). Because behavioral choice is critical to most of these risk factors, the USPSTF has suggested that clinician counseling that leads to improved personal health practices may be more valuable to patients than conventional clinical activities such as diagnostic testing. The following are general guidelines to consider when providing clinical counseling:

1. Counseling should be culturally appropriate. Present information and services in a style and format that are sensitive to the culture, values, and traditions of the patient and at a level of comprehension consistent with the age and learning skills of the patient. Use a dialect and terminology consistent with the patient's language and communication style.

2. Clinicians often cite lack of time and poor reimbursement for counseling as key barriers to patient counseling. Several measures may be taken to improve delivery of counseling:

   ■ Create an office or clinic environment that promotes preventive care.

   ■ Use a variety of resources to reinforce healthy behaviors. Display pamphlets, posters, and other materials conspicuously so that they are readily available. Patient education resources are listed at the end of each chapter of this book.

   ■ Use short patient questionnaires to quickly assess patient needs for counseling. Examples of such questionnaires are included in this book. Some are brief enough that they may be incorporated into patient intake questionnaires and history forms.

   ■ Focus interventions by assessing patients' readiness to change health-related behaviors. Research indicates that patients who are in the early stages of behavior change may benefit most from information but probably not from more intensive interventions. Patients who are ready to

---

[3]A principal finding of the US Preventive Services Task Force from US Preventive Services Task Force. *Guide to Clinical Preventive Services. 2nd ed. Washington, DC: US Department of Health and Human Services; 1996: chap xxix-xxxii.*

change may benefit from more directed, task-oriented counseling and behavior modification. Finally, those who have successfully changed behavior need support and follow-up.

- Use a team approach to provide counseling.

- Be familiar with community resources to which patients may be referred for types of counseling that cannot be provided in the practice.

- Provide repeated messages to patients. Even brief interventions, such as simple advice to stop smoking, may have a beneficial effect.

3. The USPSTF describes 12 strategies for patient education and counseling with which clinicians should be familiar (Table ii.2).

Table ii.2. US Preventive Services Task Force Patient Education/Counseling Strategies

---

1. Frame the teaching to match the patient's perceptions.
2. Fully inform patients of the purposes and expected effects of interventions and when to expect these effects.
3. Suggest small changes rather than large ones.
4. Be specific.
5. It is sometimes easier to add new behaviors than to eliminate established behaviors.
6. Link new behaviors to old behaviors.
7. Use the power of the profession.
8. Get explicit commitments from the patient.
9. Use a combination of strategies.
10. Involve office staff.
11. Refer.
12. Monitor progress through follow-up contact.

From: US Preventive Services Task Force. Patient Education/Counseling Strategies. In: *Guide to Clinical Preventive Services.* 2nd ed. Washington, DC: US Department of Health and Human Services; 1996: chap iv.

Putting Prevention into Perspective

"For some health problems, community-level interventions may be more effective than clinical preventive services."[4]

Preventive services impact the health status of individuals and populations. However, many health patterns in populations are related to an uneven distribution of societal resources. These resources encompass social, economic and political advantages such as knowledge, money, and social connections that influence people's ability to avoid risks and to minimize the consequences of disease once it occurs. The broad influence of these resources is associated with multiple risk factors and disease outcomes. Interventions such as school-based curricula, community programs, and regulatory and legislative initiatives may be effective in addressing these more global issues. Being aware of community programs, encouraging patient participation and involvement, acting as a consultant for communities implementing programs or introducing legislation, and serving as an advocate to initiate and maintain effective community interventions are suggested roles for the interested clinician. An appreciation of the link between specific risk factors and general societal factors that influence health patterns may enhance the clinicians' contribution to prevention efforts.

"It is a well-known fact that there are no social, no industrial, no economic problems which are not related to health."
     Dr. William H. Welch,
     Founder, Johns Hopkins School of Hygiene and Public Health

Summary

The concepts of prevention, as discussed in the earlier part of this section, are used to prioritize prevention strategies. These concepts include: measures of frequency and severity of the health condition; magnitude of risk associated with risk factors; accuracy of screening tests; and the strength of evidence in support and magnitude of an intervention's effectiveness. These concepts were used by some of the major authorities to direct their guideline process and to support their preventive services recommendations. These recommendations can assist the clinician in prioritizing prevention strategies for individual patients and practice population.

Preventive services for individuals may comprise a "core set" of preventive services that apply broadly to most individuals from the "average-risk" population. The average-risk approach used in the *Clinician's Handbook* stratifies individuals based on age and gender. In addition, a more targeted strategy can be offered to individuals at a relative "high-risk" based on their risk pro-

---

[4]A principal finding of the US Preventive Services Task Force from US Preventive Services Task Force. *Guide to Clinical Preventive Services. 2nd ed. Washington, DC: US Department of Health and Human Services; 1996: chap xxix-xxxii.*

file. The average-risk and high-risk strategies are complementary. Appendix A, which consists of risk tables and time lines for preventive care, illustrates the link between the two strategies. The purpose of and relationship between the risk tables and time lines are discussed further in the introduction to Appendix A.

Selected References

Frame PS and Carlson, SJ. A Critical Review of Periodic Health Screening Using Specific Screening Criteria. *J Fam Practice.* 1975;2:29-36.

McGinnis JM, Foege WH. Actual Causes of Death in the United States. *JAMA.* 1993; 270(18):2207-2212.

Rose, G. *The Strategy of Preventive Medicine.* New York, NY: Oxford University Press; 1992.

US Preventive Services Task Force. *Guide to Clinical Preventive Services.* 2nd ed. Washington, DC: US Department of Health and Human Services; 1996.

Woolf S, Jonas S, Lawrence RS. *Health Promotion and Disease Prevention in Clinical Practice.* Baltimore, Md: Williams and Wilkins; 1996.

OCCUPATIONAL AND ENVIRONMENTAL HEALTH

A comprehensive approach to preventive health care includes understanding and assessing risks related to occupational and environmental exposures. This chapter discusses the principal issues surrounding occupational health; Appendix A addresses selected occupational and environmental risks.

Every year, 6.3 million workplace injuries and over 500,000 work-related illnesses are reported to the Federal government. Many others remain unreported. Six thousand fatalities resulting from workplace trauma are reported each year, and the National Institute for Occupational Safety and Health (NIOSH) estimates that over 50,000 people die annually from work-related illnesses, most of which go unreported.

Illnesses which are often unrecognized as occupational or environmental in origin include musculoskeletal disorders of the upper extremity, irritant or allergic dermatitis, asthma, chronic obstructive lung disease, reproductive abnormalities, hearing loss, and cancers of the lung, skin, and bladder. Several of these are discussed in more detail later in this chapter.

Occupational exposures provide unique opportunities for effective disease prevention, because elimination of the exposure may prevent the disease. Unfortunately, total elimination is often difficult, and workers continue to contract preventable illnesses from exposures that have long been recognized, such as lead and silica. Clinicians may not have the opportunity to effect primary prevention efforts in the workplace but can offer important counseling to their patients.

Clinicians will see patients suffering from occupational disorders. For these patients, recognition by the health provider of the role played by workplace exposures in causing or exacerbating illnesses can have important consequences:

■ Recognition of a work-related disorder along with follow-up counseling can help prevent disease among co-workers who share the same exposures.

■ Recognition of occupational hazards along with follow-up counseling can prevent exposure of a worker's family members to substances such as lead, pesticides, and allergens, which can be carried home on a worker's clothing and contaminate the home.

- Knowledge of a patient's work activities may be important in treating non-work related conditions. Examples include deciding when a patient my safely return to work following a hospitalization, and adjusting medication dosing for patients who work night shifts.

- Failure to recognize a disorder as work-related may render treatment ineffective if the patient's work exposures are not altered.

Recognizing the important role that clinicians may have in the prevention, diagnosis, and treatment of occupational and environmental illnesses, the Institute of Medicine has recommended substantive changes in medical education: "At a minimum, all primary care [clinicians] should be able to identify possible occupationally or environmentally induced conditions and make the appropriate referrals for follow-up."[1] To achieve this minimum level of expertise, the Institute concluded that all clinicians must learn some basic principles of occupational and environmental medicine, must learn how to take an appropriate occupational and environmental history, must understand their role in worker's compensation, must know how and when to report hazards to public health and regulatory agencies, and must be aware of the legal, social, and ethical implications of diagnosing an occupational or environmental illness.

The Role of Primary Prevention in Occupational and Environmental Health

Primary prevention of occupational diseases can be achieved only through the reduction or elimination of exposures to chemical, physical, or biological hazards. Clinicians must recognize these exposures to participate meaningfully in preventive efforts. As noted below, the basic occupational history is the cornerstone of preventive efforts and needs to be obtained from each patient. Reduction of exposures can be achieved through the hierarchy of controls, listed here in descending order of importance and desirability:

1. **Elimination** of the exposure, usually through substitution of a different agent or process

2. **Engineering controls** such as noise reduction or improved ventilation

3. **Administrative controls** such as job rotation

4. **Personal Protective Equipment** such as respirators or hearing protection

---

[1]Institute of Medicine. *Role of the Primary Care Physician in Occupational and Environmental Medicine.* Washington, DC: National Academy Press; 1988.

Clinicians should inquire about exposure reduction strategies used in their patients' workplaces. When appropriate, clinicians need to urge employers and employee representatives to adopt better control measures. Clinicians need to encourage their patients to wear personal protective equipment when warranted by job exposures that are not otherwise adequately controlled.

The initial step for achieving better recognition of occupational and environmental exposures is for all clinicians to take a basic occupational history from their patients. This history should include:

- the patient's past and current job titles and industries

- a description of past and current work duties

- any known exposures to chemical, physical, or biological hazards

- the presence of any symptoms in relation to work

This initial screening history will suffice for most patients. Unfortunately, a number of studies have documented that most clinicians obtain few or no elements of the occupational history from their patients. A more detailed history is warranted in patients who report potential occupational hazards in their initial occupational screening. A number of self-administered questionnaires exist to aid the clinician in obtaining a more detailed occupational history; Table iii.1 represents one possibility.

Table iii.1. Essential Elements of the Occupational History and Questionnaire

---

Current or most recent work and exposure history
- Job title; type of industry; name of employer
- Year work started and year work finished (if not currently employed)
- Description of job (what is a typical workday), especially the parts of the job the patient believes may be potentially hazardous
- Current work hours and any shift changes
- Current exposures to dust, fumes, radiation, chemicals, biologic hazards, or physical hazards
- Protective equipment used (clothes, safety glasses, hearing protections, respirator, or gloves)
- Other employees at the workplace who have similar health problems

Earlier employment history
- Job chronology, working backward from the current or most recent jobs
  The same information as above for each job previously held

Major types of exposure associated with clinical illness
- Gases
- Corrosive substances (acids, alkalis)
- Dyes and stains
- Dusts and powders
- Asbestos, other fibers
- Infectious agents
- Insecticides and pesticides
- Metals and metal fumes
- Organic dusts (cotton, wood, biologic matter)
- Plastics
- Solvents
- Petrochemicals (coal, tar, asphalt, petroleum distillates)
- Physical factors (noise, lifting, thermal stress, vibration, repetitive motion)
- Emotional factors (stress)
- Radiation (electromagnetic fields, x-ray radiation, ultraviolet radiation)

Source: Newman, LS. Occupational illness. *N Engl J Med.* 1995;333:1128-1134. Reproduced with permission of the Massachusetts Medical Society, copyright 1997. All rights reserved.

Because workplace exposures can have additive or synergistic effects with other exposures, clinicians also need to take into account patient activities outside of work. For example, workers in noisy occupations should be counseled about the additive effects of noise exposure from work and from such avocational pursuits as shooting and the use of power tools. Counseling patients about exacerbation of occupational illness through nonemployment-related activities is not a substitute for primary prevention focused at reducing work site exposures, but does represent an additional step that clinicians can take to reduce the overall burden of occupational disease among their patients.

In addition to potentially hazardous exposures, symptoms or health conditions that have a significant likelihood of being related to occupational exposures also require a more detailed occupational history. Several such sentinel health conditions are discussed below. They do not comprise a comprehensive listing of work-related disorders, but represent some of the disorders which have been targeted by NIOSH and other authorities. Other conditions besides the ones detailed below in which occupational exposures should be evaluated include peripheral neuropathy, encephalopathy, hepatitis, nephropathy, and cancers of the skin, lung, and bladder.

Allergic and Irritant Dermatitis

The skin is an important exposure route for chemicals. Some 66,000 cases of work-related dermatitis are reported annually, though it is likely that the true number of cases is far higher. For example, almost 2% of workers surveyed in the National Health Interview Survey reported dermatitis related to work exposures. Irritant contact dermatitis can result from occupational exposures to a wide variety of compounds such as solvents and cutting fluids, while allergic contact dermatitis can result from exposure to a long list of substances, such as metals (nickel and chromium), rubber additives (epoxies and acrylates), formaldehyde and poison ivy (a common occupational and nonoccupational exposure). Rapid identification of skin problems as work related and removal of the offending exposure can hasten recovery and prevent the progression of dermatitis to a chronic skin disease.

Asthma

Mortality and morbidity from asthma is increasing in the United States, partly as a result of occupational exposures. Over 9 million workers are exposed to agents that are known sensitizers and irritants associated with asthma. As many as 28% of adult asthma cases may be attributable to work exposures, and annual costs of occupational asthma are estimated at $400 million. In addition to those who develop occupational asthma as a result of workplace exposures, there are many patients with asthma whose condition is worsened by work exposures. The morbidity of occupational asthma can be substantially reduced by early intervention. The likelihood of complete resolution of symptoms and pulmonary function abnormalities is greatest when exposures are terminated early in the course of illness, making early diagnosis a critical element for effective intervention.

Chronic Obstructive Pulmonary Disease (COPD)

A well-documented relationship exists between COPD and workplace exposures such as coal dust, grain dust, and cotton dust. Those with lung disease from other causes are especially vulnerable to occupational respiratory hazards. Although cigarette smoking is the primary cause of COPD, a substantial fraction (as much as 14%) may be attributable to environmental and occupational exposures. Occupational dust exposure provides an additional reason to encourage these workers not to smoke. All patients with lung disease should be questioned about workplace exposures as a possible contributor to their disease.

Reproductive Disorders

A few occupational and environmental exposures have been shown to contribute to reproductive disorders including birth defects, developmental disorders, spontaneous abortion, and infertility. Though a few such exposures are well known (eg, lead, high levels of ionizing radiation), the overall contribution of environmental and occupational exposures on fertility is unknown. Most chemicals in commercial use have undergone little or no reproductive testing; among the more than 1000 workplace chemicals that have been demonstrated to cause reproductive disorders in animal experiments, few have been studied in humans. Occupational exposures should be documented in pregnancy, in pre-conception counseling, and in the evaluation of infertility and adverse reproductive outcomes.

Hearing Loss

Occupational hearing loss, although largely preventable, is the most common occupational disease in the United States. It has proven difficult to convince employers and workers to adopt the appropriate preventive strategies, as hearing loss is sometimes accepted as a normal consequence of employment rather than as a preventable disorder that can seriously degrade quality of life. Millions of workers are exposed to hazardous noise and are thus at risk for hearing loss. Although hearing loss is irreversible, the prevention of further exposures can prevent worsening hearing loss. Workers in noisy settings, such as machine shops or firing ranges, should be counseled to wear hearing protection and to seek other noise-reduction strategies through their employers.

Musculoskeletal Disorders

Low back pain and upper extremity musculoskeletal disorders such as tendinitis and nerve entrapments are often related to workplace exposures. Risk factors contributing to musculoskeletal disorders include high force exertion, repetitive activities, awkward body postures, and vibration. Identification and remediation of causal or exacerbating workplace factors is often essential to providing rest to the affected area and in preventing the recurrence of these disorders.

The Role of Secondary Prevention in Occupational and Environmental Health

There is little data regarding the effectiveness of secondary prevention activities in preventing occupational diseases. For a number of specific exposures, there is federal or state mandated screening; many employers also conduct regular screening for some employee groups. Screening procedures are dependent on the specific exposures incurred by workers. Examples of screening programs include:

- periodic chest X-rays for workers exposed to asbestos

- spirometry for workers exposed to agents known to cause asthma or COPD

- periodic blood or urine testing for lead and cadmium in exposed workers

- urine cytology for workers exposed to bladder carcinogens

Probably the most widespread periodic screening is regular audiometry for workers in noisy occupations. In theory, such a program can detect early hearing loss and help to prevent further noise-induced hearing loss. However, few data exist to document the effectiveness of this and other screening programs in practice.

In summary, health care providers need to be involved in the prevention of occupational and environmental illness. Although most clinicians will find themselves limited in their ability to influence primary preventive measures at their patients' work sites or other public settings, some degree of primary prevention for the patient, patient's co-workers, and patient's family may be achieved by attending to details of the occupational history and counseling accordingly based on the potential hazardous exposures revealed, and/or by notifying the appropriate agencies when potentially hazardous conditions are suspected to exist at an employment site. Secondary prevention of occupational and environmental illness through periodic screenings targeted toward a patient's specific work and exposure history can also involve the primary care provider, although the effectiveness of such screening measures needs to be further elucidated through appropriate research.

Sources for Further Information

Agency for Toxic Substances and Disease Registry (ATSDR), 1600 Clifton Rd, NE, Atlanta GA 30333. Telephone: (404)639-6000 (Division of Toxicology); (404)639-6206 (Division of Health Education). Internet address: http://atsdr1.atsdr.cdc.gov:8080/atsdrhome.html/. Part of the US Public Health Service (USPHS), the ATSDR provides toxicologic profiles and clinically useful case studies in environmental medicine.

American College of Occupational and Environmental Medicine (ACOEM), 55 W. Seegers Rd., Arlington Heights, IL 60005-3919. Telephone: (847)228-6850. Internet address: http://www.acoem.org/. The ACOEM lists physicians who are board-certified in occupational-environmental medicine and members of the college; it also conducts educational programs on occupational health, impairment, and the worker's compensation system.

Association of Occupational and Environmental Clinics (AOEC), 1010 Vermont Ave., Suite 513, Washington, DC 20005. Telephone: (202)347-4976. Internet address: http://152.3.65.120/oem/aoec.htm. The AOEC is a network of academically based occupational-environmental medicine clinics throughout the United States. Member clinics provide professional training, community education about toxic substances, exposure and risk assessment, clinical evaluation, and consultation. Clinicians can contact the AOEC for clinical referrals to assist in the diagnosis, management, therapy, and prevention of occupational disorders.

Environmental Protection Agency (EPA), 401 M Street, SW, Washington, DC 20460. Telephone: (202)260-5922. Internet address: http://www.epa.gov/epahome/. The EPA is an independent United States federal agency whose stated mission is to protect public health and to safeguard and improve the natural environment upon which human life depends. EPA's goals include ensuring that federal environmental laws are implemented and enforced fairly and effectively and that environmental protection is an integral consideration in US policy. Their web site provides numerous sources on a wide array of environmental and health-related issues.

National Center for Environmental Health (NCEH), Centers for Disease Control and Prevention, Mail Stop F-29, 4770 Buford Highway, NE, Atlanta, GA 30341-3724. Telephone: (770)488-7030. Internet address: http://www.cdc.gov/nceh/ncehhome.htm. The NCEH is a division of the Department of Health and Human Services within the Centers for Disease Control and Prevention. Its mission is to promote health and quality of life by preventing and controlling disease, birth defects, disability, and death resulting from interactions between people and their environment. Some of its activities include: public health surveillance; applied research; dissemination of standards, guidelines, and recommendations; and technical and financial assistance to state and local health agencies.

National Institute of Environmental Health Sciences (NIEHS), P.O. Box 12233, Research Triangle Park, ND 27709. Telephone: (909)541-3345. Internet address: http://www.niehs.nih.gov/. A division of the Department of Health and Human Services within the National Institutes of Health, the NIEHS has as its stated mission to reduce the burden of human illness and dysfunction from environmental causes by understanding the interaction between environmental factors, individual susceptibility, and age. It engages in multi disciplinary biomedical research programs, prevention and intervention efforts, and communication strategies that encompass training, education, technology transfer, and community outreach.

National Institute for Occupational Safety and Health (NIOSH), Robert A. Taft Laboratories, 4676 Columbia Pkwy, Cincinnati, OH 45226-1998. Telephone: (800) 356-4674. Internet address: http://www.cdc.gov/niosh/home-page.html. A division of the Department of Health and Human Services within the Centers for Disease Control and Prevention, NIOSH provides information about substance toxicity and workplace hazards. The health-hazard evaluation program can investigate work sites at which physicians, employees, or employers suspect work-related illness and injury to have occurred. NIOSH offers training in occupational safety and health and funds continuing-medical-education courses.

Occupational Safety and Health Administration (OSHA), Department of Labor, 200 Constitution Ave., NW, Washington, DC 20210. Telephone: (202) 219-8148 (general information); (202) 219-9308 (compliance officer); (202) 219-4667 (publications). Fax: (900) 555-3400 (OSHA FAX). Internet address: http://www.osha-slc.gov/. OSHA sets US standards for health and safety in the workplace, investigates compliance, and issues citations. The publications-distribution office has articles about many occupational diseases. OSHA FAX is a fax-on-demand data-base service providing documents for a nominal telephone charge.

Selected References

Agency for Toxic Substances and Disease Registry. *Case Studies in Environmental Medicine: Taking an Exposure History.* Washington, DC: US Department of Health and Human Services, US Public Health Service, Agency for Toxic Substances and Disease Registry; 1992. Monograph No. 26.

American College of Physicians. Occupational and environmental medicine: The internist's role. *Ann Intern Med.* 1990;113(12):975-982.

American Lung Association of San Diego. Taking the occupational history. *Ann Intern Med.* 1983;99:641.

Coye MJ, Rosenstock L. The occupational health history in a family practice setting. *American Family Physician.* 1983;28(5):229-34.

Goldman R and Peters J. The occupational and environmental health history. *JAMA.* 1981; 246:2831.

Institute of Medicine. *Role of the Primary Care Physician in Occupational and Environmental Medicine.* Washington, DC: National Academy Press; 1988.

Kipen HM and Craner J. Sentinel pathophysiologic conditions: an adjunct to teaching occupational and environmental disease recognition and history taking. *Environ Res.* 1992;59:93-100.

National Institute for Occupational Safety and Health. *Report to Congress on Workers' Home Contaminations Study Conducted Under the Workers' Family Protection Act.* Washington, DC: US Department of Health and Human Services, US Public Health Service, Centers for Disease Control and Prevention, National Institute for Occupational Safety and Health; 1995.

Newman LS. Occupational illness. *N Eng J Med.* 1995;333:1128-1134.

Rosenstock L, Cullen MR, eds. *Textbook of Clinical Occupational and Environmental Medicine.* Philadelphia, Pa: W.B. Saunders; 1994.

IMPLEMENTING PREVENTIVE CARE

"Clinicians must take every opportunity to deliver preventive services, especially to those with limited access to care" [1]

Most clinicians acknowledge the importance of incorporating preventive care into their practices; however, delivery of preventive services, even those about which all authorities agree, is far from satisfactory. Providing consistent delivery of preventive care requires organizational commitment, time, and a critical analysis of the systems designed to deliver that care. Ensuring the consistent delivery of preventive services may require changes in office systems or clinic organization.

In the current health care environment, accurate documentation of the delivery of preventive services has become essential. Delivery of clinical preventive services is now one of several indicators used to rate the performance of clinicians, their practices, and health plans.

One example of such measures is the Health Plan Employer Data and Information Set (HEDIS), a set of health care quality indicators developed by the National Committee for Quality Assurance. The preventive services currently being monitored include immunizations, mammography, and smoking cessation counseling. Performance ratings in the area of preventive services serve as potential criteria for accreditation as well as the awarding of contracts.

This chapter presents practical instructions for implementing a system for delivering preventive care services. These instructions will facilitate putting prevention into *your* practice.

Assess the Need for a New System

If preventive care services are being provided, assess how well your current system works. The services provided by some practices may not require significant changes. Determining the current status of a preventive care delivery

---

[1] A principal finding of the US Preventive Services Task Force from US Preventive Services Task Force. *Guide to Clinical Preventive Services*. 2nd ed. Washington, DC: US Department of Health and Human Services; 1996: chap xxix-xxxii.

system is important before implementing big changes. The best way to assess the need for a new system is to examine clinical records. A baseline chart audit can help determine if changes are needed and can also establish a baseline for demonstrating future improvements.

Assess Readiness to Make a Systems Change

As is true about any process that requires change, assessing readiness to change is beneficial. Two commonly cited barriers to implementing preventive care in clinical practice are clinicians' attitudes about prevention and problems within office systems (eg, lack of time, staff, and resources). The effect of these barriers can be minimized if they are viewed in the context of "readiness" for change. The following questions should be addressed as part of readiness assessment:

1. Is prevention an important aspect of the care provided by this organization?

2. Is increasing the quality and consistency of preventive services a priority?

3. Are adequate resources available to incorporate preventive care services?

4. Is change feasible (in terms of time, capacity, and cost)?

5. Is the staff committed to changing the system?

6. Will the administration and key stakeholders support change?

If the answer to the majority of the questions is "yes," implementation of a preventive care system can begin. If the majority of answers is "no," attention should focus on resolving the issues associated with the questions before attempting to make a change. Use of this simple questionnaire will save significant time and energy by identifying potential barriers that need to be addressed and potential facilitators of the process and allowing time to plan for successful implementation based on information collected.

Enlist Staff Support

Communication and teamwork are critical factors to successful implementation. Involving the staff is critical to ensuring that preventive services are a routine part of office practice. Include everyone who will be impacted by the changes in the planning and implementation process. Clearly define the role of *all* staff members and include them in the planning and problem-solving. You may discover untapped resources by encouraging staff members to creatively consider their roles in prevention delivery.

Designate a Facilitator

Recent research indicates that appointing a facilitator to introduce the tools and the process for change increases the chances of successful implementation. The responsibilities of a facilitator include:

- planning and setting goals for the implementation process

- coordinating implementation activities

- ensuring good communication between all involved staff members

- helping to establish a quality-improvement process to track progress

- giving feedback on performance and encouraging progress

- facilitating creative problem-solving.

Perform a Chart Audit

1. Select a small sample of records from a specific patient population (eg, adults, children, males, females).

2. Determine which preventive care elements are to be assessed (eg, Pap testing, cholesterol screening, smoking counseling) and which guidelines to use. (Recommendations of Major Authorities in individual chapters.)

3. Use information from the health history forms, problem lists, or progress notes from the most recent visit to determine whether the client has had:
   - health-risk behavior assessed or identified in the past year
   - appropriate screening exams for age, sex, and risk in the appropriate time frame
   - documented counseling for health risk factors

4. Determine what percentage of the sample population received age- and gender-appropriate preventive care services in a timely manner.

Table iv.1 is a sample tool for performing chart audits.

Table iv.1. Sample Chart Audit Tool

Preventive Care Guideline Parameters	Documentation	Treatment or Education Provided		
Cholesterol	Current date:	Counseling done	yes	no
Women q. 5 yrs (45-65 y.o.)	_____	Prescription given	yes	no
Men q 5 yrs (35-65 y.o.)	Date of last:	Referred to outside program/class	yes	no
	_____			
	Result:_____			
Smoking Behavior	Smoker ____	Counseling done	yes	no
Assess every visit	Non-Smoker ____	Prescription given	yes	no
	Not assessed ____	Referred to outside program/class	yes	no
DTaP/DTP Immunization	Age at last visit: _____			
Children <6 y.o.	Has child received:			
5 doses	1st dose (2 mos)	yes	no	n/a
	2nd dose (4 mos)	yes	no	n/a
	3rd dose (6 mos)	yes	no	n/a
	4th dose (15-18 mos)	yes	no	n/a
	5th dose (4-6 yrs)	yes	no	n/a

Establish Preventive Care Protocols

Develop a protocol of preventive care that meets the particular needs of your specific practice and its patients. The *Clinician's Handbook* is designed to facilitate this process. Recommendations of major authorities, emphasizing age and periodicity for preventive screening, appear at the beginning of each chapter. By reviewing these recommendations, clinicians can decide which guidelines to select or can set their own standards based on current recommendations. A set of standards, even if minimal, needs to be identified and adopted as a policy. Concentrate efforts on selecting preventive services that truly can be provided in light of limited time, available staff, and other resources. Periodically examine the selected standards, updating them as needed based on current research and the changing needs of the patient population.

Once policy is set, familiarize the entire staff with the criteria and incorporate the standards into a preventive care flow sheet for tracking purposes. The flow sheet permits quick determination of a particular patient's need for preventive care services and allows the provider to deliver preventive care at all patient visits. If time limitations prevent delivery of such services during a visit, the patient may be informed of what care is needed, and a plan to obtain it can be established (eg, referral, follow-up appointment). After protocols for preventive care service are identified, the next step is to establish systems that ensure consistent, efficient delivery of these services.

Analyze Service Delivery and Patient Flow

The physical layout of a practice and the direction of patient flow can significantly influence the delivery of preventive services. Effective organization of clinic systems and patient flow, along with utilization of all staff members' skills, can improve delivery of services. Analyzing patient flow patterns can be as simple as mapping a patient's path through the office on paper, thus identifying areas where health education messages can be provided or reinforced. The analysis should consider who the patient encounters and what is done at each step. Such an analysis can provide a basis upon which clinic efficiency can be improved.

Use Basic Tools

The use of simple office tools can improve the delivery of preventive health care. The following tools are components of the Put Prevention Into Practice initiative. Many of the tools can be altered to meet individual specifications.

Preventive care flow sheets (adult, child, and child immunization)

The most basic tool for tracking and prompting preventive services is a flow sheet. For flow sheets to be useful, data must be promptly entered onto the forms. The assistance of staff in updating and maintaining chart flow sheets is very important. The entire staff must be familiar with the format of the sheets and how to use them. Over time, flow sheets prove to be useful tools for tracking and auditing the performance and results of preventive care, encouraging increased compliance with preventive care standards and early detection and treatment of preventable conditions.

Postcard reminders

Postcards or letters can be useful tools for reminding patients to come in for needed preventive care. Such reminders can easily be created by individual organizations, or preprinted cards can be obtained from outside sources. Computerized systems are capable of generating such mailed prompts. Telephone calls may also be used for reminding patients of the need for preventive care visits; however, telephone calls have been found to be less cost-effective than mailed prompts. Patient reminders can greatly increase the rate at which clients return for services.

In-office visual prompts

Use posters (eg, Put Prevention Into Practice, adult and child preventive care timelines) as visual prompts in the office and all examination rooms to remind both office staff and patients of the need for continuing preventive care services.

Patient materials: Personal Health Guide and Child Health Guide

Patients play a critical role in tracking and prompting their own preventive care. Studies have shown that patient-held (or parent-held) records, such as those used to promote childhood immunization programs, are well-received by both clinicians and patients.

The *Personal Health Guide* and the *Child Health Guide* were designed to:

- provide patients with information on a range of preventive services

- facilitate a structured dialogue between patients and providers

- assist patients in tracking their own care

When explaining how to use the *Personal Health Guide* and the *Child Health Guide*:

- let patients know that you think the information in the *Guides* is important

- discuss topics that apply to the patient's personal health behavior as well as areas in which he/she desires to make changes; instruct patients to bring the *Guides* to each visit for review and updating

- advise patients to read or review the information

- reinforce health messages and assist patients to set realistic goals for changing health behaviors

- reinforce positive behavior changes

Use other helpful tools

Other useful office tools include chart reminders, behavioral change contracts, health risk appraisals and electronic medical records.

- Chart reminders alert clinicians to the specific preventive care needs of individual patients

- Prevention prescriptions and behavioral change contracts facilitate behavior change by clearly defining the patient's and the clinician's expectations. In addition, a written plan of action, based on an agreement between the patient and the clinician, emphasizes the patient's ability and responsibility to contribute to his/her own disease prevention and health promotion. Follow-up telephone calls to determine progress are also helpful for encouraging compliance with health-related recommendations.

■ Health risk appraisals can ensure that clients are questioned about all possible risk factors, increase patient awareness of health risks, and provide the clinician with a second source of information other than the patient interview. However, health risk appraisals should be done in the proper context and with an appropriate amount of time allotted for follow-up counseling to ensure that patients understand the implications of such assessments and the steps to be taken in addressing the various risk factors revealed.

■ Computerized tracking and prompting systems are commercially available. Some features to look for include: the ability to prompt for preventive services, customize preventive care schedules, send out patient reminders, and determine a practice's performance.

Delegate Tasks and Staff Roles

The most efficient approach to implementing preventive care services is to delegate and share responsibilities among as many staff members as possible. Tasks, such as reviewing charts, administering immunizations, counseling patients, and screening, can be successfully provided by members of the office staff. Another important role for staff is facilitating patients' access to community resources, such as local mammography centers or smoking cessation support groups. Appropriate standards for assuring patient privacy must be maintained, regardless of the number of staff involved in a patient's care.

Perform Follow-up Evaluations

Follow-up chart audits will assist in evaluating both the consistency with which tools are used and the impact of tools on service delivery. Use this information as feedback in quality improvement activities in order to modify your service delivery plan.

In Summary

■ Assess your current preventive service delivery system

■ Elicit input from entire staff

■ Establish a preventive care protocol

■ Choose tools that are suited to *your* setting and system

- Personalize or adapt tools using input from all staff members involved in the process

- Ensure that all staff members understand the intent and purpose of the tools

- Distribute responsibilities across the entire staff

- Perform follow-up evaluations

Clinical Scenario

The following is one example of a systematic approach to the delivery of preventive care services:

Before a patient arrives:

- The medical record is reviewed by a designated staff member and flagged with notes or stickers for preventive care needs determined from the record

- A staff member sends a postcard or calls the patient to encourage making an appointment for preventive care services

Before a patient encounters the provider:

- The receptionist or nurse provides patient with a *Personal Health Guide* and explains how to use it; if a patient has previously received a *Personal Health Guide*, the receptionist or nurse checks to determine if he/she has brought it and reviews the *Guide*

- The nursing staff completes a health-risk assessment, elicits a health history, determines which preventive care screening exams are needed, cues the clinician to complete or order exams, and reinforces health counseling

- The nursing staff initiates health education or risk-reduction counseling

During the encounter with the provider:

- The clinician assesses health risk and health history information, verifying/updating as necessary

- The clinician questions the patient about identified health risks and his/her compliance with behavioral change contracts at every visit

- The clinician encourages the patient to ask questions about preventive health topics

- The clinician completes or orders screening services as necessary

- The clinician provides appropriate referrals

After the encounter:

- A staff member assists the patient in recording information (exam dates and test results) in the *Personal Health Guide* and encourages the patient to bring the *Guide* to every visit

- A staff member provides patient education and encourages the patient to ask questions

- A staff member provides patient-relevant health promotion literature

- A staff member reinforces recommended behavior changes, using a prevention prescription pad or a patient contract

- A staff member ensures that the patient understands any instructions and knows when to return for services

- A staff member completes follow-up with reminder postcards or telephone calls

Patient Resources

For information on how to order the Put Prevention Into Practive *Personal Health Guide* or *Child Health Guide*, write to: Put Prevention Into Practice, c/o Office of Disease Prevention and Health Promotion, Room 738G, Humphrey Building, 200 Independence Avenue, NW., Washington, DC 20201; or visit the Website at: http://www.dhhs.gov/PPIP.

Organizations may print the *Personal Health Guides* with customized covers carrying the organization's name, logo, or telephone numbers. Black and white reproducible formats for printing are available for a nominal fee from the American College of Preventive Medicine 1660 L St, NW, Washington DC 20036-5603. (202)466-2044.

Provider Resources

Copies of the "Health Risk Profile," a health risk appraisal used by the Texas Department of Health, can be obtained by calling or writing the Adult Health Program, Bureau of Chronic Disease Prevention and Control, Texas Department of Health, 1100 W 49th Street, Austin TX 78756; (512)458-7534.

For information on how to obtain Put Prevention Into Practice materials, write to: Put Prevention Into Practice, c/o Office of Disease Prevention and Health Promotion, Room 738G, Humphrey Building, 200 Independence Avenue, NW., Washington, DC 20201; or visit the Website at: http://www.dhhs.gov/PPIP.

Selected References

Burack RC, Liang J. The early detection of cancer in the primary-care setting: factors associated with the acceptance and completion of recommended procedures. *Prev Med*. 1987;16: 739-751.

Carney P, Dietrich AJ, Keller A, Landgraf J, O'Connor GT. Tools, teamwork, and tenacity: elements of a cancer control office system for primary care. *J Fam Pract*. 1992;35:388-394.

Dickey LL and Kamerow DB. Seven steps to delivering preventive care. 1994. *Family Practice Management*. 1994;1(7):32-37.

Dickey LL, Pettiti DB. A patient-held minirecord to promote adult preventive care. *J Fam Pract*. 1992;34:457-463.

Harris RP, O'Malley MS, Fletcher SW, Knight BP. Prompting physicians for preventive procedures: a five-year study of manual and computer reminders. *Am J Prev Med*. 1990;6:145-152.

Ornstein SM, Garr DR, Jenkins RG, Rust PF, Arnon AA. Computer-generated physician and patient reminders: tools to improve population adherence to selected preventive services. *J Fam Pract*. 1991;32:82-90.

Pommerenke FA, Dietrich A. Improving and maintaining preventive services: I. Applying the patient model. *J Fam Pract*. 1992;34:86-91.

Pommerenke FA and Weed DL. Physician compliance: Improving skills in preventive medicine practices. *American Family Physician*. 1991; 43(2): 560-568.

Stange, KC. One size doesn't fit all: Multimethod research yields new insights into interventions to increase prevention in family practice. *J Fam Pract*. 1996; 43(4): 358-60.

McVea, K, Crabtree, BF et al. An Ounce Of Prevention? Evaluation of the `Put Prevention Into Practice' Program. *J Fam Pract*. 1996; 43(4): 361-69.

US Preventive Services Task Force. *Guide to Clinical Preventive Services*. 2nd ed. Washington, DC: US Department of Health and Human Services; 1996.

Children and Adolescents

1

ANEMIA

Improved nutrition has eased the problem of childhood anemia in the United States. However, certain groups of children, particularly infants and adolescent girls, remain at significant risk. Factors that place infants at high risk include low socioeconomic status, consumption of cow's milk before age 1 year, consumption of formula not fortified with iron, and low birth weight. Untreated anemia can lead to fatigue, apathy, impairment of growth and development, and decreased resistance to infection.

Iron deficiency is the most common cause of anemia in children and adolescents. Hemoglobinopathies, such as sickle cell disease and thalassemia, are also significant causes. See chapters 8 and 27 for information on screening for hemoglobinopathies in newborns and adults, respectively.

Recommendations of Major Authorities

American Academy of Family Physicians (AAFP) and **US Preventive Services Task Force (USPSTF)**—Hemoglobin concentration screening should be performed between 6 and 12 months of age for infants in high-risk groups. The **AAFP** and **USPSTF** define high-risk groups as infants living in poverty; African Americans; American Indians; Alaska Natives; immigrants from developing countries; preterm and low-birthweight infants; and infants whose principal intake is unfortified cow's milk.

American Academy of Pediatrics and **Bright Futures**—Hemoglobin or hematocrit should be measured once during infancy (between 1 and 9 months) for all children and once during adolescence for all menstruating teenagers. **Bright Futures** recommends hemoglobin and hematocrit screening at age 6 months if certification for Women, Infants, and Children (WIC) is needed. **Bright Futures** also recommends annual hemoglobin and hematocrit screening for adolescent females (ages 11 to 21 years) if any of the following risk factors are present: moderate to heavy menses, chronic weight loss, nutritional deficit, or athletic activity.

Canadian Task Force on the Periodic Health Examination—
There is conflicting and insufficient evidence to recommend for or against inclusion or exclusion of routine hemoglobin measurements at 6 to 12 months of age in normal infants. However, there is fair evidence to recommend a routine measurement for high-risk infants (infants of families of low socioeconomic status, Chinese or aboriginal ethnic origin, low birth weight [<2500 grams], or fed only whole cow's milk during the first year of life).

Basics of Anemia Screening

1. Three basic methods are used to determine hemoglobin levels and hematocrits: venipuncture with analysis by automated cell counter, capillary sampling with analysis by hemoglobinometer, or capillary sampling with microhematocrit analysis by centrifuge. (**NOTE:** The microhematocrit method yields slightly higher values and is somewhat less sensitive than the automated cell counter method. The capillary methods may provide less reliable results because of greater variation in sampling technique than venipuncture.)

2. In general, do not screen for anemia in a child who has had fever or infection during the preceding 2 to 3 weeks.

3. If the capillary method is used, observe the following principles of collection:

    In infants, the best sites are the medial and lateral aspects of the plantar surface of the heel. In older children, the best sites are the medial and lateral aspects of the pulp of a finger; make the puncture perpendicular to the skin and across the dermal ridges.

    To increase blood flow and accuracy of the test, make sure the heel or finger is warm.

    Before puncture, clean the site with an antiseptic and allow it to dry.

    Use sterile, disposable lancets with tips less than 2.5 mm long for infants aged 6 months or younger. Lancets with longer tips (up to 5 mm) may be used for older children.

    Wipe away the first two to three drops of blood, which contain tissue fluids, with a dry gauze.

    Do not milk or squeeze the puncture site, because this may cause hemolysis and admixture of tissue fluids with the specimen.

4. Table 1.1 shows hemoglobin and hematocrit cut points for the diagnosis of anemia in children, which are derived from the Second National Health and Nutrition Examination Survey (NHANES II) conducted from 1976

Table 1.1. Hemoglobin and Hematocrit Cut Points for Anemia in Children 1 Year of Age or Older

Gender	Age, years	Hemoglobin, g/dL	Hematocrit, %
Both Genders	1-1.9	11.0	33.0
	2-4.9	11.2	34.0
	5-7.9	11.4	34.5
	8-11.9	11.6	35.0
Female	12-14.9	11.8	35.5
	15-17.9	12.0	36.0
	≥18	12.0	36.0
Male	12-14.9	12.3	37.0
	15-17.9	12.6	38.0
	≥18	13.6	41.0

From: Centers for Disease Control. CDC criteria for anemia in children and childbearing-aged women. MMWR. 1989;38:400-404.

through 1980. Although NHANES II did not provide data for children younger than 1 year of age, the cut points for 6-month-old children determined by extrapolation are only a fraction of a unit less than those for 1-year-old children.

Cut points for anemia should be adjusted upward for children and adolescents who live at high altitudes or smoke (See Tables 27.1 and 27.2).

Patient Resources

Sickle Cell Anemia (New Hope for People With). FDA Office of Consumer Affairs. HFE 88 Rm 1675, 5600 Fishers Ln, Rockville, MD 20857; (800)532-4440.

Provider Resources

Bright Futures: Guidelines for Health Supervision of Infants, Children and Adolescents; Bright Futures Pocket Guide; Bright Futures Anticipatory Guidance Cards. Available from the National Center for Education in Maternal and Child Health, 2000 15th Street North, Suite 701, Arlington, VA 22201-2617; (703)524-7802. Internet address: http://www.brightfutures.org

Selected References

American Academy of Family Physicians. *Summary of Policy Recommendations for Periodic Health Examination.* Kansas City, Mo: American Academy of Family Physicians; 1997.

American Academy of Pediatrics, Committee on Nutrition. *Pediatric Nutrition Handbook*. 3rd ed. Elk Grove Village, Il: American Academy of Pediatrics; 1993.

American Academy of Pediatrics, Committee on Practice and Ambulatory Medicine. Recommendations for pediatric preventive health care. *Pediatrics*. 1995;96:373-374.

Canadian Task Force on the Periodic Health Examination. Prevention of iron deficiency anemia in infants. In: *The Canadian Guide to Clinical Preventive Health Care*. Ottawa, Canada: Minister of Supply and Services; 1994: chap 23.

Centers for Disease Control. CDC criteria for anemia in children and childbearing-aged women. *MMWR*. 1989;38:400-404.

Dallman PR. Has routine screening of infants for anemia become obsolete in the United States? *Pediatrics*. 1987;80:439-441.

Dallman PR. New approaches to screening for iron deficiency. *J Pediatr*. 1977;90:678-681.

Dallman PR, Yip R, Johnson C. Prevalence and causes of anemia in the United States, 1976 to 1980. *Am J Clin Nutr*. 1984;39:437-445.

Green M, ed. *Bright Futures: Guidelines for Health Supervision of Infants, Children, and Adolescents*. Arlington, Va: National Center for Education in Maternal and Child Health, 1994.

Lozoff B, Brittenham GM, Wolf AW, et al. Iron deficiency anemia and iron therapy effects on infant developmental test performance. *Pediatrics*. 1987;79:981-995.

Meites S, Levitt MJ. Skin-puncture and blood-collecting techniques for infants. *Clin Chem*. 1979;25:183-189.

Randolph VS. Considerations for the clinical laboratory serving the pediatric patient. *Am J Med Technol*. 1982;48:7.

Reeves JD, Yip R, Kiley VA, Dallman PR. Iron deficiency in infants: the influence of mild antecedent infection. *J Pediatr*. 1984;105:874-879.

Thomas WJ, Collins TM. Comparison of venipuncture blood counts with microcapillary measurement in screening for anemia in one-year-old infants. *J Pediatr*. 1982;101:32-35.

US Preventive Services Task Force. Screening for iron deficiency anemia. In: *Guide to Clinical Preventive Services*. 2nd ed. Washington, DC: US Department of Health and Human Services; 1996: chap 22.

Yip R, Binkin NJ, Fleshood L, Trowbridge FL. Declining prevalence of anemia among low-income children in the United States. *JAMA*. 1987;258:1619-1623.

Young PC, Hamill BH, Wasserman RC, Dickerman JD. Evaluation of the capillary microhematocrit as a screening test for anemia in pediatric office practice. *Pediatrics*. 1986;78:206-209.

2

BLOOD PRESSURE

Important changes have occurred in the measurement, epidemiology, and significance of childhood blood pressure since the publication of the first edition of the *Clinician's Handbook*. These changes were summarized in an update from The National High Blood Pressure Education Program Working Group on Hypertension Control in Children and Adolescents (October, 1996). Current understanding of childhood blood pressure not only recognizes the importance of identification of children with hypertension due to secondary conditions but also the realization that mild elevations in blood pressure during childhood (and particularly adolescence) are more common than previously thought. Elevated blood pressure in some children may represent the early onset of essential hypertension.

Blood pressure varies throughout the day in children and adults because of normal diurnal fluctuation and other factors such as physical activity and emotional stress. Body size is the most important determinant of blood pressure in children. New tables of blood pressure percentiles (Tables 2.1 and 2.2) have been released; these tables consider height in addition to age and sex.

Hypertension is defined as average systolic or diastolic blood pressure greater than or equal to the 95th percentile for age, sex, and height measured on at least three separate occasions. Elevated blood pressure must be confirmed on repeated visits before characterizing an individual as having hypertension. A more precise characterization of an individual's blood pressure level is an average of multiple measurements taken over weeks to months. With repeated measurement using standardized techniques, only about 1% of children and adolescents will be diagnosed with hypertension.

Table 2.1. Blood Pressure Levels for the 90th and 95th Percentiles of Blood Pressure for Boys Aged 1 to 17 Years by Percentiles of Height

Age, y	Blood Pressure Percentile*	Systolic Blood Pressure by Percentile of Height, mm Hg †							Diastolic Blood Pressure by Percentile of Height, mm Hg †						
		5%	10%	25%	50%	75%	90%	95%	5%	10%	25%	50%	75%	90%	95%
1	90th	94	95	97	98	100	102	102	50	51	52	53	54	54	55
	95th	98	99	101	102	104	106	106	55	55	56	57	58	59	59
2	90th	98	99	100	102	104	105	106	55	55	56	57	58	59	59
	95th	101	102	104	106	108	109	110	59	59	60	61	62	63	63
3	90th	100	101	103	105	107	108	109	59	59	60	61	62	63	63
	95th	104	105	107	109	111	112	113	63	63	64	65	66	67	67
4	90th	102	103	105	107	109	110	111	62	62	63	64	65	66	66
	95th	106	107	109	111	113	114	115	66	67	67	68	69	70	71
5	90th	104	105	106	108	110	112	112	65	65	66	67	68	69	69
	95th	108	109	110	112	114	115	116	69	70	70	71	72	73	74
6	90th	105	106	108	110	111	113	114	67	68	69	70	70	71	72
	95th	109	110	112	114	115	117	117	72	72	73	74	75	76	76
7	90th	106	107	109	111	113	114	115	69	70	71	72	72	73	74
	95th	110	111	113	115	116	118	119	74	74	75	76	77	78	78
8	90th	107	108	110	112	114	115	116	71	71	72	73	74	75	75
	95th	111	112	114	116	118	119	120	75	76	76	77	78	79	80
9	90th	109	110	112	113	115	117	117	72	73	73	74	75	76	77
	95th	113	114	116	117	119	121	121	76	77	78	79	80	80	81
10	90th	110	112	113	115	117	118	119	73	74	74	75	76	77	78
	95th	114	115	117	119	121	122	123	77	78	79	80	80	81	82
11	90th	112	113	115	117	119	120	121	74	74	75	76	77	78	78
	95th	116	117	119	121	123	124	125	78	79	79	80	81	82	83
12	90th	115	116	117	119	121	123	123	75	75	76	77	78	78	79
	95th	119	120	121	123	125	126	127	79	79	80	81	82	83	83
13	90th	117	118	120	122	124	125	126	75	76	76	77	78	79	80
	95th	121	122	124	126	128	129	130	79	80	81	82	83	83	84
14	90th	120	121	123	125	126	128	128	76	76	77	78	79	80	80
	95th	124	125	127	128	130	132	132	80	81	81	82	83	84	85
15	90th	123	124	125	127	129	131	131	77	77	78	79	80	81	81
	95th	127	128	129	131	133	134	135	81	82	83	83	84	85	86
16	90th	125	126	128	130	132	133	134	79	79	80	81	82	82	83
	95th	129	130	132	134	136	137	138	83	83	84	85	86	87	87
17	90th	128	129	131	133	134	136	136	81	81	82	83	84	85	85
	95th	132	133	135	136	138	140	140	85	85	86	87	88	89	89

*Blood pressure percentile was determined by a single measurement.

†Height percentile was determined by standard growth curves.

From: National High Blood Pressure Education Program Working Group on Hypertension Control in Children and Adolescents. Update on the 1987 task force report on high blood pressure in children and adolescents: a working group report from the National High Blood Pressure Education Program. Pediatrics. 1996;98(4):649-658.

Table 2.2. Blood Pressure Levels for the 90th and 95th Percentiles of Blood Pressure for Girls Aged 1 to 17 Years by Percentiles of Height

Age, y	Blood Pressure Percentile*	Systolic Blood Pressure by Percentile of Height, mm Hg †							Diastolic Blood Pressure by Percentile of Height, mm Hg †						
		5%	10%	25%	50%	75%	90%	95%	5%	10%	25%	50%	75%	90%	95%
1	90th	97	98	99	100	102	103	104	53	53	53	54	55	56	56
	95th	101	102	103	104	105	107	107	57	57	57	58	59	60	60
2	90th	99	99	100	102	103	104	105	57	57	58	58	59	60	61
	95th	102	103	104	105	107	108	109	61	61	62	62	63	64	65
3	90th	100	100	102	103	104	105	106	61	61	61	62	63	63	64
	95th	104	104	105	107	108	109	110	65	65	65	66	67	67	68
4	90th	101	102	103	104	106	107	108	63	63	64	65	65	66	67
	95th	105	106	107	108	109	111	111	67	67	68	69	69	70	71
5	90th	103	103	104	106	107	108	109	65	66	66	67	68	68	69
	95th	107	107	108	110	111	112	113	69	70	70	71	72	72	73
6	90th	104	105	106	107	109	110	111	67	67	68	69	69	70	71
	95th	108	109	110	111	112	114	114	71	71	72	73	73	74	75
7	90th	106	107	108	109	110	112	112	69	69	69	70	71	72	72
	95th	110	110	112	113	114	115	116	73	73	73	74	75	76	76
8	90th	108	109	110	111	112	113	114	70	70	71	71	72	73	74
	95th	112	112	113	115	116	117	118	74	74	75	75	76	77	78
9	90th	110	110	112	113	114	115	116	71	72	72	73	74	74	75
	95th	114	114	115	117	118	119	120	75	76	76	77	78	78	79
10	90th	112	112	114	115	116	117	118	73	73	73	74	75	76	76
	95th	116	116	117	119	120	121	122	77	77	77	78	79	80	80
11	90th	114	114	116	117	118	119	120	74	74	75	75	76	77	77
	95th	118	118	119	121	122	123	124	78	78	79	79	80	81	81
12	90th	116	116	118	119	120	121	122	75	75	76	76	77	78	78
	95th	120	120	121	123	124	125	126	79	79	80	80	81	82	82
13	90th	118	118	119	121	122	123	124	76	76	77	78	78	79	80
	95th	121	122	123	125	126	127	128	80	80	81	82	82	83	84
14	90th	119	120	121	122	124	125	126	77	77	78	79	79	80	81
	95th	123	124	125	126	128	129	130	81	81	82	83	83	84	85
15	90th	121	121	122	124	125	126	127	78	78	79	79	80	81	82
	95th	124	125	126	128	129	130	131	82	82	83	83	84	85	86
16	90th	122	122	123	125	126	127	128	79	79	79	80	81	82	82
	95th	125	126	127	128	130	131	132	83	83	83	84	85	86	86
17	90th	122	123	124	125	126	128	128	79	79	79	80	81	82	82
	95th	126	126	127	129	130	131	132	83	83	83	84	85	86	86

*Blood pressure percentile was determined by a single measurement.

†Height percentile was determined by standard growth curves.

From: National High Blood Pressure Education Program Working Group on Hypertension Control in Children and Adolescents. Update on the 1987 task force report on high blood pressure in children and adolescents: a working group report from the National High Blood Pressure Education Program. Pediatrics. 1996;98(4):649-658.

Figure 2.1. Determination of proper cuff size: step 1. The cuff bladder width should be approximately 40% of the circumference of the arm measured at a point midway between the olecranon and acromion.

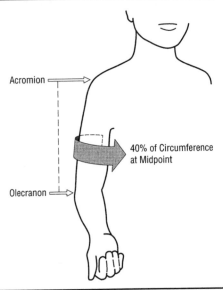

From: National Institutes of Health, National Heart, Lung, and Blood Institute. Update on the Task Force Report (1987) on High Blood Pressure in Children and Adolescents: a Working Group Report From the National High Blood Pressure Education Program. Bethesda, Md: National Institutes of Health; 1996. NIH Publication No. 96-3790.

Recommendations of Major Authorities

American Academy of Pediatrics and **Bright Futures**—Blood pressure should be measured in children at 3, 4, 5, 6, and 8 years of age, and annually beginning at 10 years of age.

American Medical Association—During adolescence, blood pressure should be measured annually.

National Heart, Lung, and Blood Institute Task Force on Blood Pressure Control in Children—Blood pressure should be measured annually beginning at 3 years of age.

US Preventive Services Task Force—Measurement of blood pressure during office visits is recommended for children and adolescents. Beginning age and periodicity are not specified. This recommendation is based on the proven benefits of early detection of treatable causes of secondary hypertension.

Figure 2.2. Determination of proper cuff size: step 2. The cuff bladder should cover 80% to 100% of the circumference of the arm.

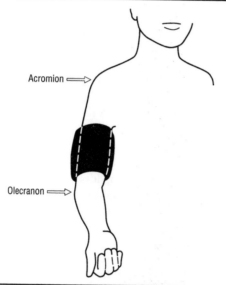

Acromion ⟹

Olecranon ⟹

From: National Institutes of Health, National Heart, Lung, and Blood Institute. Update on the Task Force Report (1987) on High Blood Pressure in Children and Adolescents: a Working Group Report From the National High Blood Pressure Education Program. Bethesda, Md: National Institutes of Health; 1996. NIH Publication No. 96-3790.

Basics of Blood Pressure Screening

1. Advise patients, especially adolescents, not to smoke or otherwise use to-bacco or ingest caffeine, including cola products, for at least 30 minutes before the measurement.

2. Perform the measurement in a controlled area and after 3 to 5 minutes of rest with the child in the seated position. The right arm should be fully ex-posed and the cubital fossa supported at heart level.

3. The mercury column sphygmomanometer is preferred over the calibrated aneroid manometer.

4. Choose an appropriately sized cuff. The bladder width should be 40% of the arm circumference measured at midpoint between the olecranon and acromion (Figure 2.1). This usually translates into a cuff that covers 80% to 100% of the circumference of the arm without impinging on the antecu-bital fossa (Figure 2.2). Use of a cuff that is too small will result in falsely elevated measurements. Use of a cuff that is too large will result in falsely low measurements.

5. Place the bell of the stethoscope lightly on the antecubital fossa over the brachial artery. Applying too much pressure may lead to inaccurate measurements. Rapidly inflate the cuff to approximately 20 mm Hg above the point at which the pulse is no longer audible. Then deflate the cuff at a rate of 2 to 3 mm Hg per second. The onset of a tapping sound (the first Korotkoff sound) is used to determine systolic blood pressure, and the disappearance of Korotkoff sounds determines the diastolic blood pressure.

6. Documentation of the patient's position, limb used, and cuff size may be required for consistency of repeated blood pressure measurements.

7. The systolic and diastolic blood pressures corresponding to the 90th and 95th percentiles according to gender, age, and percentile of height are shown in Tables 2.1 and 2.2. The height percentile is determined from the standard growth charts. A child is considered normotensive if the blood pressure is below the 90th percentile. Blood pressures in the 90th through 94th percentiles are considered high normal, and those at or above the 95th percentile are considered elevated.

8. Standards for systolic and diastolic BP for infants younger than 1 year are available. In children of this age, systolic BP is used to define hypertension.

Patient Resources

Eat Right to Lower Your High Blood Pressure; High Blood Pressure: Treat it for Life; Check Your Healthy Heart IQ; High Blood Pressure and What You Can Do About It; Six Good Reasons to Control Your High Blood Pressure. National Heart, Lung, and Blood Institute Information Center, PO Box 30105, Bethesda, MD 20824-0105; (301)251-1222 (English and Spanish). Internet address: http://www.nhlbi.nih.gov/nhlbi/nhlbi.htm

Provider Resources

The Fifth Report of the Joint National Committee on Detection, Evaluation, and Treatment of High Blood Pressure. National Heart, Lung, and Blood Institute Information Center, PO Box 30105, Bethesda, MD 20824-0105; (301)251-1222 (English and Spanish). Internet address: http://www.nhlbi.nih.gov/nhlbi/nhlbi.htm

Bright Futures Guidelines for Health Supervision of Infants, Children and Adolescents; Bright Futures Pocket Guide; Bright Futures Anticipatory Guidance Cards. Available from the National Center for Education in Maternal and Child Health, 2000 15th Street North, Suite 701, Arlington, VA 22201-2617. (703)524-7802. Internet address: http://www.brightfutures.org

Selected References

American Academy of Pediatrics, Committee on Practice and Ambulatory Medicine. Recommendations for pediatric preventive health care. *Pediatrics.* 1995;96:373-374.

American Medical Association. Rationale and recommendation: hypertension. In: *AMA Guidelines for Adolescent Preventive Services (GAPS): Recommendations and Rationale.* Chicago, Il: American Medical Association; 1994: chap 8.

DeSwiet M, Dillon MJ. Hypertension in children. *Br Med J.* 1989;299(6697):469-470.

Fixler DE, Laird WP. Validity of mass blood pressure screening in children. *Pediatrics.* 1983;72:459-463.

Green M, ed. *Bright Futures: Guidelines for Health Supervision of Infants, Children, and Adolescents.* Arlington, Va: National Center for Education in Maternal and Child Health; 1994.

Joint National Committee on Detection, Evaluation, and Treatment of High Blood Pressure. *The Fifth Report of the Joint National Committee on the Detection, Evaluation, and Treatment of High Blood Pressure.* Bethesda, Md: National Institutes of Health; 1993. US Department of Health and Human Services publication NIH 93-1088. (See also, *Arch Intern Med.* 1993;153:154-183.)

Lauer RM, Burns TL, Clarke WR. Assessing children's blood pressure—considerations of age and body size: the Muscatine study. *Pediatrics.* 1985;75:1081-1090.

Mehta SK. Pediatric hypertension: a challenge for pediatricians. *Am J Dis Child.* 1987;141:893-894.

National High Blood Pressure Education Program Working Group on Hypertension Control in Children and Adolescents. *Update on the 1987 task force report on high blood pressure in children and adolescents: a working group report from the National High Blood Pressure Education Program.* Bethesda, Md: National Institutes of Health; 1996. US Department of Health and Human Services publication NIH 96-3790.

Sinaiko AR, Gomez-Marion O, Prineas RJ. Prevalence of "significant" hypertension in junior high school-aged children: the Children and Adolescent Blood Pressure Program. *J Pediatr.* 1989;114:664-669.

Task Force on Blood Pressure Control in Children. Report of the Second Task Force on Blood Pressure Control in Children—1987. *Pediatrics.* 1987;79:1-25.

US Preventive Services Task Force. Screening for hypertension. In: *Guide to Clinical Preventive Services.* 2nd ed. Washington, DC: US Department of Health and Human Services; 1996: chap 3.

3

BODY MEASUREMENT

Body measurement of infants and children helps clinicians recognize significant childhood problems, including growth retardation, malnutrition, obesity, and developmental abnormalities. Measurement of head circumference can identify abnormal brain development in infants, including hydrocephalus. In older children and adolescents, body measurement can identify those who are overweight and those with possible eating disorders. Both of these conditions are targets for screening in this population. The prevalence of overweight in children is increasing and has been associated with development of heart disease and Type 2 diabetes mellitus in adulthood.

Recommendations of Major Authorities

American Academy of Family Physicians and US Preventive Services Task Force—Measure height and weight periodically.

American Academy of Pediatrics and **Bright Futures**—Height, weight, and head circumference should be measured at birth, at 2 to 4 weeks, and at 1, 2, 4, 6, 9, 12, 15, 18, and 24 months of age. Height and weight should also be measured at 3, 4, 5, 6, and 8 years of age, and annually beginning at 10 years of age. **Bright Futures** also recommends scoliosis and sexual maturity ratings as part of a complete physical exam for adolescents (ages 10 to 21).

American Medical Association—All adolescents should be screened annually for eating disorders and obesity by measuring weight and stature and by asking about body image and dieting patterns.

Canadian Task Force on the Periodic Health Examination—There is fair evidence for the inclusion of serial measurements of height, weight, and head circumference in the periodic health examination of infants and children.

Basics of Body Measurement

1. To ensure accurate measurements of infants and young children, use an assistant, and if necessary, take measurements more than once, particularly when children are very young or uncooperative.

2. Determine the height of children younger than 2 years of age by measuring their length while they are recumbent. Use a measuring board with a stationary headboard and a sliding vertical foot piece, if one is available. Otherwise, use a horizontal surface, a stationary vertical surface, a movable vertical-surfaced object, and a measuring tape. The general principles for taking the measurement are the same, regardless of the apparatus used:

   - Have the child lie flat on his/her back along the center of the board or examining table with all parts of the body touching the board

   - Position the child's head against the headboard, with eyes looking upward

   - Fully extend the hips and knees

   - Move the foot piece until it rests firmly against the child's heels with feet flat

   - Record measurements to the nearest 1/8 inch (0.3 cm)

3. Obtain the standing height of children beginning at 2 years of age. Use of a stadiometer, an instrument specifically designed for height measurements, is preferred. However, accurate measurements may be obtained by using a graduated ruler or tape attached to a wall and placing a flat-surfaced object horizontally on top of the child's head. Height-measuring rods that are attached to weight scales tend to become inaccurate with use; in general, do not use them unless they are checked frequently for accuracy. The general principles for taking the measurement are as follows:

   - Have the child remove his/her shoes before being measured

   - Have the child stand with the head, shoulder blades, buttocks, and heels touching the wall

   - Make sure the knees are straight and the feet are flat on the floor

   - Ask the child to look straight ahead

   - Lower the flat-surfaced object (or movable headboard) until it touches the crown of the child's head, compressing the hair

4. Use a balance-beam or electronic scale to weigh infants and children. Spring-type scales are not sufficiently accurate for this use. Check the scale before each use to ensure that it is zeroed. The infant or child should wear only a dry diaper or light undergarment while being weighed. Check scales regularly for accuracy, and make an effort to use the same scale on subsequent visits.

5. Measure a child's head circumference by extending a nonstretchable measuring tape (disposable paper tapes are better than cloth) around the most prominent part of the occiput to the middle of the forehead. Tighten the tape to compress the hair.

6. Plot measurements on age- and gender-specific National Center for Health Statistics (NCHS) growth charts for comparison with NCHS reference values. Recording serial measurements over time provides an accurate record of growth; large or sustained deviations signal a potential problem. Interpret measurements within the context of the individual child's family and growth history. If a child's measurements fall within the 10th through 25th percentile range or the 75th through 90th percentile range, assess past growth patterns and genetic and environmental factors to determine if follow-up is necessary. Recheck measurements that are below the 5th percentile or above the 95th percentile. If these measurements are confirmed, further medical evaluations may be needed.

NOTE: Disagreement exists about the validity of using a single set of reference standards for all subpopulations of children in the United States. Although measurements should be assessed within the context of genetic and environmental factors, most authorities support use of the NCHS reference standards. Exceptions include children with genetic conditions such as Down's, Turner's, Marfan's, and fragile X syndromes, achondroplasia, sickle cell disease, and neurofibromatosis. Separate growth charts have been developed for some of these conditions. Growth charts also have been developed for use with infants born prematurely (See Selected References).

7. Some authorities, including the American Medical Association, recommend using body mass index (BMI) calculation to assess the weight of adolescents. (See chapter 29 for information about the calculation and use of BMI.) However, because of the lack of standardized recommended values to assess BMI in adolescents, growth charts are the preferred method for assessing their weight.

Patient Resources

Health Diary: Myself, My Baby. This booklet contains information about pregnancy and early childhood development. To order, contact the Superintendent of Documents, Government Printing Office, Washington, DC 20402-9325.

The Child Health Record. This material includes growth charts and other record forms. *Rx for Good Health Growth Chart.* This 8-1/2" x 33" poster contains information on growth for children from birth to 10 years of age. *Your Child's*

Growth: Developmental Milestones. Presents guidelines to gauge normal stages of development in children 3 months to 6 years of age. To order, contact the American Academy of Pediatrics, PO Box 927, Elk Grove Village, IL 60009-0927; (800)433-9016. Internet address: http://www.aap.org

Your Growing Baby. This pamphlet includes information on growth. To order, contact Ross Laboratories, Dept L-1120, Columbus, OH 43260; (800)227-5767.

Provider Resources

Growth Charts: Mead Johnson Nutritional Division. For the name and telephone number of an area representative, call: (812)429-5000.

Growth Charts: Ross Laboratories, Dept L-1120, Columbus, OH 43260; (800)227-5767.

Bright Futures: Guidelines for Health Supervision of Infants, Children and Adolescents; Bright Futures Pocket Guide; Bright Futures Anticipatory Guidance Cards. Available from the National Center for Education in Maternal and Child Health, 2000 15th Street North, Suite 701, Arlington, VA 22201-2617; (703)524-7802. Internet address: http://www.brightfutures.org

Selected References

American Academy of Family Physicians. *Summary of Policy Recommendations for Periodic Health Examination.* Kansas City, Mo: American Academy of Family Physicians; 1997.

American Medical Association. Rationale and recommendation: dietary habits, eating disorders, and obesity. In: *AMA Guidelines for Adolescent Preventive Services (GAPS): Recommendations and Rationale.* Chicago, Ill: American Medical Association; 1994: chap 5.

American Academy of Pediatrics, Committee on Practice and Ambulatory Medicine. Recommendations for pediatric preventive health care. *Pediatrics.* 1995;96:373-374.

Babson SG, Benda GI. Growth graphs for the clinical assessment of infants of varying gestational age. *J Pediatr.* 1976;89:814-820.

Canadian Task Force on the Periodic Health Examination. Screening for childhood obesity. In: *The Canadian Guide to Clinical Preventive Health Care.* Ottawa, Canada: Minister of Supply and Services; 1994: chap 30.

Canadian Task Force on the Periodic Health Examination. Well baby care in the first 2 years of life. In: *The Canadian Guide to Clinical Preventive Health Care.* Ottawa, Canada: Minister of Supply and Services; 1994: chap 24.

Casey PH, Kraemer HC, Bernbaum J, et al. Growth patterns of low birth weight preterm infants: an analysis of a large, varied sample. *J Pediatr.* 1990;117:289-307.

Chinn S, Price CE, Rona RJ. Need for new reference curves for height. *Arch Dis Child.* 1989;64:1545-1553.

Cronk C, Crocker AC, Pueschel SM, et al. Growth charts for children with Down syndrome: 1 month to 18 years of age. *Pediatrics.* 1988;81:102-110.

Dine MS, Gartside PS, Glueck CJ, et al. Relationship of head circumference to length in the first 400 days of life. *Pediatrics.* 1981;67:506-507.

Green M, ed. *Bright Futures: Guidelines for Health Supervision of Infants, Children, and Adolescents.* Arlington, Va: National Center for Education in Maternal and Child Health, 1994.

Hamill PVV, Drizd TA, Johnson CL, et al. Physical growth: National Center for Health Statistics percentiles. *Am J Clin Nutr.* 1979;32:607-629.

Lohman TG, Roche AF, Martorell R. *Anthropometric Standardization Reference Manual.* Champaign, Ill: Human Kinetics Books; 1988.

Moore WM, Roche AF. *Pediatric Anthropometry.* Columbus, Oh: Ross Laboratories; 1982.

Naeraa RW, Nielsen J. Standards for growth and final height in Turner's syndrome. *Acta Paediatr Scand.* 1990;79:182-190.

Nutritional Screening of Children: A Manual for Screening and Followup. Washington, DC: US Department of Health and Human Services, Public Health Service, Health Services Administration, Bureau of Community Health Services, Office of Maternal and Child Health; 1981. US Department of Health and Human Services publication HSA 81-5114.

National Center for Health Statistics Growth Charts. *Monthly Vital Statistics Report.* Hyattsville, Md: US Department of Health, Education, and Welfare; 1976;25:1-22. USHEW publication HRA 76-1120.

US Preventive Services Task Force. Screening for obesity. In: *Guide to Clinical Preventive Services.* 2nd ed. Washington, DC: US Department of Health and Human Services; 1996: chap 21.

Vaughn VC. On the utility of growth curves. *JAMA.* 1992;267:975-976.

Yip R, Scanlon K, Trowbridge F. Improving the growth status of Asian refugee children in the United States. *JAMA.* 1992;267:937-940.

CHOLESTEROL

Coronary heart disease (CHD) is the major cause of death in the United States. The atherosclerotic process that leads to CHD often begins in childhood. Because unfavorable lipoprotein levels are linked to early atherosclerotic changes in children, and because children with high cholesterol levels are at increased risk of having high cholesterol levels as adults, identifying such children and intervening to decrease their cholesterol levels have been suggested as a means of preventing CHD in adulthood.

Children from higher risk families (with a pattern of hypercholesterolemia or premature CHD in the adult members) who have elevated serum cholesterol levels appear to be at a particularly increased risk for CHD when they reach adulthood. This association is the basis for some of the recommendations made by major authorities for the selective screening of children for elevated cholesterol. For the general pediatric population over age 2 years, counseling to encourage a reduced intake of dietary fat, especially saturated fats, is recommended.

Children identified with high cholesterol levels may be considered for dietary or drug interventions to lower their cholesterol level. In the Dietary Intervention Study in Children (DISC), diet produced a significant reduction in cholesterol levels without adverse effects on growth and development, but the effects of drug treatment over periods of 40 years or more have not been established.

See chapter 20 for information on nutrition counseling in children/adolescents.

Recommendations of Major Authorities

Canadian Task Force on the Periodic Health Examination—
There is insufficient evidence to recommend for or against routine cholesterol screening of children and adolescents. Individual clinical judgment should be exercised to determine the need for screening.

National Heart, Lung, and Blood Institute's National Cholesterol Education Program Expert Panel on Blood Cholesterol Levels in Children and Adolescents; American Academy of Pediatrics; Bright Futures; and **American Medical Association**— Universal screening of children and adolescents for cholesterol levels is not recommended. Children older than 2 years of age who have a parent with a total cholesterol level of 240 mg/dL or greater should be screened for both total serum cholesterol and HDL cholesterol levels. Children (older than age 2 years) and adolescents with a family history of premature cardiovascular disease (ie, a parent or grandparent who, at age 55 years or younger, had a documented myocardial infarction, angina pectoris, peripheral vascular disease, cerebrovascular disease, or sudden cardiac death, or underwent diagnostic coronary arteriography and was found to have atherosclerosis, or underwent coronary artery bypass surgery or angioplasty) should be screened for lipoprotein levels after a 12-hour fast. In children whose family history is not obtainable, screening may be indicated, especially if risk factors for coronary artery disease are present (eg, high blood pressure, smoking, overweight, or excessive consumption of saturated fat and cholesterol).

US Preventive Services Task Force—There is insufficient evidence to recommend screening of children and adolescents. For adolescents who have a family history of very high cholesterol, premature CHD in a first-degree relative (before age 50 years in men or age 60 years in women), or major nonlipid risk factors for CHD (eg, smoking, hypertension, diabetes), screening may be recommended on other grounds, because of the greater absolute risk attributable to high cholesterol levels in such persons and the potential long-term benefits of early lifestyle interventions in young persons with high cholesterol levels. Recommendations against screening of children may be made on other grounds, including the costs and inconvenience of screening and follow-up, greater potential for adverse effects of treatment, and the uncertain long-term benefits of small reductions in childhood cholesterol levels.

Basics of Cholesterol Screening

1. Children may eat a normal diet before total cholesterol screening. Children undergoing lipoprotein analysis should fast, ingesting nothing but water for 12 hours before the blood sample is taken.

2. Do not screen children who are acutely ill, including those with infectious diseases. Do not screen pregnant adolescents.

3. A venous sample obtained with the patient in the sitting position yields the most accurate results; recumbency lowers lipid levels. Documentation of position is important when comparing follow-up measurements.

4. Take into account the cholesterol-raising effect of certain medications, including corticosteroids, isotretinoin, thiazides, anticonvulsants, beta blockers, and certain anabolic steroids. If a patient meeting screening criteria takes one of these drugs, a potential strategy is to perform the test, and if the result is elevated, consider the magnitude of the elevation and the ease and safety of suspending medication for retesting in the absence of drugs.

5. The laboratory used for analysis should participate in a program of external standardization to ensure compliance with standards of precision and accuracy. The National Cholesterol Education Program's Laboratory Standardization Panel recommends that bias not exceed ±5% from the true value and that the intralaboratory coefficient of variation not exceed ±5%.

6. The National Cholesterol Education Program has recommended protocols for assessing cholesterol levels in the screening of children (Figures 4.1 and 4.2).

Figure 4.1. Assessment and Follow-up of Total Cholesterol Measurements

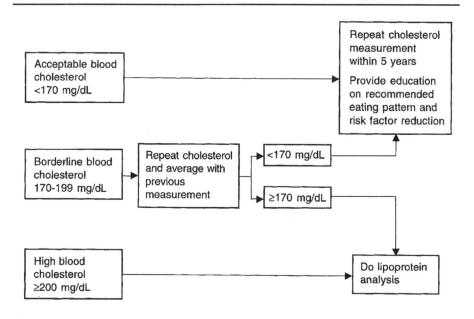

From: National Cholesterol Education Program. Report of the Expert Panel on Blood Cholesterol Levels in Children and Adolescents. Bethesda, Md: National Institutes of Health, National Heart, Lung, and Blood Institute; 1991. US Department of Health and Human Services publication NIH 91-2732.

Figure 4.2. Assessment and Follow-up of Lipoprotein Analysis

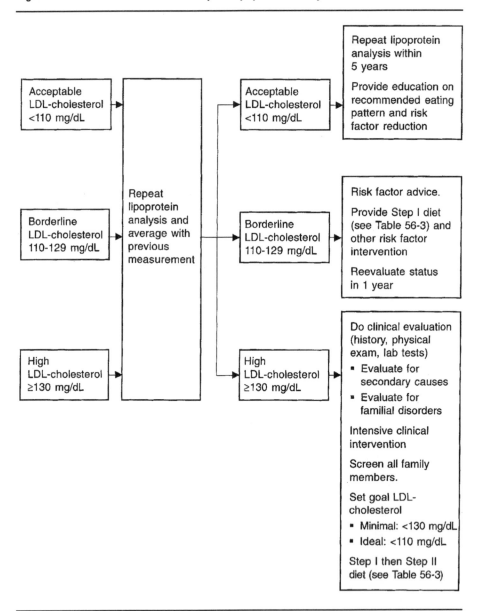

From: National Cholesterol Education Program. Report of the Expert Panel on Blood Cholesterol Levels in Children and Adolescents. Bethesda, Md: National Institutes of Health, National Heart, Lung, and Blood Institute; 1991. US Department of Health and Human Services publication NIH 91-2732.

Patient Resources

Step by Step: Eating to Lower Your High Blood Cholesterol; So You Have High Blood Cholesterol; Parents Guide: Cholesterol in Children—Healthy Eating is a Family Affair. National Heart, Lung, and Blood Institute Information Center, PO Box 30105, Bethesda, MD 20824-0105; (301)251-1222 (English and Spanish). Internet address: http://www.nhlbi.nih.gov/nhlbi/nhlbi.htm

Growing up Healthy: Fat, Cholesterol, and More. This brochure provides health and eating guidelines for children 2 to 6 years old. American Academy of Pediatrics, PO Box 927, Elk Grove Village, IL 60009-0927; (800)433-9016.

Provider Resources

Bright Futures: Guidelines for Health Supervision of Infants, Children and Adolescents; Bright Futures Pocket Guide; Bright Futures Anticipatory Guidance Cards. Available from the National Center for Education in Maternal and Child Health, 2000 15th Street North, Suite 701, Arlington, VA 22201-2617; (703)524-7802. Internet address: http://www.brightfutures.org

Selected References

American Academy of Pediatrics. Prudent life-style for children: dietary fat and cholesterol. *Pediatrics.* 1986;78:521-525.

American Academy of Pediatrics. *Pediatric Nutrition Handbook.* 3rd ed. Elk Grove Village, IL: American Academy of Pediatrics; 1993.

American Academy of Pediatrics, Committee on Nutrition. Statement on cholesterol. *Pediatrics.* 1992;90:469-473.

American Medical Association. Rationale and recommendation: hyperlipidemia. In: *AMA Guidelines for Adolescent Preventive Services (GAPS): Recommendations and Rationale.* Chicago, Il: American Medical Association; 1994: chap 9.

Bao W, Srinivasan SR, Wattigney WA, Bao W, Berenson GS. Usefulness of childhood low-density lipoprotein cholesterol level in predicting adult dyslipidemia and other cardiovascular risks. *Arch Intern Med.* 1996;156:1315-20.

Canadian Task Force on the Periodic Health Examination. Lowering the blood total cholesterol level to prevent coronary heart disease. In: *The Canadian Guide to Clinical Preventive Health Care.* Ottawa, Canada: Minister of Supply and Services; 1994: chap 54.

The Dietary Intervention Study In Children Collaborative Research Group. Efficacy and safety of lowering dietary intake of fat and cholesterol in children with elevated low-density lipoprotein cholesterol. *JAMA.* 1995;273:1429-35.

Diller PM, Huster GA, Leach AD, Laskamziski PM, Sprecher DL. Definition and application of the discretionary screening indicators according to the National Cholesterol Education Program for children and adolescents. *J Pediatr.* 1995;426:345-52.

Garcia RE, Moodie DS. Routine cholesterol surveillance in childhood. *Pediatrics.* 1989;84:751-755.

Green M, ed. *Bright Futures: Guidelines for Health Supervision of Infants, Children, and Adolescents.* Arlington, Va: National Center for Education in Maternal and Child Health, 1994.

Kuehl KS. Cholesterol screening in childhood. Targeted versus universal approaches. *Ann NY Acad Sci.* 1991;623:193-199.

National Cholesterol Education Program. *Recommendations for Improving Cholesterol Measurement.* Bethesda, MD: National Institutes of Health, National Heart, Lung, and Blood Institute; 1990. US Department of Health and Human Services, Public Health Service publication NIH 90-2964.

National Cholesterol Education Program, Expert Panel on Blood Cholesterol Levels in Children and Adolescents. *Report of the Expert Panel on Blood Cholesterol Levels in Children and Adolescents.* Bethesda, MD: National Institutes of Health, National Heart, Lung, and Blood Institute; 1991. US Department of Health and Human Services, Public Health Service publication NIH 91-2732.

Newman WP, Wattigney W, Berenson G. Autopsy studies in United States children and adolescents. Relationship of risk factors to atherosclerotic lesions. *Ann NY Acad Sci.* 1991;623:17-25.

Newman TB, Browner W, Hulley SB. The case against childhood cholesterol screening. *JAMA.* 1990;264:3039-3043.

Resnicow K, Berenson G, Shea S, Srinivasan S, et al. The case against the "case against childhood cholesterol screening." *JAMA.* 1991;265:3003-3005.

Resnicow K, Morley-Kotchen J, Wynder E. Plasma cholesterol levels of 6585 children in the United States; results of the know your body screening in five states. *Pediatrics.* 1989;84:969-976.

US Preventive Services Task Force. Screening for blood cholesterol. In: *Guide to Clinical Preventive Services.* 2nd ed. Washington, DC: US Department of Health and Human Services; 1996: chap 2.

5

DEPRESSION AND SUICIDE

Depression in children and adolescents is a significant health problem in the United States and is often overlooked or misdiagnosed in the primary care setting. The incidence of major depressive disorders in children is approximately 2% to 4% and increases two- to threefold during adolescence.

A family history of depression, particularly parental, is a major risk factor for childhood depression, but no other specific risk factors have been consistently identified. The following factors may be associated with a variety of adverse mental health outcomes in children, including depression: a history of verbal, physical, or sexual abuse; frequent separation from or loss of a loved one; attention deficit disorder; hyperactivity; chronic illness; poverty; and mental retardation. Complications of depression in childhood and adolescence include poor school performance, poor peer relations, alcohol and drug use, promiscuity, teenage pregnancy, other psychiatric illness, and suicide.

Suicide is the third leading cause of death among persons aged 15 to 24 years, following unintentional injuries and homicide. The rate of suicide among young males is five times that among young females. Firearms are the most common method of suicide for young males and females. Among young females, attempted suicide is reported more frequently than is completed suicide, although no national data are available.

Risk factors for suicide frequently occur in combination. The strongest risk factors for both attempted and completed suicide by children and adolescents are mental disorders, especially clinical depression and conduct problems, and substance abuse. Other risk factors include a family history of mental or addictive disorders or suicide, family violence, previous suicide attempts, and availability and accessibility of firearms in the home. Acute adverse life events such as incarceration or the breakup of a relationship, in association with an underlying psychiatric disorder or other risk factors, and the presence of a firearm in the home can be a potentially dangerous combination leading to suicide.

Recommendations of Major Authorities

American Academy of Pediatrics and **Bright Futures**—Behavioral assessment should be a routine part of health supervision throughout childhood and adolescence. Adolescents and their parents should be asked about suicidal thoughts or threats.

American Medical Association—Because of the pervasive nature of mood disorders, all adolescents should be screened annually for signs and symptoms of recurrent or severe depression. Special attention should be directed at adolescents who are performing poorly in school, who use alcohol or drugs, or who have had a deteriorating relationship with parents and peers. Physicians should also screen adolescents annually to identify those at risk for suicide. Parents or other adult care-givers of adolescents with suicidal intent should be counseled to remove weapons and potentially lethal medications from the home.

Canadian Task Force on the Periodic Health Examination—Routine screening for depression is not recommended, but physicians should maintain a high level of clinical sensitivity. Evaluation of suicide risk is recommended for persons at high risk: those with a history of psychiatric illness, depression, or drug and alcohol abuse, especially those living in isolation; those with chronic terminal illness; Native and Aboriginal people, especially young males; those with a family history of suicide; and first-generation immigrant women.

US Preventive Services Task Force—There is insufficient evidence to recommend for or against performance of routine screening tests for depression in asymptomatic patients in the primary care setting. Clinicians should, however, maintain an especially high index of suspicion for depressive symptoms in adolescents and young adults, persons with a family or personal history of depression, those with chronic illness, those who perceive or have experienced a recent loss, and those with sleep disorders, chronic pain, or multiple unexplained somatic complaints. There is also insufficient evidence to recommend for or against routine screening by primary care clinicians to detect suicide risk in asymptomatic persons. Clinicians should be alert to evidence of suicidal ideation when the history reveals risk factors for suicide, such as depression, alcohol or other drug abuse, other psychiatric disorders, prior attempted suicide, recent divorce, separation, unemployment, and recent bereavement.

Basics of Screening for Depression and Suicide

Depression

1. Become familiar with the risk factors for and symptoms of depression (See Recommendations of Major Authorities and Table 5.1).

2. Identify any risk factors or symptoms indicating the need for in-depth evaluation by a mental health professional.

Suicide

1. Become familiar with the risk factors for suicide (See Recommendations of Major Authorities).

2. Inquire about suicidal thoughts in a direct, straightforward manner.

3. Question those with suicidal thoughts about the extent and specificity of plans for suicide. Immediate referral to a mental health professional is advisable, especially for individuals with serious intent.

4. Counsel parents about the importance of restricting the access of children and adolescents to dangerous prescription drugs and firearms in the home.

Table 5.1. Symptoms of Major Depression

Depressed mood (or irritable mood in children and adolescents)

Markedly diminished interest or pleasure in activities

Significant weight loss or gain when not dieting, or decrease/increase in appetite (in children, consider failure to make expected weight gains), insomnia or hypersomnia

Psychomotor agitation or retardation

Fatigue or loss of energy, indecisiveness

Feelings of worthlessness or excessive or inappropriate guilt

Diminished ability to think or concentrate, problems at school

Recurrent thoughts of death, recurrent suicidal ideation

Adapted from: American Psychiatric Association, Committee on Nomenclature. Diagnostic and Statistical Manual of Mental Disorders, Third Edition, Revised. Washington, DC: American Psychiatric Association; 1987. Reproduced by permission of the publisher; copyright © 1987.

Patient Resources

Facts for Families: The Depressed Child; Teen Suicide; Children and Grief; Manic Depressive Illness in Teens. American Academy of Child and Adolescent Psychiatry, 3615 Wisconsin Ave, NW, Washington, DC 20016-3007; (202)966-7300; E-mail: 74003.264@compuserve.com

Surviving: Coping with Adolescent Depression and Suicide; Caring for Your Adolescent: Age 12 to 21; Divorce and Children. American Academy of Pediatrics, PO Box 927, Elk Grove Village, IL 60000-0927; (800)443-9016. Internet address: http://www.aap.org

Provider Resources

Bright Futures: Guidelines for Health Supervision of Infants, Children and Adolescents; Bright Futures Pocket Guide; Bright Futures Anticipatory Guidance Cards. Available from the National Center for Education in Maternal and Child Health, 2000 15th Street North, Suite 701, Arlington, VA 22201-2617; (703)524-7802. Internet address: http://www.brightfutures.org

The Classification of Child and Adolescent Mental Diagnosis in Primary Care. American Academy of Pediatrics, PO Box 927, Elk Grove Village, IL 60009-0927; (800)433-9016. Internet address: http://www.aap.org

Prevention in Child and Adolescent Psychiatry; Prevention of Mental Disorders, Alcohol and Other Drug Use in Children and Adolescents. American Academy of Child and Adolescent Psychiatry, 3615 Wisconsin Ave, NW, Washington, DC 20016-3007; (202)966-7300; E-mail 74003.264@compuserve.com

National Institute of Mental Health, 5600 Fishers Ln, Room 14C-02, Rockville, MD 20857; (800)421-4211. Internet address: http://www.nimh.nih.gov

National Mental Health Association, 1021 Prince St, Alexandria, VA 22314; (800)969-6642.

Selected References

American Academy of Pediatrics, Committee on Adolescence. Suicide and suicide attempts in adolescents and young adults. *Pediatrics.* 1988;81:322-324.

Angold A, Costello EJ. The epidemiology of depression in children and adolescents. In: Goodyer IM, ed. *The Depressed Child and Adolescent: Developmental and Clinical Perspectives.* Cambridge Ma: Cambridge University Press; 1995:127-147.

American Academy of Pediatrics, Committee on Psychosocial Aspects of Child and Family Health. *Guidelines for Health Supervision.* Elk Grove Village, Ill: American Academy of Pediatrics; 1988.

American Medical Association. Rationale and recommendation: depression (severe and recurrent) and suicide. In: *AMA Guidelines for Adolescent Preventive Services (GAPS): Recommendations and Rationale*. Chicago, Il: American Medical Association; 1994: chap 12.

American Psychiatric Association: *Diagnostic and Statistical Manual of Mental Disorders, Fourth Edition*. Washington, DC: American Psychiatric Association; 1994.

Brent DA, Perper JA, Goldstein CE, et al. Risk factors for adolescent suicide. *Arch Gen Psychiatry*. 1988;45:581-587.

Canadian Task Force on the Periodic Health Examination. Early detection of depression. In: *The Canadian Guide to Clinical Preventive Health Care*. Ottawa, Canada: Minister of Supply and Services; 1994: chap 39.

Canadian Task Force on the Periodic Health Examination. Prevention of suicide. In: *The Canadian Guide to Clinical Preventive Health Care*. Ottawa, Canada: Minister of Supply and Services; 1994: chap 40.

Chang G, Warner V, Weissman MM. Physicians' recognition of psychiatric disorders in children and adolescents. *Am J Dis Child*. 1988;142:736-739.

Costello EJ, Angold A. Scales to assess child and adolescent depression: checklists, screens, and nets. *J Am Acad Child Adolesc Psychiatry*. 1988;27:726-737.

Green M, ed. *Bright Futures: Guidelines for Health Supervision of Infants, Children, and Adolescents*. Arlington, Va: National Center for Education in Maternal and Child Health, 1994.

Grayson P, Carlson G. The utility of a DSM-III-R-based checklist in screening child psychiatric patients. *J Am Acad Child Adolesc Psychiatry*. 1991;30:669-673.

Kashani J, Sherman D. Childhood depression: epidemiology, etiological models, and treatment implications. *Integr Psychiatry*. 1988;6:1-21.

Lewinsohn PM, Rohde P, Seeley JR. Adolescent suicidal ideation and attempts: Prevalence, risk factors, clinical implications. *Clinical Psychology: Science and Practice*. 1996;3:25-46.

Moscicki EK. Epidemiology of suicidal behavior. *Suicide and life-threatening behavior: Suicide Prevention: Toward the year 2000 (Special Issue)*. 1995;25:22-35.

Roberts N, Vargo B, Ferguson HB. Measurement of anxiety and depression in children and adolescents. *Psychiatr Clin North Am*. 1989;12:837-860.

Slap G, Vorters D, Khalid N, Margulies S, Forke C. Adolescent suicide attempters: do physicians recognize them? *J Adolesc Health*. 1992;13:286-292.

US Preventive Services Task Force. Screening for depression. In: *Guide to Clinical Preventive Services*. 2nd ed. Washington, DC: US Department of Health and Human Services, 1996: chap 49.

US Preventive Services Task Force. Screening for suicide risk. In: *Guide to Clinical Preventive Services*. 2nd ed. Washington, DC: US Department of Health and Human Services, 1996: chap 50.

HEARING

An estimated 1% to 2% of infants and children in the United States suffer from hearing impairment. Approximately half of these cases are congenital or are acquired during infancy. Severe or profound hearing loss affects one of every 750 live births. Approximately 5% of infants in neonatal intensive care units have evidence of significant hearing loss. Some 8 million school-aged children experience temporary hearing loss, which usually occurs as a complication of otitis media with middle ear effusion.

Hearing is necessary for normal development of speech and language and is also important for acquiring psychosocial skills during infancy and childhood. Because most speech and language development occurs between birth and 3 years of age, early detection of hearing impairment in infants and children and initiation of medical and educational interventions are critical.

Refer to chapter 35 for information on hearing screening in adults.

Recommendations of Major Authorities

Normal-Risk Children

> **American Academy of Pediatrics** and **Bright Futures** endorse the recommendation by the Joint Committee on Infant Hearing and also recommend that pure-tone audiometry be performed at 3, 4, 5, 10, 12, 15, and 18 years of age. Subjective assessment of hearing should be performed at other ages.

> **American Speech-Language-Hearing Association**—Annual pure-tone audiometry should be performed for children functioning at a developmental level of age 3 years to grade 3 and for any high-risk children, including those above grade 3.

Canadian Task Force on the Periodic Health Examination—Repeated examination of hearing is recommended for young children, especially during the first year of life. Suggested guidelines for this examination include checking the startle or turning response to a novel noise produced outside the infant's field of vision at birth and 6 months of age and checking for the absence of babbling at 6 months of age. Screening using auditory brainstem responses or evoked otoacoustic emission by 3 months of age is not recommended pending further evaluation. Routine hearing assessment of asymptomatic preschoolers using history-taking, audiometry, tympanometry, or acoustic reflexometry is not recommended.

Joint Committee on Infant Hearing (American Speech-Language Hearing Association, American Academy of Pediatrics, American Academy of Otolaryngology-Head and Neck Surgery, American Academy of Audiology, American Academy of Pediatrics and the Directors of Speech and Hearing Programs in State Health and Welfare Agencies) and **Bright Futures**—endorse the goal of universal detection of infants with hearing loss as early as possible using auditory brainstem response or otoacoustic emissions. All infants should be screened before 3 months of age.

US Preventive Services Task Force—There is insufficient evidence to recommend for or against routine screening of asymptomatic neonates for congenital hearing loss using evoked otoacoustic emission (EOE) testing or auditory brainstem response (ABR). Routine hearing screening of asymptomatic children beyond age 3 years is not recommended. There is insufficient evidence to recommend for or against routinely screening asymptomatic adolescents for hearing impairment. However, screening of workers for noise-induced hearing loss should be performed in the context of existing worksite programs and occupational medicine guidelines.

High-Risk Children

American Academy of Pediatrics and **American Speech-Language-Hearing Association (ASHA)**—Children with frequently recurring otitis media or middle ear effusion, or both, should have audiology screening and monitoring of communication skills development. **ASHA** recommends annual pure-tone audiometry testing for all children at high risk for hearing impairment.

Joint Committee on Infant Hearing (American Speech-Language Hearing Association, American Academy of Pediatrics, American Academy of Otolaryngology-Head and Neck Surgery, American Academy of Audiology, American Academy of Pediatrics and the Directors of Speech and Hearing Programs in State Health and Welfare Agencies)—Neonates (birth to 28 days of age) with one or more of the neonatal risk criteria should have audiology screening, preferably before hospital discharge but no later than 3 months of age.

> *Neonatal Risk Criteria:* Family history of hereditary sensorineural hearing loss; in utero infection (eg, cytomegalovirus, rubella, syphilis, herpes, or toxoplasmosis); craniofacial anomalies, including those with morphological abnormalities of the pinna and ear canal; birth weight less than 1500 grams (3.3 lbs); hyperbilirubinemia at a serum level requiring exchange transfusion; ototoxic medications, including but not limited to aminoglycosides, used in multiple courses or in combination with loop diuretics; bacterial meningitis; Apgar scores of 0 to 4 at 1 minute or 0 to 6 at 5 minutes; mechanical ventilation lasting 5 days or longer; and stigmata or other findings associated with a syndrome known to include a sensorineural and/or conductive hearing loss.

Infants and children less than 2 years of age with one or more of the following risk criteria should have audiology screening.

> *Risk Criteria for Ages 29 days to 2 Years:* Parent/care-giver concern regarding hearing, speech, language, and/or developmental delay; bacterial meningitis or other infections associated with sensorineural hearing loss; head trauma associated with loss of consciousness or skull fracture; stigmata or other findings associated with a syndrome known to include a sensorineural and/or conductive hearing loss; ototoxic medications, including but not limited to aminoglycosides, used in multiple courses or in combination with loop diuretics; recurrent or persistent otitis media with effusion for at least 3 months associated with hearing loss; anatomic deformities and other disorders that affect eustachian tube function; neurofibromatosis type II and neurodegenerative disorders.

Infants and children with the following risk factors for delayed-onset hearing loss require hearing evaluation every 6 months until 3 years of age.

> *Risk Factors for Delayed-Onset Hearing Loss:* Family history of hereditary childhood hearing loss; in utero infection, such as cytomegalovirus, rubella, syphilis, herpes, or toxoplasmosis; neurofibromatosis type II and neurodegenerative disorders; recurrent or persistent otitis media with effusion, anatomic deformities, and other disorders that affect eustachian tube function; neurodegenerative disorders.

US Preventive Services Task Force—Screening for hearing impairment in high-risk infants can be recommended based on the relatively high prevalence of hearing impairment, parental anxiety, and the potential beneficial effect on language development from early treatment of infants with moderate or severe hearing loss. Refer to neonatal risk criteria listed above under Joint Committee on Infant Hearing. Clinicians examining any infant or young child should remain alert for symptoms or signs of hearing impairment, including parent/care-giver concern regarding hearing, speech, language, and/or developmental delay.

Basics of Hearing Screening

1. Assess the family and medical history of every child for risk factors for hearing impairment.

2. Ask parents about the auditory responsiveness and speech and language development of young children. Any parental reports of impairment should be seriously evaluated.

3. In infants, assessment of hearing by observational techniques is very imprecise. Consider referring all infants and young children with suspected hearing difficulties to an audiologist.

4. When performing physical examinations, remain alert for structural defects of the ear, head, and neck. Remain alert for abnormalities of the ear canal (inflammation, cerumen impaction, tumors, or foreign bodies) and the eardrum (perforation, retraction, or evidence of effusion).

5. Children as young as 6 months of age, depending on how cooperative they are, may be screened by pure-tone audiometry. Two screening methods are suggested as the most appropriate tools for children who are functioning at 6 months to 3 years developmental age: visual reinforcement audiometry (VRA) and conditioned play audiometry (CPA). For children from approximately 6 months through 2 years of age, VRA is the recognized method of choice. As children mature beyond their second birthday, CPA may be attempted. For those children who can be conditioned for VRA, screen using earphones (conventional or insert), with 1000, 2000, and 4000 Hz tones at 30 dB HL. For those children who can be conditioned for play audiometry, screen using earphones (conventional or insert), with 1000, 2000, and 4000 Hz tones at 20 dB HL. Hand-held audiometers are of unproven effectiveness in screening children.

   After 6 months of age, any child may be screened for middle ear dysfunction using tympanometry. Perform tympanometry with a low frequency (220, 226 Hz) probe tone and a positive to negative air pressure sweep. Middle ear pressure peaks between -150 mmhos and $+150$ mmhos are considered normal. Patients with pressure peaks outside this range or lack of any identifiable pressure peak should be referred for otologic follow-up.

6. Repeat screening to substantiate audiometric evidence of hearing impairment. Remove and reposition the earphones and carefully repeat the instructions to the child to assure proper understanding and attention to the test. Referral to a qualified specialist (ie, audiologist, otolaryngologist) is recommended for confirmation and work-up of hearing impairment.

Patient Resources

Is My Baby's Hearing Normal? American Academy of Otolaryngology-Head and Neck Surgery, Order Department, 1 Prince St, Alexandria, VA 22314; (703)836-4444.

Answers to Questions About Otitis Media, Hearing, and Language Development; How Does Your Child Hear and Talk?; Recognizing Communication Disorders. American Speech-Language-Hearing Association, 10801 Rockville Pike, Rockville, MD 20852. For general information, call: (800)638-8255. To order, call: (301)897-5700, ext 218; Internet address: http://www.asha.org

Middle Ear Fluid in Young Children: Parent Guide; Ear Infection in Children. The American Academy of Pediatrics, PO Box 927, Elk Grove Village, IL 60009-0927; (800)433-9016. Internet address: http://www.aap.org

Provider Resources

Bright Futures: Guidelines for Health Supervision of Infants, Children and Adolescents; Bright Futures Pocket Guide; Bright Futures Anticipatory Guidance Cards. Available from the National Center for Education in Maternal and Child Health, 2000 15th Street North, Suite 701, Arlington, VA 22201-2617; (703)524-7802. Internet address: http://www.brightfutures.org

National Institute on Deafness and Other Communication Disorders. Internet address: http://www.nih.gov/nidcd

American Speech-Language-Hearing Association.
Internet address: http:// www.asha.org

Selected References

American Academy of Otolaryngology-Head and Neck Surgery, Joint Committee on Infant Hearing. 1990 position statement. *American Academy of Otolaryngology-Head and Neck Surgery Bulletin.* March 1991:15-18.

American Academy of Pediatrics, Committee on Practice and Ambulatory Medicine. Recommendations for pediatric preventive health care. *Pediatrics.* 1995;96:373-374.

American Academy of Pediatrics. Managing otitis media with effusion in young children. *Pediatrics.* 1994;94:766-773.

American Academy of Pediatrics. Joint Committee on Infant Hearing position statement 1982. In: *Policy Reference Guide: A Comprehensive Guide to AAP Policy Statements through December 1991.* Elk Grove Village, Ill: American Academy of Pediatrics; 1991;333-334.

American Academy of Pediatrics. Middle ear disease and language development. In: *Policy Reference Guide: A Comprehensive Guide to AAP Policy Statements through December 1991.* Elk Grove Village, Ill: American Academy of Pediatrics; 1991;418.

American Speech-Language-Hearing Association. Guidelines for the audiologic assessment of children from birth through 36 months of age. *ASHA.* 1991;33(suppl 5):37-43.

American Speech-Language-Hearing Association. Guidelines for audiologic screening of newborn infants who are at risk for hearing impairment. *ASHA.* 1989;31(3):89-92.

American Speech-Language-Hearing Association. Guidelines for identification audiometry. *ASHA.* 1985;May:49-53.

American Speech-Language-Hearing Association. Guidelines for screening for hearing impairment and middle-ear disorders. *ASHA.* 1990;32(suppl 2):17-24.

American Speech-Language-Hearing Association. Preferred practice patterns for the professions of speech-language pathology and audiology. Rockville, MD: *ASHA.* In press.

American Speech-Language-Hearing Association. The prevention of communication disorders tutorial. *ASHA.* 1991;33(suppl 6):15-41.

Canadian Task Force on the Periodic Health Examination. Routine preschool screening for visual and hearing problems. In: *The Canadian Guide to Clinical Preventive Health Care.* Ottawa, Canada: Minister of Supply and Services; 1994: chap 27.

Canadian Task Force on the Periodic Health Examination. Well-baby care in the first 2 years of life. In: *The Canadian Guide to Clinical Preventive Health Care.* Ottawa, Canada: Minister of Supply and Services; 1994: chap 24.

Green M, ed. *Bright Futures: Guidelines for Health Supervision of Infants, Children, and Adolescents.* Arlington, Va: National Center for Education in Maternal and Child Health, 1994.

Joint Committee on Infant Hearing. Joint Committee on Infant Hearing 1994 position statement. *Pediatrics.* 1995;95:152-156.

National Institutes of Health. *Early Identification of Hearing Impairment in Infants and Young Children.* Bethesda, Md: National Institutes of Health. In press.

Thompson MD, Thompson G. Early identification of hearing loss: listen to parents. *Clin Pediatr.* 1991;30:77-80.

US Preventive Services Task Force. Screening for hearing impairment. In: *Guide to Clinical Preventive Services.* 2nd ed. Washington, DC: US Department of Health and Human Services; 1996: chap 35.

Watkin PM, Baldwin M, Laoide S. Parental suspicion and identification of hearing impairment. *Arch Dis Child.* 1990;65:846-850.

7

LEAD

Childhood lead poisoning is one of the most common, preventable health problems in the United States. From 1991 to 1994, an estimated 890,000 US children aged 1 to 5 years (4.4% of all children in this age group) had blood lead levels greater than or equal to 10 µg/dL, the current definition of lead toxicity. Although rates of lead poisoning are higher among low-income, inner-city children, no socioeconomic group, geographic area, or racial or ethnic population is spared.

Studies have shown that blood lead levels as low as 10 to 15 µg/dL are associated with diminished intelligence, impaired neurobehavioral development, decreased hearing acuity, and growth inhibition. Higher levels can cause severe damage to the central nervous, renal, and hematopoietic systems and can be fatal.

Children at risk for lead poisoning who are screened can be followed or treated based on their blood lead levels. If lead poisoning is diagnosed, the clinician needs to call the appropriate local health authority to help determine the lead source. In several states, reporting to the local health department is required. Local public health departments may initiate community-wide educational programs and environmental assessments in response to such reports. Expert consultation for treating and following lead toxicity should be obtained by contacting the state or local health department, a university medical center, or a certified regional poison control center.

Recommendations of Major Authorities

American Academy of Family Physicians—Determination of lead levels is recommended for infants at 12 months of age who live in communities in which the prevalence of lead levels requiring intervention is high or undefined; live in or frequently visit a home built before 1950 with dilapidated paint or with recent or ongoing renovation or remodeling; have close contact with a person who has an elevated lead level; live near lead industry or heavy traffic; live with someone whose job or hobby involves lead exposure; use lead-based pottery; or take traditional remedies that contain lead.

American Academy of Pediatrics—Pediatric-care providers should increase their efforts to screen children for lead exposure. Blood lead screening should be a part of routine health supervision of children and can best be addressed by increasing children's access to health care. Because lead is ubiquitous in the US environment, this screening should occur at about 9 to 12 months of age and, if possible, again at about 24 months of age. The Centers for Disease Control and Prevention has raised the possibility that there may be low-risk communities that do not require screening, but no explicit guidance has been developed for determining a community's risk. As more data are collected, it may become evident that there are locales where selective screening of children is more appropriate than routine screening.

Canadian Task Force on the Periodic Health Examination—There is insufficient evidence to recommend for or against universal lead screening of children to detect mild or moderate lead exposure. Screening is recommended for children at high risk: children who live in or regularly visit homes built before 1960 with deteriorating paint or recent, ongoing, or planned renovation or remodeling; who have a sibling, housemate, or playmate known to have had lead poisoning; who live with an adult whose job or hobby involves exposure to lead; or who live near lead industries or busy highways.

Centers for Disease Control and Prevention (CDC)—(**NOTE:** Revised guidelines are expected to be published in the fall of 1997. Revisions to the CDC guidelines were being considered at the time of this publication. Please consult Provider Resources below for information on how to obtain current recommendations.) CDC's draft guidelines recommend that state and local health officials make screening recommendations that are based on an assessment of local lead exposure sources and on blood lead screening data. Where risk is widespread, universal screening should be recommended; where risk is less or confined to small pockets, targeted screening should be recommended. Screening should be focused on children at 12 and at 24 months of age. A targeted screening recommendation would call for screening of children who meet criteria established by the health department. Likely criteria include: residence in a high-risk zip code or neighborhood, poverty, or response to a personal-risk questionnaire that is tailored to local conditions. An example of one such basic questionnaire is presented in Table 7.1. Health departments will be expected to tailor the questionnaire to make it appropriate to local sources of exposure.

US Preventive Services Task Force—Screening for elevated lead levels by measuring blood lead at least once at about 12 months of age is recommended for all children at increased risk of lead exposure. All children with identifiable risk factors should be screened, as should children living in communities in which the prevalence of blood lead levels requiring individual intervention, including chelation therapy or residential lead hazard control, is high or undefined. If capillary blood is used, elevated lead levels should be confirmed by measurement of venous blood lead. The optimal frequency of screening for lead exposure in children, or for repeated testing of children previously found to have elevated blood lead levels, is unknown and is left to clinical discretion; consideration should be given to the degree of elevation, the interventions provided, and the natural history of lead exposure, including the typical peak in lead levels at 18 to 24 months of age. In communities where the prevalence of blood lead levels requiring individual intervention is low, a strategy of targeted screening, possibly using locale-specific questionnaires of known and acceptable sensitivity and specificity, can be used to identify high-risk children who should have blood lead testing. There is currently insufficient evidence to recommend an exact population prevalence below which targeted screening can be substituted for universal screening. Clinicians should seek guidance from their local or state health department.

Basics of Lead Screening

1. Begin risk assessment and counseling during prenatal visits and continue after birth during regular office visits until the child is at least 6 years of age. Counsel parents against sanding old lead paint while remodeling during pregnancy.

2. Evaluate each child's risk of lead toxicity. Use of a structured set of questions such as that developed by CDC (Table 7.1) can be very helpful. If the answer to any of the questions is positive, consider the child at high risk for exposure.

3. Measurement of the blood lead level is more sensitive and specific than measurement of the erythrocyte protoporphyrin (EP) level.

Table 7.1. Recommended Questions for Assessing Lead Exposure Risk

Does your child live in or regularly visit a house built before 1950? (Including daycare centers, preschools, homes of baby-sitters or relatives)

Does your child live in or regularly visit a house built before 1978 (the year lead-based paint was banned for residential use) with recent, ongoing, or planned renovation or remodeling?

Does your child have a sibling, housemate, or playmate being followed or treated for lead poisoning (blood lead level 15 μg/dL)?

Adapted from: Centers for Disease Control and Prevention. Screening Young Children for Lead Poisoning. Expected date of publication: 1997.

4. Screening blood lead levels may be obtained from capillary sampling. Follow the precautions listed in Table 7.2 to minimize the chance of contamination from environmental sources. Confirm elevated blood lead test results (15 µg/dL or greater) obtained on capillary specimens by using venous blood. A child with a capillary lead level of 70 µg/dL or greater requires immediate retesting using a venous sample.

Table 7.2. Recommendations for Minimizing the Contamination of Capillary Blood Samples Obtained by Finger Stick

---

Personnel who collect specimens should be well trained in and completely familiar with the collection procedure and observe universal precautions.

Puncturing the fingers of infants younger than 1 year of age is not recommended. The heel is a more suitable site for these children.

If examination gloves are coated with powder, rinse them with tap water.

Thoroughly wash the child's hands or heel with soap and water, and then dry with a clean, low-lint towel.

Once the finger or heel to be punctured is washed, clean it with alcohol; do not allow it to come into contact with any surface, including the child's other fingers.

Although its effectiveness in reducing contamination is under study, silicone spray can be used to form a protective layer between the skin and blood droplets.

Use sterile gauze or a cotton ball to wipe off the first droplet of blood, which contains tissue fluids.

Do not collect blood that has run down the finger or onto the fingernail.

Avoid contact between the skin and the collection container.

Adapted from: Centers for Disease Control. Preventing Lead Poisoning in Young Children: A Statement by the Centers for Disease Control. Atlanta, GA: Centers for Disease Control; 1991.

5. Interpret and manage blood lead test results according to the CDC recommendations listed in Table 7.3. Several states require primary care providers and persons in charge of lead screening programs to report both presumptive and confirmed cases of lead toxicity to the appropriate health agency.

Table 7.3. CDC Recommendations for Follow-up of Blood Lead Measurements

Blood Lead Level (BLL) (μg/dL)	Action
≤9	Reassess or rescreen in 1 year. No additional action necessary unless exposure sources change
10-14	Family lead education Follow-up testing Social services, if necessary
15-19	Family lead education Follow-up testing Social services, if necessary If BLLs persist (ie, 2 venous BLLs in this range at least 3 months apart) or worsen, proceed according to actions for BLLs 20-44
20-44	Coordination of care (case-management) Clinical management* Environmental investigation Lead-hazard reduction
45-69	Within 48 hours, begin coordination of care (case management), clinical management*, environmental investigation, lead hazard reduction
≥70	Hospitalize child and begin medical treatment immediately. Begin coordination of care (case management), clinical management*, environmental investigation and lead-hazard reduction immediately

* Refer to CDC source publication, Screening Young Children for Lead Poisoning, for description of clinical management.

Adapted from: Centers for Disease Control. Screening Young Children for Lead Poisoning. Expected date of publication: 1997.

6. Laboratories where blood is tested for lead levels must participate in a blood-lead proficiency testing program, such as the collaborative program between the Health Resources and Services Administration and CDC. Information on this program is available by calling the Wisconsin State Hygiene Laboratory (608)262-1146.

7. Because iron deficiency can enhance lead absorption and toxicity, test all children with blood lead levels of 20 μg/dL or greater for iron deficiency.

8. Provide guidance to parents about creating an environment safe from lead exposure for their children. Include advice on eliminating peeling or chipping paint, decreasing the lead content of water, preventing contact via hobbies or contaminated work clothing, remaining alert for pica behavior, and assuring good hygiene. (See Patient Resources for publications to aid in counseling.)

Patient Resources

Department of Housing and Urban Development, Office of Lead-Based Paint. Internet access: htp://www.hud.gov/lea

National Lead Information Center of the National Safety Council; (800)LEADFYI.

What Everyone Should Know About Lead Poisoning. To obtain individual copies, contact: Alliance to End Childhood Lead Poisoning, 600 Pennsylvania Ave SE, Suite 100, Washington, DC 20003. To obtain bulk copies, contact: Channing L. Bete Co, Inc, 200 State Rd, South Deerfield, MA 01373; (800)628-7733.

Protect your family from lead in your home. Centers for Disease Control and Prevention, Lead Poisoning Prevention Program, 1600 Clifton Rd NE, Atlanta, GA 30333; (770)488-7330.

Provider Resources

Preventing Lead Poisoning in Young Children: A Statement by the Centers for Disease Control; The Strategic Plan for the Elimination of Lead Poisoning; Nutrition and Childhood Lead Poisoning Prevention. Centers for Disease Control and Prevention, Lead Poisoning Prevention Program, 1600 Clifton Rd NE, Atlanta, GA 30333; (770)488-7330.

Case Studies in Environmental Medicine: Lead Toxicity. Agency for Toxic Substances and Disease Registry, Division of Health Education, Mailstop E33, 1600 Clifton Rd NE, Atlanta, GA 30333; (404)639-6205.

Selected References

Agency for Toxic Substances and Disease Registry. *Case Studies in Environmental Medicine: Lead Toxicity.* Atlanta, Ga: Agency for Toxic Substances and Disease Registry, Centers for Disease Control; September 1992. US Department of Health and Human Services.

American Academy of Family Physicians. *Summary of Policy Recommendations for Periodic Health Examination.* Kansas City, Mo: American Academy of Family Physicians; 1997.

Canadian Task Force on the Periodic Health Examination. Screening children for lead exposure in Canada. In: *The Canadian Guide to Clinical Preventive Health Care.* Ottawa, Canada: Minister of Supply and Services; 1994: chap 25.

Centers for Disease Control and Prevention. Update: Blood Lead Levels—United States, 1991-1994. *MMWR.* 1997;46(7):141-144.

Centers for Disease Control. *Preventing Lead Poisoning in Young Children: A Statement by the Centers for Disease Control.* Atlanta, GA: Centers for Disease Control; 1991. US Department of Health and Human Services.

Crocetti AF, Mushak P, Schwartz J. Determination of numbers of lead-exposed US children by areas of the United States: an integrated summary of a report to the US Congress on childhood lead poisoning. *Environ Health Perspect.* 1990;89:109-120.

DeBaun MR, Sox HC. Setting the optimal erythrocyte protoporphyrin screening decision threshold for lead poisoning: a decision analytic approach. *Pediatrics.* 1991;88:121-131.

Mahaffey KR, Annest JL, Roberts J, Murphy RS. National estimates of blood lead levels: United States, 1976-1980. *N Engl J Med.* 1982;307:573-579.

Needleman HL. The persistent threat of lead: a singular opportunity. *Am J Public Health.* 1989;79:643-645.

Needleman HL, Schell A, Bellinger D, Leviton A, Allred EN. The long-term effects of exposure to low doses of lead in childhood: an 11-year follow-up report. *N Engl J Med.* 1990;322:83-88.

Ratcliffe SD, Lee J, Lutz LJ, Woolley FR, et al. Lead toxicity and iron deficiency in Utah migrant children. *Am J Public Health.* 1989;79:631-633.

Ruff HA, Bijur PE, Markowitz M, Yeou-Cheng M, Rosen JF. Declining blood lead levels and cognitive changes in moderately lead-poisoned children. *JAMA.* 1993;269:1641-1654.

US Preventive Services Task Force. Screening for elevated lead levels in childhood and pregnancy. In: *Guide to Clinical Preventive Services.* 2nd ed. Washington, DC: US Department of Health and Human Services; 1996: chap 23.

NEWBORN SCREENING

Virtually all states require screening of newborns for congenital hypothy-roidism and phenylketonuria (PKU). Testing for galactosemia and hemoglobinopathies is required in a majority of states, and some states re-quire screening of newborns for maple syrup urine disease, homocystinuria, biotinidase deficiency, tyrosinemia, congenital adrenal hyperplasia, cystic fi-brosis, and toxoplasmosis. Table 8.1 provides a state-by-state listing of new-born screening policies.

HYPOTHYROIDISM

Most children with congenital hypothyroidism who are not identified and treated promptly suffer the irreversible mental retardation, growth failure, deafness, and neurologic abnormalities characteristic of the syndrome of cre-tinism. The incidence of this disorder is 1 per 3600 to 1 per 5000 live births. Infants who receive adequate treatment with thyroxine within the first weeks of life have normal or near-normal intellectual performance at 4 to 7 years of age.

PHENYLKETONURIA (PKU)

Phenylketonuria is an autosomal recessive aminoacidopathy that leads to se-vere, irreversible mental retardation (IQ below 50) if it is not treated during infancy. The incidence of this disorder is 1 per 10,000 to 1 per 15,000 live births. Most children who undergo early screening, diagnosis, and optimal treatment with dietary restriction of phenylalanine will be in the normal range of intelligence.

GALACTOSEMIA

Galactosemia presents following milk feeding with vomiting, diarrhea, failure to thrive, and Escherichia coli septicemia (which is often fatal). Continued expo-sure to galactose results in liver disease (manifested by hepatomegaly, jaundice, and cirrhosis), cataracts, and irreversible mental retardation. The incidence of galactosemia is 1 per 60,000 to 1 per 80,000 live births. Treatment is directed to the elimination of dietary lactose by avoiding galactose in breast milk, cow's milk, and infant formulas. Treatment can lead to dramatic improvement in all clinical features except for central nervous system dysfunction.

HEMOGLOBINOPATHIES

Sickle cell disease and other hemoglobinopathies, such as thalassemia and hemoglobin E, are most common in persons of African, Mediterranean, Asian, Caribbean, and South and Central American ancestry. Affected individuals may have overwhelming sepsis, chronic hemolytic anemia, episodic vascular occlusive crises, hyposplenism, periodic splenic sequestration, and bone marrow aplasia. Carriers (genetic heterozygotes) do not suffer significant morbidity. Early detection of sickle cell disease in newborns allows prophylactic use of penicillin to prevent septicemia and prompt clinical intervention for infection and sequestration crises.

Recommendations of Major Authorities

American Academy of Pediatrics and **Bright Futures** —Newborn screening should be performed according to each state's regulations.

National authorities have made recommendations for the following specific conditions:

Hypothyroidism

American Academy of Family Physicians—Neonatal screening for thyroid function abnormalities is recommended.

American Academy of Pediatrics (AAP), American Thyroid Association (ATA), Canadian Task Force on the Periodic Health Examination (CTFPHE), and US Preventive Services Task Force—All neonates should be screened for congenital hypothyroidism between 2 and 6 days of life. Care should be taken to assure that infants born at home, ill at birth, or transferred between hospitals in the first week of life are screened before 7 days of life. According to the **CTFPHE**, it is better to obtain a specimen within 24 hours of birth than no specimen at all. According to the **AAP** and **ATA**, blood should be obtained from infants before discharge from the hospital or after 48 hours of age.

Phenylketonuria (PKU)

American Academy of Family Physicians—Neonatal screening for PKU is recommended.

Canadian Task Force on the Periodic Health Examination (CTFPHE) and US Preventive Services Task Force (USPSTF)—

All infants should be screened for PKU before discharge from the nursery. Premature infants and those with illness should be tested at or near 7 days of age. Infants tested before 24 hours of age should receive a repeat screening. According to the **CTFPHE**, this should occur between 2 and 7 days of age; according to the **USPSTF**, this should occur by 2 weeks of age.

Hemoglobinopathies

American Academy of Family Physicians—Neonatal screening for hemoglobinopathies is recommended.

Canadian Task Force on the Periodic Health Examination and **US Preventive Services Task Force (USPSTF)**—Neonatal screening for sickle hemoglobinopathies is recommended. Whether such screening should be universal or targeted to high-risk groups will depend on the proportion of high-risk individuals in the screening area. All screening must be accompanied by comprehensive counseling and treatment services. There is insufficient evidence to recommend for or against screening for hemoglobinopathies in adolescents and young adults in order to help them make informed reproductive decisions. According to the **USPSTF**, such screening may be justified on the basis of burden of suffering and patient preference.

Sickle Cell Disease Guideline Panel of the Agency for Health Care Policy and Research, US Public Health Service—Universal screening for sickle cell disease should be conducted on all newborns. This recommendation has been endorsed by the **American Academy of Pediatrics**, the **American Nurses Association**, and the **National Medical Association.**

Basics of Newborn Screening

Schedule[1]

1. For the full-term, well neonate, obtain the specimen as close as possible to the time of discharge from the nursery and in no case later than 7 days of age. If the initial specimen is obtained earlier than 24 hours after birth, obtain a second specimen at 1 or 2 weeks of age to decrease the probability that PKU and other disorders with metabolite accumulation will be missed.

2. For any premature infant, any infant receiving parenteral feeding, or any neonate being treated for illness, obtain a specimen for screening at or near the seventh day of life if a specimen has not been obtained before that time, regardless of feeding status. For infants requiring transfusion or

1 Adapted from: American Academy of Pediatrics, Committee on Genetics. Issues in newborn screening. Pediatrics. 1992;89:345-349. Reproduced by permission of Pediatrics; copyright ©1992.

dialysis before the standard time for obtaining a specimen, obtain the sample for screening before transfusion or dialysis, if the neonate's condition is amenable. If a sample cannot be obtained beforehand, ensure that an adequate specimen is obtained at a time when the plasma or red blood cells, or both, will again reflect the child's own metabolic processes or phenotype.

Collection Technique[2]

1. Apply the same standards and techniques for the collection of blood specimens for neonatal screening programs for all of the congenital diseases. State screening agencies hold individual hospitals accountable for instituting policies that assure proper collection of filter-paper blood samples.

2. Enter the required information on the specimen collection kit with a ballpoint pen, not a soft-tip pen or typewriter.

3. Universal precautions: Use all appropriate precautions, including wearing gloves, when handling blood, and dispose of used lancets in a biohazard container for sharp objects.

4. Site Selection: The source of blood must be the most lateral surface of the plantar aspect (walking surface) of the infant's heel. Skin punctures to obtain blood specimens must not be performed on the central area of the newborn's foot (area of the arch) or on the fingers of newborns. Puncturing the heel on the posterior curvature will permit blood to flow away from the puncture, making proper spotting difficult. Do not lance a previous puncture site.

5. Site Preparation: Warm the puncture site to increase blood flow. Place a warm, moist towel at a temperature no higher than 42°C (108°F) on the site for 3 minutes. Holding the infant's leg in a position lower than the heart will increase venous pressure.

6. Cleaning the Site: Clean the infant's heel with 70% isopropyl alcohol (rubbing alcohol). Wipe away excess alcohol with a dry sterile gauze or cotton ball, and allow the heel to air-dry thoroughly. Failure to wipe off alcohol residue may dilute the specimen and adversely affect test results.

7. Puncture: To ensure sufficient blood flow, puncture the plantar surface of the infant's heel with a sterile lancet to a depth of 2.0 to 2.4 mm or with an automated lancet device. Wipe away the first drop of blood with sterile gauze. In small premature infants, the heel bone may be no more than 2.4 mm beneath the plantar heel skin surface and half this distance at the pos-

2 Adapted from: National Committee for Clinical Laboratory Standards. Blood Collection on Filter Paper for Neonatal Screening Programs—Second Edition; Approved Standard. Villanova, Pa: National Committee for Clinical Laboratory Standards; 1992. Permission to use portions of NCCLS document LA4-A2 has been granted by the National Committee for Clinical Laboratory Standards; copyright ©1992.

terior curvature of the heel. Puncturing deeper may risk bone damage. Do not milk or squeeze the puncture site, as this may cause hemolysis and admixture of tissue fluids with the specimen.

8. Filter Paper Handling and Application: Avoid touching the area within the printed circle on the filter paper before collection. Gently touch the filter paper against a large drop of blood and, in one step, allow a sufficient quantity of blood to soak through to completely fill the circle on the filter paper. Do not press the paper against the puncture site on the heel. Apply blood to only one side of the filter paper. Examine both sides of the filter paper to assure that the blood penetrates and saturates the paper. Do not layer successive drops of blood within the circle. If blood flow diminishes so that the circle is incompletely filled, repeat the sampling steps at a different site. Do not touch the blood sample after collection; do not allow water, feeding formulas, antiseptic solutions, or any other contaminant to come into contact with the sample. Allow the sample to dry thoroughly before insertion into the envelope. Insufficient drying can adversely affect test results.

9. Hemostasis: After blood has been collected from the heel of the newborn, elevate the foot above the body and press a sterile gauze pad or cotton ball against the puncture site until the bleeding stops.

Documentation

Ensure that children receive proper newborn screening and that test results are reviewed. Be aware of patients who are at increased risk for not being screened. Such patients include sick or premature neonates, neonates undergoing adoption or being transferred within or between hospitals, infants born at home, children of transient or homeless families, and infants born outside the United States and Canada. Document newborn screening results in an easily accessible part of the patient record for future reference.

Follow-up

Confirm all abnormal results with retesting. With certain rare exceptions (eg, galactosemia and maple syrup urine disease), do not initiate treatment until a confirmatory test result has been obtained. Prompt physical examination of patients with abnormal results is important. Start all patients with sickle cell disease on penicillin prophylaxis as soon as the diagnosis is confirmed.

Counseling

Provide appropriate counseling to all parents of children with abnormal test results. Provide information about the significance of the results and the need for retesting, the implications for the child's health, treatment regimens, symptoms to be alert for, and genetic issues for future childbearing.

Table 8.1. Newborn Screening By State

STATE	MANDATED	BIO	CAH	CF	GAL	HGB	HCU	HYPO	MSUD	PKU	TOXO	TYR
ALABAMA	•		•		•	•		•		•		
ALASKA	•	•	•		•			•	•	•		
ARIZONA	•	•			•	•	•	•	•	•		
ARKANSAS	•				•	•		•		•		
CALIFORNIA	•				•	•		•		•		
COLORADO	•	•		•	•	•		•		•		
CONNECTICUT	•	•		•	•	•	•	•	•	•		
DELAWARE	•	•			•	•		•		•		
FLORIDA	•		•		•	•		•		•		
GEORGIA	•		•		•	•	•	•	•	•		•
HAWAII	•							•		•		
IDAHO	•	•			•		•	•	•	•		
ILLINOIS	•	•	•		•	•		•		•		
INDIANA	•				•	•	•	•	•	•		
IOWA	•		•		•	•		•		•		
KANSAS	•				•	•		•		•		
KENTUCKY	•				•	•		•		•		
LOUISIANA	•					•		•		•		
MAINE	•				•	•	•	•	•	•		
MARYLAND	•	•			•	•	•	•	•	•		•
MASSACHUSETTS	•	•	•		•	•	•	•	•	•	•	
MICHIGAN	•	•	•		•	•		•	•	•		
MINNESOTA	•		•		•	•		•		•		
MISSISSIPPI	•				•	•		•		•		
MISSOURI	•				•	•		•		•		
MONTANA	•			•	•			•		•		•
NEBRASKA	•	•			•	•		•		•		
NEVADA	•	•			•	•		•	•	•		
NEW HAMPSHIRE	•				•	•	•	•	•	•	•	
NEW JERSEY	•				•	•		•		•		
NEW MEXICO	•	•			•	•		•		•		
NEW YORK	•	•			•	•	•	•	•	•		
NORTH CAROLINA	•		•		•	•		•		•		

continued

Table 8.1. Newborn Screening By State—*Continued*

STATE	MANDATED	BIO	CAH	CF	GAL	HGB	HCU	HYPO	MSUD	PKU	TOXO	TYR
NORTH DAKOTA	•		•		•			•		•		
OHIO	•				•	•	•	•		•		
OKLAHOMA	•				•	•		•		•		
OREGON	•	•			•	•		•	•	•		
PENNSYLVANIA	•					•		•	•	•		
RHODE ISLAND	•	•	•		•	•	•	•	•	•		
SOUTH CAROLINA	•		•		•			•		•		
SOUTH DAKOTA	•				•			•		•		
TENNESSEE	•				•	•		•		•		
TEXAS	•		•		•	•		•		•		
UTAH	•				•			•		•		
VERMONT	•	•			•	•	•	•	•	•		
VIRGINIA	•	•			•	•	•	•	•	•		
WASHINGTON	•		•			•		•		•		
WASHINGTON, DC	•				•	•	•	•	•	•		
WEST VIRGINIA	•				•	•		•		•		
WISCONSIN	•	•	•	•	•	•		•		•		
WYOMING	•	•		•	•	•		•		•		

Key

BIO	Biotinidase Deficiency	HYPO	Congenital Hypothyroidism
CAH	Congenital Adrenal Hyperplasia	MSUD	Maple Syrup Urine Disease
CF	Cystic Fibrosis	PKU	Phenylketonuria
GAL	Galactosemia	TOXO	Toxoplasmosis
HGB	Hemoglobinopathies	TYR	Tyrosinemia
HCU	Homocystinuria		

Adapted from: Illinois Department of Public Health. An Overview of Newborn Screening Programs in the United States and Canada. Springfield, Ill, Illinois Department of Public Health; 1996.

Patient Resources

Sickle Cell Disease: Guide for Parents. Agency for Health Care Policy and Research Publications Clearinghouse, PO Box 8547, Silver Spring, MD 20907; (800)358-9295.

Sickle Cell Anemia (New Hope for People With). FDA Office of Consumer Affairs. HFE 88 Room 1675, 5600 Fishers Ln, Rockville, MD 20857; (800)532-4440.

Understanding PKU. PKU Clinic, Children's Hospital Medical Center, 300 Longwood Ave, Boston, MA 02115; (617)355-6394.

Provider Resources

Sickle Cell Disease: Clinical Practice Guideline; Sickle Cell Disease: Guideline Report; Sickle Cell Disease: Quick Reference Guide. Agency for Health Care Policy and Research Publications Clearinghouse, PO Box 8547, Silver Spring, MD 20907; (800)358-9295.

Blood Collection on Filter Paper for Neonatal Screening Programs—Second Edition; Approved Standard. National Committee for Clinical Laboratory Standards (NCCLS), 940 W Valley Rd, Suite 1400, Wayne, PA 19087-1898. An educational videotape depicting the LA4-A2 collection procedure is also available.

Management and Therapy of Sickle Cell Disease. NIH publication No. 96-2117. NHLBI Information Center, PO Box 30105, Bethesda, MD 20814-0105.

New England Connection for PKU and Allied Disorders, 16 Angelina Ln, Mansfield, MA 02048. Various brochures on PKU, maple syrup urine disease, homocystinuria, tyrosinemia, urea cycle disorders, and organic acidemias are available; (508)261-1291.

Bright Futures: Guidelines for Health Supervision of Infants, Children and Adolescents; Bright Futures Pocket Guide; Bright Futures Anticipatory Guidance Cards. Available from the National Center for Education in Maternal and Child Health, 2000 15th Street North, Suite 701, Arlington, VA 22201-2617; (703)524-7802. Internet address: http://www.brightfutures.org

Selected References

American Academy of Family Physicians. *Summary of Policy Recommendations for Periodic Health Examination.* Kansas City, Mo: American Academy of Family Physicians; 1997.

American Academy of Pediatrics, Committee on Genetics. Issues in newborn screening. *Pediatrics.* 1992;89:345-349.

American Academy of Pediatrics, Committee on Genetics. Health supervision for children with sickle cell diseases and their families. *Pediatrics.* 1996;98:467-472.

American Academy of Pediatrics, Committee on Genetics. Health supervision for children with achondroplasia. *Pediatrics.* 1995;95:443-451.

American Academy of Pediatrics, Committee on Genetics. Health supervision for children with Down's syndrome. *Pediatrics.* 1994;93:855-859.

American Academy of Pediatrics, Committee on Genetics. Newborn screening fact sheets. *Pediatrics.* 1989;83:449-464.

American Academy of Pediatrics, Committee on Genetics. Prenatal genetic diagnosis for pediatricians. *Pediatrics.* 1994;93:1010-1015.

American Academy of Pediatrics, Committee on Genetics. Health supervision for children with fragile X syndrome. *Pediatrics.* 1996;98:297-300.

American Academy of Pediatrics, Committee on Genetics. Health supervision for children with Marfan syndrome. *Pediatrics.* 1996;98:978-982.

American Academy of Pediatrics, Committee on genetics. Health supervision for children with neurofibromatosis. *Pediatrics*. 1995;96:368-372.

American Academy of Pediatrics, Committee on Genetics. Health supervision for children with Turner syndrome. *Pediatrics*. 1995;96:1166-1173.

American Academy of Pediatrics, Section on Endocrinology and Committee on Genetics, American Thyroid Association, Committee on Public Health. Newborn screening for congenital hypothyroidism: recommendations for guidelines. *Pediatrics*. 1993;91:1203-1209.

Canadian Task Force on the Periodic Health Examination. Screening for congenital hypothyroidism. In: *The Canadian Guide to Clinical Preventive Health Care*. Ottawa, Canada: Minister of Supply and Services; 1994: chap 18.

Canadian Task Force on the Periodic Health Examination. Screening for hemoglobinopathies in Canada. In: *The Canadian Guide to Clinical Preventive Health Care*. Ottawa, Canada: Minister of Supply and Services; 1994: chap 20.

Canadian Task Force on the Periodic Health Examination. Screening for phenylketonuria. In: *The Canadian Guide to Clinical Preventive Health Care*. Ottawa, Canada: Minister of Supply and Services; 1994: chap 17.

Donnell G, ed. *Galactosemia: New Frontiers in Research*. Bethesda, MD: National Institutes of Health, National Institute of Child Health and Development; 1993.

Green M, ed. *Bright Futures: Guidelines for Health Supervision of Infants, Children, and Adolescents*. Arlington, Va: National Center for Education in Maternal and Child Health, 1994.

Illinois Department of Public Health. *An Overview of Newborn Screening Programs in the United States and Canada*. Springfield, Ill: Illinois Department of Public Health; 1996.

National Committee for Clinical Laboratory Standards. *Blood Collection on Filter Paper for Neonatal Screening Programs—Second Edition; Approved Standard*. Villanova, Pa: National Committee for Clinical Laboratory Standards; 1992.

National Institutes of Health. *Newborn Screening for Sickle Cell Disease and Other Hemoglobinopathies*. National Institutes of Health Consensus Development Conference Statement. 1987;6(9):1-22.

National Screening Status Report. *Infant Screening*. 1993;16(1):7.

Sickle Cell Disease Guideline Panel, Agency for Health Care Policy and Research. *Sickle Cell Disease: Screening, Diagnosis, Management, and Counseling in Newborns and Infants*. Clinical Practice Guideline No. 6. Rockville, Md: US Department of Health and Human Services; April 1993. DHHS publication AHCPR 93-0562.

Therrell BL, ed. *Methods for Neonatal Screening*. Washington, DC: American Public Health Association, 1993.

US Preventive Services Task Force. Screening for congenital hypothyroidism. In: *Guide to Clinical Preventive Services*. 2nd ed. Washington, DC: US Department of Health and Human Services; 1996: chap 45.

US Preventive Services Task Force. Screening for hemoglobinopathies. In: *Guide to Clinical Preventive Services*. 2nd ed. Washington, DC: US Department of Health and Human Services; 1996: chap 43.

US Preventive Services Task Force. Screening for phenylketonuria. In: *Guide to Clinical Preventive Services*. 2nd ed. Washington, DC: US Department of Health and Human Services; 1996: chap 44.

9

TUBERCULOSIS (Including Prophylaxis and BCG Vaccination)

Tuberculosis (TB) continues to be a public health problem in the United States for both children and adults. Although the number of new TB cases in the United States among children younger than 15 years of age declined steadily from 1953 (when national surveillance for TB began) until 1988, the number of new cases increased 51% between 1988 and 1992 (from 1133 to 1708). Despite a drop in new TB cases in children between 1992 and 1995, 38% more new cases occurred in 1995 compared with 1988. Factors contributing to the increase in the number of TB cases include adverse social and economic conditions, the epidemic of human immunodeficiency virus (HIV) infection, immigration of individuals with *Mycobacterium tuberculosis* infection, and noncompliance of clinicians and patients with recommended screening and treatment regimens. The recent emergence of multiple-drug-resistant strains of *M. tuberculosis* has added urgency to the need for improved preventive efforts to combat the disease.

Of additional concern is that the number of TB cases among children younger than age 2 years is twice that among older children. Young children, in whom early TB disease may go unrecognized because their TB skin tests may be negative and because they may have few symptoms of disease, are more likely to develop severe disease such as meningitis or miliary tuberculosis than older children or adults. Young children are also more likely to progress from primary TB infection to active disease in a shorter time period than older children and adults.

The diagnosis of TB disease in a child is a sentinel event, signifying recent and ongoing transmission of *M. tuberculosis* in the community. In most states, the clinician is responsible for reporting cases of TB to the appropriate local or state health department, in order to initiate an epidemiologic investigation to identify and to treat infectious cases and contacts in the community.

Pediatric populations at high risk for TB disease include foreign born, African American, and Hispanic children. General populations at high risk of tuberculous infection include: 1) close contacts of persons known or suspected to have TB; 2) persons infected with HIV; 3) persons who inject illicit drugs or other locally identified high-risk substance abusers (eg, crack cocaine users); 4) persons who have medical risk factors known to increase the risk for TB disease if infection occurs; 5) residents and employees of high-risk congregate settings (eg, correctional institutions, nursing homes, mental institutions, other long-term residential facilities, and shelters for the homeless); 6) health-care workers who serve high-risk clients; 7) foreign-born persons, including children, who have arrived within 5 years from countries with a high incidence or prevalence of TB; and 8) some medically underserved, low-income populations.

Conditions and chronic diseases that predispose patients to development of TB disease include HIV infection, diabetes mellitus, end-stage renal disease, and hematologic and reticuloendothelial diseases; history of intestinal bypass or gastrectomy, chronic malabsorption syndromes, silicosis, cancers of the upper gastrointestinal tract or oropharynx, prolonged steroid use, and immunosuppressive therapy; and being 10% or more below desirable body weight.

Screening for TB consists of an intradermal injection of purified protein derivative (Mantoux test). A positive skin reaction (Table 9.1) necessitates additional work-up (chest x-rays, sputum smears and cultures) to differentiate between TB infection and TB disease. A drug regimen based on this evaluation will either be a prophylactic treatment of TB infection or a multi-drug treatment of TB disease (based on the organism's antibiotic sensitivities).

Isoniazid prophylaxis has been shown to be effective in preventing the progression of TB infection to clinical TB disease. When isoniazid is taken for 12 months, it reduces the occurrence of TB disease by 54% to 88%. The efficacy of isoniazid is directly related to the length of prophylaxis, the extent of patient compliance with the prophylactic regimen, and the susceptibility of the infecting organism to isoniazid.

In the United States, the use of Bacillus of Calmette and Guérin (BCG) vaccine to prevent TB infection is rarely indicated; however, new recommendations have been developed in light of two meta-analyses of BCG vaccine clinical trials, as well as the increase in TB cases and the outbreaks of multi-drug-resistant TB. The meta-analyses of BCG protective efficacy indicated that the vaccine efficacy for preventing serious forms of TB in children (meningeal and miliary) was high (>80%). (See Basics of: BCG Vaccination.)

Tuberculosis disease is currently designated as an infectious disease notifiable at the national level. Refer to Appendix C for further information on nationally notifiable diseases.

Table 9.1. Definition of a Positive Mantoux Skin Test (5 Tuberculin Units of Purified Protein Derivative) in Children*

Reaction ≥ 5 mm

Children in close contact with known/suspected infectious cases of TB

(Households with active or previously active cases if treatment cannot be verified as adequate before exposure, treatment was initiated after the child's contact, or reactivation is suspected.)

Children suspected to have TB disease

(Chest x-ray consistent with active or previously active TB; clinical evidence of TB)

Children receiving immunosuppressive therapy or with immunosuppressive conditions, including HIV infection

---

Reaction ≥ 10 mm

Children at increased risk of disseminated disease

(Age <4 years; other medical risk factors including: diabetes mellitus, chronic renal failure, malnutrition)

Children with increased environmental exposure

(Born, or whose parents were born, in high-prevalence regions; frequently exposed to adults who are HIV infected, homeless, users of illicit drugs, medically indigent city dwellers, residents of nursing homes, incarcerated or institutionalized persons, and migrant workers; travel and exposure to high-prevalence regions)

Reaction ≥ 15 mm

Children ≥ 4 years of age without any risk factors

---

* The recommendations should be considered regardless of previous BCG administration.

Adapted from: American Academy of Pediatrics, Committee on Infectious Disease. Update on tuberculosis skin testing of children. Pediatrics. 1996;97:282-284. Reproduced with permission of the publisher, copyright 1996.

Recommendations of Major Authorities

Screening

All major authorities, including **American Academy of Pediatrics (AAP), American Academy of Family Physicians, American Medical Association, American Thoracic Society, Canadian Task Force on the Periodic Health Examination, Centers for Disease Control and Prevention,** and **US Preventive Service Task Force (USPSTF)**—Tuberculin testing should be performed on children and adolescents at high risk of disease. **AAP** has recommended annual TB testing for infants and children with HIV and incarcerated adolescents; testing every 2 to 3 years for children exposed to individuals in certain high-risk groups (HIV infected, homeless, residents of nursing homes, institutionalized adolescents or adults, users of illicit drugs, incarcerated adolescents or adults and migrant farm workers); and testing at ages 4 to 6 years and 11 to 16 years for children without specific risk factors who reside in high prevalence areas and for children whose parents immigrated from regions with a high prevalence of TB or with continued potential exposure by travel to the endemic areas and/or household contact with persons from the endemic areas with unknown skin test status. The **USPSTF** has stated that the frequency of skin testing is a matter of clinical discretion.

Prophylaxis

American Academy of Pediatrics (AAP), American Thoracic Society (ATS), and **Centers for Disease Control and Prevention (CDC)**—Children with a positive Mantoux test and without active disease should receive prophylaxis with isoniazid. Certain children with a negative Mantoux test should be considered for isoniazid prophylaxis (See Basics of Prophylaxis: Indications). The **AAP** has also suggested prophylaxis for patients who are anergic and from a population with a high prevalence of TB. Recommendations for the duration of isoniazid prophylaxis vary among authorities. The **ATS** and **CDC** recommend a minimum of 6 months of prophylaxis; the **AAP** recommends a minimum of 9 months of prophylaxis. According to **AAP** recommendations, newborn prophylaxis may be discontinued at 3 months of age if a Mantoux test at that time is negative; if all known adult contacts have negative sputum samples and are compliant with anti-TB medications; and if a repeat Mantoux test is performed at 6 months of age. The **ATS** and **CDC** recommend maintaining newborn prophylaxis until a negative PPD test is obtained at 6 months of age. Patients who are HIV-positive or who have evidence of prior TB on chest radiograph should receive isoniazid prophylaxis for 12 months. In the latter case, a 4-month course of isoniazid combined with rifampin can also be used.

BCG Vaccination

Advisory Committee on Immunization Practices (ACIP), Advisory Council for the Elimination of Tuberculosis, American Academy of Pediatrics (AAP), Centers for Disease Control and Prevention (CDC), and **US Preventive Services Task Force (USPSTF)**—BCG vaccination should be considered for an infant or child who has a negative TB skin-test result if the following circumstances are present:

the child is exposed continually to an untreated or ineffectively treated patient who has infectious pulmonary TB, and the child cannot be separated from the presence of the infectious patient or given long-term primary preventive therapy

OR

the child is exposed continually to a patient who had infectious pulmonary TB caused by *M. tuberculosis* strains resistant to isoniazid and rifampin, and the child cannot be separated from the presence of the infectious patient.

The **AAP** and **USPSTF** also recommend consideration of BCG vaccination for infants and children in groups in which an excessive rate of new infections is present (eg, >1%) and the usual surveillance and treatment have failed or are not feasible (eg, in groups without a source of regular health care). In the United States, BCG vaccination is rarely indicated. Physicians considering the use of BCG vaccine for their patients are encouraged to consult the TB control programs in their area or the CDC's Division of Tuberculosis Elimination at (404)639-8120.

Basics of Tuberculosis Screening

NOTE: Persons who are not likely to be infected with *M. tuberculosis* generally should not undergo skin testing, because the predictive value of a positive skin test in low-risk populations is poor.

1. The Mantoux test is the standard method of testing. Multiple-puncture tests should not be used to determine whether a person is infected.

2. For the Mantoux test, use 0.1 mL of purified protein derivative (PPD) containing 5 tuberculin units. Administer PPD using a disposable tuberculin syringe, with the bevel of the needle facing upward. Administer the injection intradermally on the volar surface of the forearm to produce a pale, discrete elevation of the skin (weal) 6 to 10 mm in diameter. The weal disappears shortly after the test is administered.

3. Read the test 48 to 72 hours after injection by measuring the diameter of induration (not erythema) transverse to the long axis of the forearm. Record the actual millimeters of induration. Do not consider the erythema that may surround the area of induration.

4. The definition of a positive skin test reaction depends on the likelihood of tuberculosis infection and the risk of tuberculosis disease if infection has occurred. A positive skin reaction can be expected 2 to 10 weeks after infection with TB has occurred.

5. Do not retest patients who have a documented history of a positive Mantoux test; such testing has no diagnostic utility.

6. Live-virus vaccines, such as measles-mumps-rubella (MMR), varicella (VCV), and oral polio vaccine (OPV), may interfere with a response to a tuberculin skin test. The tuberculin skin test should either be administered on the same day as the live-virus vaccinations, or postponed until 4 to 6 weeks after the vaccinations.

Basics of Tuberculosis Prophylaxis

1. Indications

A child with a positive Mantoux test result but without active disease is a candidate for isoniazid prophylaxis. Active disease is excluded by a normal chest radiograph and a lack of symptoms suggesting TB disease. See Table 43.1 for more information on general indications for prophylaxis.

Special pediatric cases should be considered candidates for isoniazid prophylaxis even if they lack documentation of a positive Mantoux test:

■ Newborn prophylaxis: Infants whose mothers have active disease (even if noncontagious) and infants whose mothers have a positive Mantoux test but do not have active disease (preventive therapy can be discontinued after the entire family is demonstrated to have negative tuberculin skin tests)

■ Children who are both anergic or HIV-positive and from populations where the prevalence of TB infection is higher than 10% (eg, injection drug users, homeless persons, migrant laborers, and individuals from Asia, Africa, or Latin America)

■ Children who have had close contact within the past 3 months with a person with infectious TB.

2. Dosage and Administration

The recommended dosage of isoniazid is 10 to 15 mg/kg (up to a maximum of 300 mg) given orally once daily. For noncompliant patients, 15 mg/kg (to a maximum of 900 mg) may be given twice weekly under the direct observation of a health professional.

3. Duration

Continue isoniazid prophylaxis for 6 to 12 months. Recommendations regarding the duration of isoniazid prophylaxis vary (See Recommendations of Major Authorities: Prophylaxis).

4. Precautions

Patients receiving isoniazid prophylaxis must be monitored monthly for signs and symptoms of hepatotoxicity, including loss of appetite, nausea, vomiting, persistent dark urine, jaundice, fever, and abdominal tenderness (especially in the right upper quadrant). Isoniazid should be discontinued at the first sign of hepatotoxicity, and the patient evaluated for the cause of hepatitis. If isoniazid is not the cause of hepatotoxicity, consider reinstating isoniazid preventive therapy once the patient is clinically stable. In otherwise healthy children, the incidence of hepatitis during isoniazid therapy is low enough that routine screening with liver function testing is not required. Peripheral neuritis and convulsions caused by inhibition of pyridoxine metabolism by isoniazid have rarely occurred. When neuritis or convulsions occur during isoniazid treatment, consider accidental overdosage as a possible cause. Pyridoxine supplementation may be considered on an individual basis for breast-feeding children, children with deficient diets (particularly those low in meat and milk), and pregnant women.

Basics of BCG Vaccination

1. Indications

Recommendations differ slightly among authorities. (See Recommendations of Major Authorities.)

2. Vaccine Types

One BCG vaccine (Tice®) is available in the United States. Other BCG preparations that are available for the treatment of bladder cancer are not intended for use as vaccines. Other vaccines are in use in Canada and Mexico.

3. Dose and Administration

≥30 days old: Drop 0.3 mL of the vaccine on the cleansed surface of the skin in the lower deltoid area. Administer the vaccine percutaneously by applying a multiple-puncture disc through the vaccine; the vaccine should flow into the puncture wounds and dry. A dressing is not required, but advise the patient to keep the site dry for 24 hours.

<30 days old: Administer only half the usual dose to infants younger than 30 days old. If an infant's indications for vaccination persist (ie, the TB skin test result is <5 mm induration), administer a full dose of vaccine at 1 year of age.

4. Contraindications

Until the risks and benefits of BCG vaccination in immunocompromised populations are defined, BCG vaccination should not be administered to persons with impaired immune responses (ie, HIV infection, congenital immunodeficiency, leukemia, lymphoma, or generalized malignancy) or suppressed immune responses (from steroids, alkylating agents, antimetabolites, or radiation.) Although no harmful effects to the fetus have been associated with BCG vaccination, its use is not recommended during pregnancy.

5. Adverse reactions

A bluish-red pustule usually forms at the site within 2 to 3 weeks. After 6 weeks, the pustule ulcerates and forms a lesion approximately 5 mm in diameter. Healing is usually complete within 3 months, but a permanent scar usually occurs at the site. Keep draining lesions clean and bandaged. Hypertrophic scars occur in 28% to 33% of vaccinated persons, and keloid scars occur in 2% to 4% of vaccinees.

Although BCG vaccination often results in local adverse effects, serious or long-term complications are rare. Moderate axillary or cervical lymphadenopathy, induration and subsequent pustule formation at the injection site can be expected. More severe local reactions include ulceration at the site and regional suppurative lymphadenitis. Disseminated BCG infection is a rare occurrence, but it is the most serious complication of the vaccine, and can occur from 4 months to 2 years after the vaccination.

6. Interactions

BCG vaccination can cause false-positive Mantoux reactions, but these tuberculin skin test reactions decrease with time after vaccination, and reactions of 15 mm induration or larger are rare. The presence or size of a post-vaccination tuberculin skin-test reaction does not predict whether BCG will provide any protection against TB disease. In general, consider BCG-vaccinated individuals with positive Mantoux test results to have true infection with *M. tuberculosis*.

7. Follow-up

Perform tuberculin skin testing 3 months after BCG vaccination; record test results, in millimeters of induration, in the patient's medical record. The vaccinated person may continue to participate in ongoing skin-testing programs if results remain negative (<5 mm induration). Vaccinees who have positive skin-test results (≥5 mm induration) after vaccination should not be retested unless exposed to a person with infectious TB. A diagnosis of TB infection and the use of preventive therapy should be considered for any BCG-vaccinated person who has a tuberculin skin-test reaction of 10 mm of induration, particularly if any of the following circumstances are present:

- The vaccinated person is a contact of another person who has infectious TB, particularly if the infectious person has transmitted TB to others

- The vaccinated person was born or has resided in a country in which the prevalence of TB is high

- The vaccinated person is exposed continually to populations in which the prevalence of TB is high

Patient Resources

Facts About the TB Skin Test; Facts About Tuberculosis. American Lung Association, 1740 Broadway, New York, NY 10019-4374; (212)315-8700.

TB: Get the Facts; Tuberculosis: Connection between TB and HIV. Centers for Disease Control and Prevention, Attn: Information Technology and Services, Mailstop E-06, 1600 Clifton Rd NE, Atlanta, GA 30333; (404)639-1819.

Provider Resources

Core Curriculum on Tuberculosis. Centers for Disease Control and Prevention; 1994. Centers for Disease Control and Prevention, Attn: Information Technology and Services, Mailstop E-06, 1600 Clifton Rd NE, Atlanta, GA 30333; (404)639-1819.

Initial Therapy for TB in the Era of Multiple Drug Resistance; Mantoux Tuberculin Skin Testing (videotape). Centers for Disease Control and Prevention, Attn: Information Services Office, 1600 Clifton Rd NE, Atlanta GA 30333; (404)639-8135.

Selected References

American Academy of Family Physicians. *Summary of Policy Recommendations for Periodic Health Examination. Kansas City, Mo: American Academy of Family Physicians; 1997.*

American Academy of Pediatrics, Committee on Infectious Diseases. Tuberculosis. In: 1994 *Red Book: Report of the Committee on Infectious Diseases.* Elk Grove Village, Ill: American Academy of Pediatrics; 1994:480-500.

American Academy of Pediatrics, Committee on Infectious Diseases. Update on tuberculosis skin testing of children. *Pediatrics.* 1996;97(2):282-284.

American Medical Association. Rationale and recommendation: Infectious diseases. In: *AMA Guidelines for Adolescent Preventive Services (GAPS): Recommendations and Rationale.* Chicago, Ill: American Medical Association; 1994: chap 15.

American Thoracic Society. Control of tuberculosis in the United States. *Am Rev Respir Dis.* 1992;146:1623-1633.

American Thoracic Society/Centers for Disease Control. Diagnostic standards and classification of tuberculosis. *Am Rev Respir Dis.* 1990;142:725-735.

American Thoracic Society. Treatment of tuberculosis and tuberculosis infection in adults and children. *Am J Respir Crit Care Med.* 1994;149:1359-1374.

Canadian Task Force on the Periodic Health Examination. Screening and isoniazid prophylactic therapy for tuberculosis. In: *The Canadian Guide to Clinical Preventive Health Care.* Ottawa, Canada: Minister of Supply and Services; 1994: chap 62.

Centers for Disease Control. Prevention and control of tuberculosis in US communities with at-risk minority populations and prevention and control of tuberculosis among homeless persons. *MMWR.* 1992;4:1-23.

Centers for Disease Control and Prevention. Screening for tuberculosis and tuberculous infection in high-risk populations: recommendations of the Advisory Committee for the Elimination of Tuberculosis. *MMWR.* 1995;44(RR-11):19-34.

Centers for Disease Control and Prevention. Guidelines for preventing the transmission of Mycobacterium tuberculosis in health care facilities, 1994. *MMWR.* 1994;43(RR-13).

Centers for Disease Control and Prevention. Essential components of a tuberculosis prevention and control program; and Screening for tuberculosis and tuberculosis infection in high-risk populations; recommendations of the Advisory Council for the Elimination of Tuberculosis. *MMWR.* 1995;44(RR-11).

Centers for Disease Control and Prevention. The role of BCG vaccine in the prevention and control of tuberculosis in the United States: a joint statement by the Advisory Council for the Elimination of Tuberculosis and the Advisory Committee on Immunization Practices. *MMWR.* 1996;45(RR-4):1-18.

Colditz GA, Brewer TF, Berkey CS, et al. Efficacy of BCG vaccine in the prevention of tuberculosis: meta-analysis of published literature. *JAMA.* 1994;271:698-702.

Huebner RE, Schein MF, Bass JB. The tuberculin skin test. *Clin Infect Dis.* 1993;17:968-975.

Physician's Desk Reference. Oradell, NJ: Medical Economics Company; 1993:898-899; 1689-1692.

Pust, RE. Tuberculosis in the 1990s: resurgence, regimens, and resources. *South Med J.* 1992;85:584-593.

US Preventive Services Task Force. Screening for tuberculosis infection (including BCG immunization). In: *Guide to Clinical Preventive Services*. 2nd ed. Washington, DC: US Department of Health and Human Services; 1996: chap 25.

Ussery XT, Valway SE, McKenna M, Cauthen GM, McCray E, Onorato IM. Epidemiology of tuberculosis among children in the United States: 1985 to 1994. *Pediatr Infect Dis J*. 1996;15:697-704.

10

URINALYSIS

Urinalysis can detect many abnormalities in the urine, including the presence of glucose, protein, red and white blood cells, bacteria, and bacterial breakdown products. Screening the urine of asymptomatic children for the presence of red blood cells and protein is generally not productive, because the causative disorders tend to be transient and benign. Screening for glucosuria is also of questionable value, because renal thresholds for glucose spillage vary, and the interval between onset of glucosuria and onset of the symptoms of diabetes mellitus is short. Screening for indicators of occult infection, such as white blood cells and bacteria, may be beneficial as a means of promoting early treatment.

During infancy, the prevalence of asymptomatic bacteriuria is higher among boys (2.5%) than among girls (0.9%), in part because boys have structural abnormalities of the urinary tract more frequently than girls. After infancy, the prevalence of asymptomatic bacteriuria is much higher among girls (1% to 2%) than among boys (<0.1%). Asymptomatic bacteriuria develops into symptomatic urinary tract infections in fewer than 10% of cases. Urinary tract infections can lead to renal scarring and permanent renal damage. Such damage generally occurs in children before 2 to 3 years of age, when screening is difficult because of problems of specimen collection. Treatment of asymptomatic bacteriuria with antibiotics may alter the composition of body flora and lead to infection with resistant bacteria.

Asymptomatic sexually transmitted diseases, particularly infection with *Chlamydia trachomatis*, are common in adolescents and young adults. The prevalence of asymptomatic chlamydial urethral infection in young males ranges from 6% to 11%. These infections can be passed to female partners, resulting in pelvic inflammatory disease, ectopic pregnancy, and infertility. Recently, dipstick urinalysis has been advocated as a noninvasive initial screening technique for detecting such occult infections in sexually active young males. Such testing has moderate sensitivity and low specificity, necessitating additional follow-up testing of patients with positive results. The FDA has not approved these tests for screening for sexually transmitted diseases including *C. trachomatis*.

Recommendations of Major Authorities

American Academy of Family Physicians and **US Preventive Services Task Force (USPSTF)**—Routine screening of males and most females for asymptomatic bacteriuria is not recommended; there is insufficient evidence for or against routine screening of diabetic women (including children and adolescents). **The Canadian Task Force on the Periodic Health Examination** and the **USPSTF** recommend against screening for asymptomatic bacteriuria with urinalysis in infants, children, and adolescents.

American Academy of Pediatrics—Urinalysis should be performed once at 5 years of age. Also, dipstick leukocyte esterase testing to screen for sexually transmitted diseases should be performed once in adolescence, preferably at 14 years of age.

American Medical Association and **Bright Futures**—Sexually active adolescent males should be screened yearly for gonorrhea and chlamydia by urinalysis with a dipstick leukocyte esterase test.

Basics of Urinalysis

1. To obtain urine from infants and young children, apply a plastic urine bag to the perineum. This method is associated with a relatively high rate of false-positive results (up to 30%) because of contamination. Positive test results of urine obtained by bag collection should be confirmed by catheterization or suprapubic aspiration.

2. In screening children and adolescents for bacteriuria, obtain specimens using midstream "clean catch" techniques. This method permits follow-up culture testing of dipstick-positive specimens. The vulva of girls and the glans of boys should be cleansed well with a mild soap solution. Do not use antiseptic solutions because of the potential for suppressing bacterial growth in the sample. During urination, the labia of girls should be held open to avoid impinging on the flow of urine. This may be accomplished without manual holding by having the girl sit backward with legs astride a toilet seat. The foreskin of uncircumcised boys should be retracted to avoid impinging on the flow of urine.

3. The sensitivity of screening for bacteriuria may be improved by obtaining a specimen from the first void of the day, which is more concentrated and contains higher amounts of bacteria and bacterial breakdown products compared with subsequent voids. Specimen collection from later voids is acceptable and may be more practical.

4. The dipstick leukocyte esterase test is the most efficient way to screen specimens for bacteriuria. The sensitivity and specificity of both this test and

the more labor-intensive microscopic analysis are roughly equivalent (approximately 80%). The nitrite test is also available on many dipsticks, but its low sensitivity, approximately 30%, makes it an inadequate screening tool if used alone. A positive nitrite test result, however, is approximately 99% specific for significant bacteriuria.

5. To screen males for sexually transmitted diseases, collect a urine sample from the first 15 to 20 mL of a void and test the unspun sample with a leukocyte esterase dipstick. Because of the poor specificity and relatively high cost of this test, as well as the potential morbidity associated with treatment, confirm positive test results with more specific techniques, such as enzyme immunoassay and/or culture. Negative results from symptomatic males should always be confirmed by enzyme immunoassay and/or culture.

Provider Resources

Bright Futures: Guidelines for Health Supervision of Infants, Children and Adolescents; Bright Futures Pocket Guide; Bright Futures Anticipatory Guidance Cards. Available from the National Center for Education in Maternal and Child Health, 2000 15th Street North, Suite 701, Arlington, VA 22201-2617. (703)524-7802. Internet address: http://www.brightfutures.org

Selected References

American Academy of Family Physicians. *Summary of Policy Recommendations for Periodic Health Examination.* Kansas City, Mo: American Academy of Family Physicians; 1997.

American Academy of Pediatrics, Committee on Practice and Ambulatory Medicine. Recommendations for pediatric preventive health care. *Pediatrics.* 1995;96:373-374.

American Medical Association. Guidelines for adolescent preventive services. In: *AMA Guidelines for Adolescent Preventive Services (GAPS): Recommendations and Rationale.* Chicago, Ill: American Medical Association; 1994:xxix-xxxviii.

Aronson MD, Phillips RS. Screening young men for Chlamydia infection. *JAMA.* 1993;270:2097-2098.

Boehm JJ, Haynes JL. Bacteriology of "midstream catch" urines. *Am J Dis Child.* 1966;111:366-369.

Canadian Task Force on the Periodic Health Examination. Screening for urinary infection in asymptomatic infants and children. In: *The Canadian Guide to Clinical Preventive Health Care.* Ottawa, Canada: Minister of Supply and Services; 1994: chap 21.

Canadian Task Force on the Periodic Health Examination. The periodic health examination 1979. *Can Med Assoc J.* 1979;121:1193-1254.

Dodge WF. Cost effectiveness of renal disease screening. *Am J Dis Child.* 1977;131:1274-1280.

Edelman CM, Ogwo JE, Fine BP, Martinez AB. The prevalence of bacteriuria in full-term and premature newborn infants. *J Pediatr.* 1973;82:125-132.

Genc M, Ruusuvaara, Mardh PA. An economic evaluation of screening for Chlamydia trachomatis in adolescent males. *JAMA.* 1993;270:2057-2064.

Goldsmith BM, Campos JM. Comparison of urine dipstick, microscopy, and culture for the detection of bacteriuria in children. *Clin Pediatr*. 1990;29:214-218.

Green M, ed. *Bright Futures: Guidelines for Health Supervision of Infants, Children, and Adolescents*. Arlington, Va: National Center for Education in Maternal and Child Health, 1994.

Lindberg U. Asymptomatic bacteriuria in school girls: V. The clinical course and response to treatment. *Acta Paediatr Scand*. 1975;64:718-724.

Lohr JA, Donowitz LG, Dudley SM. Bacterial contamination rates for non-clean-catch and clean-catch midstream urine collections in boys. *J Pediatr*. 1986;109:659-660.

Lohr JA, Donowitz LG, Dudley SM. Bacterial contamination rates in voided urine collections in girls. *J Pediatr*. 1989;114:91-93.

Kemper KJ, Avner ED. The case against screening urinalyses for asymptomatic bacteriuria in children. *Am J Dis Child*. 1992;146:343-346.

Kunin CM. *Detection, Prevention and Management of Urinary Tract Infections*. 4th ed. Philadelphia, Pa: Lea & Febiger, 1987.

Mitchell N, Stapleton FB. Routine admission urinalysis examination in pediatric patients: a poor value. *Pediatrics*. 1990;86:345-349.

Quinn C, Gaydos C, Shepherd M, Bobo L, et al. Epidemiologic and microbiologic correlates of Chlamydia trachomatis infection in sexual partnerships. *JAMA*. 1996;276:1727-1742.

Schlager TA, Dunn ML, Dudley SM, Lohr JA. Bacterial contamination rate of urine collected in a urine bag from healthy non-toilet-trained male infants. *J Pediatr*. 1990;116:738-739.

Shafer M, Schachter J, Moncada J, et al. Evaluation of urine-based screening strategies to detect Chlamydia trachomatis among sexually active asymptomatic young males. *JAMA*. 1993;270:2065-2070.

US Preventive Services Task Force. Screening for asymptomatic bacteriuria. In: *Guide to Clinical Preventive Services*. 2nd ed. Washington, DC: US Department of Health and Human Services; 1996: chap 31.

Zhanel GG, Harding GKM, Guay DRP. Asymptomatic bacteriuria. Which patients should be treated? *Arch Intern Med*. 1990;150:1389-1396.

11

VISION

Refractive errors are the most common vision disorders in children, occurring in 20% of children by age 16 years. Amblyopia ("lazy eye") develops in 2% to 5% of children, and the risk of developing this disorder is greatest during the first 2 to 3 years of life. The potential for its development exists, however, until visual development is complete at 9 years of age. Untreated amblyopia may result in irreversible visual deficits. Strabismus, one of the primary causes of amblyopia, occurs in 2% of children. Other eye diseases occurring during infancy and childhood include cataracts (1 per 1000 live births), congenital glaucoma (1 per 10,000 live births), and retinoblastoma (1 per 20,000 live births).

Through careful history, examination, vision testing, and appropriate referral, amblyopia and other ophthalmologic disorders can be detected and visual impairment can be lessened or averted. Early detection and prompt intervention are essential.

Recommendations of Major Authorities

Normal-Risk Children

American Academy of Family Physicians—Children should be screened for amblyopia and strabismus at 3 to 4 years of age.

American Academy of Pediatrics and **Bright Futures**—Visual acuity testing should first be performed at 3 years of age. If the child is uncooperative, retesting should occur 6 months later. Subsequent testing should occur at 4, 5, 10, 12, 15, and 18 years of age. Subjective assessment by history should occur at visits at all other ages. All infants should be examined by 6 months of age to evaluate fixation preference, alignment, and presence of any eye disease. Children should again be medically evaluated for these problems by 3 to 4 years of age.

American Academy of Ophthalmology (AAO), American Association for Pediatric Ophthalmology and Strabismus (AAPOS), and **American Optometric Association (AOA)**—Eye and vision screening should be performed at birth and at approximately 6 months, 3 years, and 5 years of age. **AAO** has published recommendations regarding screening methods and indications for referral to be used by primary care clinicians in screening preschool children (Table 11.1). **AAO** and **AAPOS** recommend that screening after 5 years of age be carried out at routine school checks or after the appearance of symptoms. **AOA** recommends optometric examinations every 2 years throughout school years.

Canadian Task Force on the Periodic Health Examination—Repeat examination of the eyes for strabismus is recommended during well-baby visits, especially during the first 6 months of life. There is fair evidence to include testing of visual acuity in the periodic health examination of preschool children.

US Preventive Services Task Force—All children should have testing for amblyopia and strabismus once before entering school, preferably at 3 to 4 years of age. Stereoacuity testing may be more effective than visual acuity testing in detecting these conditions. There is insufficient evidence to recommend for or against routine screening for diminished visual acuity among asymptomatic school children. Recommendations against such screening can be made on other grounds, including the inconvenience and cost of routine screening and the fact that refractive errors can be readily corrected when they produce symptoms. Clinicians should be alert for signs of ocular misalignment when examining all newborns, infants, and children.

High-Risk Children

American Academy of Ophthalmology—Asymptomatic children should have a comprehensive examination by an ophthalmologist if they are at high risk because of health and developmental problems that make screening by the primary care clinician difficult or inaccurate (eg, retinopathy of prematurity or diagnostic evaluation of a complex disease with ophthalmic manifestations); a family history of conditions that cause or are associated with eye or vision problems (eg, retinoblastoma, significant hyperopia, strabismus [particularly accommodative esotropia], amblyopia, congenital cataract, or glaucoma); multiple health problems, systemic disease, or use of medications that are known to be associated with eye disease and vision abnormalities (eg, neurodegenerative disease, juvenile rheumatoid arthritis, systemic steroid therapy, systemic syndromes with ocular manifestations, or developmental delay with visual system manifestations).

American Optometric Association—The primary care clinician should remain alert for visual/ocular abnormalities associated with the following high-risk groups: infants who are premature, with low birth weight, or whose mothers have had rubella, venereal disease, AIDS-related infection or a history of substance abuse or other medical problems during pregnancy, and children failing to progress educationally or exhibiting reading and/or learning disabilities. The presence of high refractive error or a family history of eye disease, crossed eyes, or congenital eye disorders also places infants and children at risk. Infants at risk should be examined by a doctor of optometry by 6 months of age. Children at risk should be examined at 3 years of age and annually beginning at 6 years of age. All infants and children may be referred to an optometrist for a comprehensive eye and/or vision examination.

Basics of Vision Screening

1. History

When screening for present or potential visual disorders, consider the following factors:

- Family history of vision or eye problems

- History of maternal, intrapartum, or neonatal conditions that may place the child at high risk for visual disorders (See High-Risk Children)

- Parental concerns about a child's visual functioning

- Worsening grades and other school difficulties

2. Physical Examination

A comprehensive examination of the eye includes the lids, lashes, tear ducts, orbit, conjunctiva, sclera, cornea, iris, pupillary responsiveness, range of motion, anterior chamber, lens, vitreous, retina, and optic nerve and vessels. Gaining the cooperation of a young child with an ophthalmoscopic examination can be difficult. It may be helpful to demonstrate the examination procedure on the parent beforehand and to have the child sit on the parent's lap.

Table 11.1. Eye and Vision Examination Recommendations for Primary Care Clinicians

Age	Screening Method	Indicators Requiring Further Evaluation
Newborn to 3 months old	Red reflex	Abnormal or asymmetric
	Corneal light reflex	Asymmetric
	Inspection	Structural abnormality
6 months to 1 year old	Red reflex	Abnormal or asymmetric
	Corneal light reflex	Asymmetric
	Differential occlusion	Failure to object equally to covering each eye
	Fix and follow with each eye	Failure to fix and follow
	Inspection	Structural abnormality
3 years old (approximately)	Visual acuity*	20/50 or worse or difference of 2 lines between eyes
	Red reflex	Abnormal or asymmetric
	Corneal light reflex/cover-uncover	Asymmetric/ocular refixation movements
	Stereoacuity†	Failure to appreciate random dot or Titmus stereogram
	Inspection	Structural abnormality
5 years old (approximately)	Visual acuity*	20/30 or worse
	Red reflex	Abnormal or asymmetric
	Corneal light reflex/cover-uncover	Asymmetric/ocular refixation movements
	Stereoacuity†	Failure to appreciate random dot or Titmus stereogram
	Inspection	Structural abnormality

* Allen figures, HOTV, Tumbling E, or Snellen

† Optional, sometimes advocated in lieu of visual acuity; Random Dot E game (RDE), Titmus stereograms, Randot stereograms

From: American Academy of Ophthalmology, Quality of Care Committee, Pediatric Ophthalmology Panel. Comprehensive Pediatric Eye Evaluation. San Francisco, Calif. American Academy of Ophthalmology; 1992. Reproduced by permission of the publisher; copyright 1992.

3. Testing Procedures

Red Reflex: Perform this exam with an ophthalmoscope or other light source. In a darkened room, hold the light source at arm's length from the infant, and draw the infant's attention to look directly at the light. Both retinal reflexes should be red or red-orange and of equal intensity.

Corneal Light Reflex: To detect strabismus, perform this test with an ophthalmoscope or other light source. Corneal light reflections should fall symmetrically on corresponding points of the patient's eyes. Improper alignment will appear as asymmetry of reflections.

Differential Occlusion: Gently cover the infant's eyes, one at a time. Aversion to the occlusion is normal. This test may give a false-positive result and is generally less accurate than the corneal light reflex test for detecting strabismus.

Fixation: Hold a light or a small object in front of the infant. Normal eyes will be aligned in the same direction, without deviation.

Cover/Uncover: Have the child focus on a stationary target. Place a hand or cover in front of one eye, and observe the other eye. Movement of the observed eye is abnormal and demonstrates the presence of strabismus. As the covered eye is uncovered, observe it for movement. Movement is abnormal and indicates the presence of heterophoria.

Stereo testing: To detect stereopsis (binocular depth perception), use a stereo testing technique, such as the Random Dot E stereogram. While wearing polarized glasses, the child views test cards that contain fields of random dots. If stereopsis is present, the child will see a form stand out from the background of the cards.

Visual Acuity: Several eye charts are available to test visual acuity in children. In order of decreasing cognitive difficulty, these are: Snellen Letters, Snellen Numbers, Tumbling E, HOTV, Allen Figures, and LH (Leah Hyvarinen) Test. Use the test with the highest level of difficulty that the child is capable of performing. In general, the Snellen tests are too advanced for preschool-aged children. Test for visual acuity at 10, 15, or 20 feet using the appropriate chart. Using a distance of 10 feet for young children may result in better compliance because of closer interaction with the examiner. To ensure that a young child does not "peek" with the eye not being tested, hold the occluder for the child or use an adhesive occluder. Give a passing score for each line on which the child gives more than 50% correct responses. Recommended criteria for referral to an ophthalmologist or optometrist vary slightly. In general, refer any child with a difference between eye scores of two or more lines; children younger than age 5 years who score 20/40 or worse in either eye; and children aged 5 years or older who score 20/30 or worse in either eye.

4. Safety Counseling

Counsel parents and children about eye safety and the appropriate use of protective equipment. Children who participate in school shop or science labs or in certain sports (ie, racquetball, squash) should wear safety lenses and safety frames approved by the American National Standards Institute. Children with good vision in only one eye should wear safety lenses and safety frames to protect the good eye, even if they do not otherwise need to wear glasses.

Patient Resources

Amblyopia: Is it Affecting Your Child's Sight?; Cataracts in Children: Eye Safety and Children; Eyeglasses for Infants and Children; Home Eye Test for Strabismus. American Academy of Ophthalmology, PO Box 7424, San Francisco, CA 94120. Send a business-size, self-addressed, stamped envelop with your request.

Your Child's Eyes. American Academy of Pediatrics, 141 Northwest Point Blvd, PO Box 927, Elk Grove Village, IL 60009-0927; (800)433-9016. Internet address: http://www.aap.org

Answers to Your Questions About: Lazy Eye, Nearsightedness, Astigmatism, Eye Coordination, Color Deficiency, Crossed-Eyes; Signs of a Child's Vision Problems; Toys, Games and Your Child's Vision; Your Child's Eyes; Your Preschool Child's Eyes; Your School-Aged Child's Eyes. American Optometric Association, 243 N Lindbergh Blvd, St. Louis, MO 63141; (314)991-4100. Internet address: http://www.aoanet.org/aoanet

Provider Resources

Bright Futures: Guidelines for Health Supervision of Infants, Children and Adolescents; Bright Futures Pocket Guide; Bright Futures Anticipatory Guidance Cards. Available from the National Center for Education in Maternal and Child Health, 2000 15th Street North, Suite 701, Arlington, VA 22201-2617; (703)524-7802. Internet address: http://www.brightfutures.org

Policy Statement: Frequency of Ocular Examinations; National Eyecare Project (for those who do not have an eye doctor); Glaucoma 2001 Project (for people at risk for glaucoma). American Academy of Ophthalmology, PO Box 7424, San Francisco, CA 94120. Send a business-size, self-addressed, stamped envelope with your request.

Pediatric Eye and Vision Examination, Care of the Patient with Amblyopia, and other clinical practice guidelines. American Optometric Association, 243 N Lindbergh Blvd, St. Louis, MO 63141; (800)262-2210. Internet address: http://www.aoanet.org/aoanet/members

Selected References

American Academy of Family Physicians. *Sumary of Policy Recommendations for Periodic Health Examination.* Kansas City, Mo: American Academy of Family Physicians; 1997.

American Academy of Ophthalmology. *Infant and Children's Vision Screening: Policy Statement.* San Francisco, Calif: American Academy of Ophthalmology; 1991.

American Academy of Ophthalmology, Quality of Care Committee, Pediatric Ophthalmology Panel. *Comprehensive Pediatric Eye Evaluation.* San Francisco, Calif: American Academy of Ophthalmology; 1992.

American Optometric Association. *Guidelines for Preventive Eye Care.* St. Louis, Mo: American Optometric Associaiton; 1993.

American Optometric Association. *Pediatric Eye and Vision Examination.* St. Louis, Mo: American Optometric Association; 1994.

American Academy of Pediatrics, Committee on Practice and Ambulatory Medicine. Recommendations for pediatric preventive health care. *Pediatrics.* 1995;96:373-374.

Canadian Task Force on the Periodic Health Examination. The periodic health examination. *Can Med Assoc J.* 1979;121:1194-1254.

Canadian Task Force on the Periodic Health Examination. Periodic health examination: 2; 1989 update. *Can Med Assoc J.* 1989;141:4-24.

Canadian Task Force on the Periodic Health Examination. Routine preschool screening for visual and hearing problems. In: *The Canadian Guide to Clinical Preventive Health Care.* Ottawa, Canada: Minister of Supply and Services; 1994: chap 27.

Canadian Task Force on the Periodic Health Examination. Well baby care in the first 2 years of life. In: *The Canadian Guide to Clinical Preventive Health Care.* Ottawa, Canada: Minister of Supply and Services; 1994: chap 24.

Gaynon MW. Retinopathy of prematurity. *Pediatrician.* 1990;17:127-133.

Green M, ed. *Bright Futures: Guidelines for Health Supervision of Infants, Children, and Adolescents.* Arlington, Va: National Center for Education in Maternal and Child Health, 1994.

Hope C. Random dot stereogram E in vision screening of children. *Austr N Zea J Ophthalmol.* 1990;18:319-324.

Romano PE. Advances in vision and eye screening: screening at six months of age. *Pediatrician.* 1990;17:134-141.

Romano PE. Vision/eye screening: Test twice and refer once. *Pediatr Annals.* 1990;19:359-367.

US Preventive Services Task Force. Screening for visual impairment. In: *Guide to Clinical Preventive Services.* 2nd ed. Washington, DC: US Department of Health and Human Services, 1996: chap 33.

12

DIPHTHERIA, TETANUS AND PERTUSSIS

Diphtheria is an acute infectious disease caused by *Corynebacterium diphtheriae*. It is characterized by a local inflammatory lesion, usually in the respiratory tract, and a toxic reaction that primarily affects the heart valves and peripheral nerves. Diphtheria is a rare occurrence in the United States. During the past decade, only 0 to 5 cases of diphtheria were reported each year.

Tetanus (lockjaw) is an acute and often fatal disease caused by an exotoxin produced in a wound by *Clostridium tetani*. Approximately 50 cases of tetanus are reported each year in the United States.

Pertussis (whooping cough) is an acute respiratory infection caused by *Bordetella pertussis*. Prior to the availability of a vaccine, more than 100,000 cases of pertussis were reported annually in the United States. In 1995, 5137 cases of pertussis were reported; 36% of these cases occurred in children under 1 year of age.

Diphtheria, tetanus, and pertussis are currently designated as infectious diseases notifiable at the national level. Refer to Appendix C for further information on nationally notifiable diseases.

See chapter 52 for information on tetanus and diphtheria immunization and prophylaxis in adults.

Recommendations of Major Authorities

Most major authorities, including **Advisory Committee on Immunization Practices, American Academy of Family Physicians, American Academy of Pediatrics, American College of Preventive Medicine, Bright Futures,** and **US Preventive Services Task Force—** All children should receive immunization against diphtheria, tetanus, and pertussis: 5 doses total by their seventh birthday (3 doses of primary series at 2, 4 and 6 months of age and 2 doses of booster vaccine at 15 to 18 months and 4 to 6 years of age). All US authorities recommend that a booster dose of Td (tetanus-diphtheria toxoid for adult use) be given at 11 to 16 years of age.

Canadian Task Force on the Periodic Health Examination—All children should receive immunization against diphtheria, tetanus, and pertussis at 2, 4, 6 and 18 months.

Basics of Diphtheria, Tetanus, and Pertussis Immunization

1. Vaccine Types

Diphtheria, tetanus, acellular pertussis (DTaP)/diphtheria, tetanus, pertussis (DTP):

> There are two types of diphtheria, tetanus and pertussis vaccines: DTaP and whole-cell DTP. DTaP, in which the pertussis portion of the vaccine is acellular, has fewer side effects and is preferred for all five vaccinations in the series. However, during the period of transition from use of DTP to DTaP, whole-cell DTP is an acceptable alternative to DTaP. Three acellular pertussis vaccines are currently licensed for administration to infants: Tripedia®, Connaught Laboratories; ACEL-IMUNE®, Wyeth-Lederle Pediatric Vaccines; and Infanrix®, SmithKline Beecham. Four whole-cell vaccines are currently licensed for administration to infants. They are produced by: Lederle, Connaught Laboratories, Massachusetts Public Health Biologic Laboratories, and Michigan Biologic Products.

Combined vaccines:

> A combined whole-cell DTP and Haemophilus influenzae type b (DTP-HbOC) vaccine (TETRAMUNE®, Lederle) has been licensed for the first four doses of the childhood vaccination series to prevent diphtheria, tetanus and pertussis, and H. influenzae type b (Hib).

> The Food and Drug Administration has approved reconstituting H. influenzae type b conjugate vaccine (ActHIB®, Connaught Laboratories, or OmniHIB®, SmithKline Beecham) with the DTP vaccine produced by Connaught Laboratories for the first four doses of the diphtheria, tetanus and pertussis series. The DTaP vaccine Tripedia® produced by Connaught Laboratories can be reconstituted with either ActHIB®, Connaught Laboratories, or OmniHIB®, SmithKline Beecham, and administered for the fourth dose.

Tetanus toxoid:

> There are two forms of tetanus toxoid: adsorbed and fluid. Tetanus toxoid adsorbed contains aluminum, which enhances the immune response and, for this reason, is the preferred form. Tetanus toxoid fluid vaccine can be

used as an alternative in cases where there is a known hypersensitivity to aluminum, which is found in the adsorbed type. Generally, the tetanus toxoid in vaccinations such as DTP, DTaP, DT, and Td are adsorbed. Check the Physician's Desk Reference for further information.

2. Schedule

The Advisory Committee on Immunization Practices (ACIP), the American Academy of Pediatrics, and the American Academy of Family Physicians currently recommend the following schedule for diphtheria, tetanus, and pertussis vaccination (Table 12.1):

Table 12.1. Schedule for Diphtheria, Tetanus, Pertussis Vaccination

Dose	Age	Notes
Dose 1[a]	2 months	Administer first 3 doses a minimum of 4 weeks apart.
Dose 2	4 months	
Dose 3	6 months	
Dose 4[b]	15 - 18 months	Administer dose 4 at least 6 months after the third dose.
Dose 5[c]	4-6 years	

a May be given as early as 6 weeks of age

b If the interval between the third and fourth doses is greater than 6 months and the child is not likely to return for a visit at the recommended age, the fourth dose of either DTaP or DTP may be administered as early as 12 months of age.

c Fifth vaccination is not necessary if the fourth vaccination was given when the child was 4 years of age or older.

3. Dose and Administration

The recommended dose of DTaP, DTP, DTP-HbOC, DT, Td, and the single-antigen adsorbed preparations is 0.5 mL, given intramuscularly.

For infants younger than 12 months of age: The preferred site is the anterolateral thigh. Bunch the thigh muscle, using the free hand, and inject the needle (22- to 25-gauge, 7/8" to 1" in length) inferiorly at an angle to reach the muscle but avoid contact with neurovascular structures or bone. DTaP or DTP may be given simultaneously with other childhood vaccinations, but avoid giving other vaccinations in the same limb with DTaP or DTP.

For toddlers and older children: Vaccination may be given in the deltoid (if muscle mass appears adequate) using a 22- to 25-gauge needle that is 5/8" to 1-1/4" in length. DTaP or DTP may be given simultaneously with other childhood vaccinations, but avoid giving other vaccinations in the same limb with DTaP or DTP.

4. Contraindications/Precautions

There are few, true contraindications to administering vaccinations. See Appendix B, Table B.3 for a listing of valid contraindications. Table 12.2 lists contraindications specific to DTaP/DTP vaccination.

- Pertussis vaccine is contraindicated in children over 7 years of age.

- Because of the high diphtheria toxoid content of DT, it is not recommended for use in children over the age of 7; vaccinate children over 7 years of age with Td.

5. Adverse Reactions

Local side effects, including redness, swelling, or pain, along with mild systemic reactions (fever less than 40.5°C [104.9°F], drowsiness, fretfulness, vomiting, or anorexia) can commonly occur. These side effects occur much less frequently with the acellular DTaP vaccine than with the DTP vaccine. Acetaminophen or ibuprofen given at the time of DTP vaccination and every 4 hours for the next 24 hours may help prevent or relieve minor side effects (eg, fever, pain).

Moderate to severe systemic events include the following: fever of 40.5°C (104.9°F) within 48 hours; persistent inconsolable crying for 3 hours or more; an unusual, high-pitched cry within 48 hours; collapse or shock-like state (hypotonic-hyporesponsive episode) within 48 hours; and convulsions with or without fever occurring within 72 hours of vaccination. These side effects are rare following DTP vaccination and are very rare following DTaP vaccination.

Severe adverse events are very rare following DTP vaccination and are expected to be extremely rare following DTaP. These reactions include anaphylaxis (severe allergic hypersensitivity) and acute encephalopathy.

All adverse side effects should be reported to the Vaccine Adverse Event Reporting System (VAERS). Refer to Table B.4 for a detailed listing of adverse events. VAERS forms and instructions are available in the FDA Drug Bulletin (Food and Drug Administration) and the Physician's Desk Reference or by calling the 24-hour VAERS information recording, (800)822-7967. Refer to Appendix B for details.

Table 12.2. Contraindications for Administration of DTP and DTaP Vaccines

True Contraindications	NOT Contraindications (vaccines may be given)
History of anaphylaxis or anaphylactic shock within 24 hours	Temperature <40.5°C (104.9°F) following a previous dose of DTaP/DTP
Encephalopathy within 7 days of administration of previous dose of DTP/DTaP	Personal or family history of convulsions†
	Family history of sudden infant death syndrome
	Family history of an adverse event following DTP/DTaP administration

Precautions

Fever ≥40.5°C (104.9°F) within 48 hours after vaccination with a previous dose of DTP/DTaP*

Collapse or shock-like state (hypotonic-hyporesponsive episode) within 48 hours of receiving a previous dose of DTP/DTaP*

Seizures within 3 days of receiving a previous dose of DTP/DTaP*

Persistent, inconsolable crying lasting 3 hours within 48 hours of receiving a previous dose of DTP/DTaP*

*Precautions should be carefully reviewed. The benefits and risks of administering a specific vaccine to a child under the circumstances should be considered. If the risks are believed to outweigh the benefits, withhold immunization; if the benefits are believed to outweigh the risks (eg, during an outbreak or foreign travel), administer vaccine.

†Pertussis vaccination is not a contraindication for children with a family history of seizures. The ACIP recommends that DTaP should be the vaccine of choice, when pertussis vaccination is considered for children with personal history of seizures. Infants with evolving neurologic conditions should not be vaccinated until a treatment regimen has been established and the condition has stabilized.

Adapted from: National Vaccine Advisory Committee. Standards for Pediatric Immunization Practices. Atlanta, Ga: Centers for Disease Control and Prevention; 1993.

6. Special Cases

If pertussis vaccine is contraindicated in a child younger than age 7 years for reasons other than acute anaphylaxis, replace DTaP or DTP with DT in the immunization schedule.

If a nonimmunized child is 7 years of age or older, administer three doses of Td. Give the second dose 4 to 8 weeks after the first, and administer the third dose 6 to 12 months after the second dose.

If at least 5 years have elapsed since the last dose of DTaP, DTP, DTP-HbOC, or DT, give a booster immunization with Td at 11 to 16 years of age.

7. Patient Education

The National Childhood Vaccine Injury Act requires health care providers to provide the following information to (parents of) patients prior to administering DTP/DTaP: (1) a concise description of the benefits of the vaccine, (2) a concise description of the risks associated with the vaccine, and (3) notice of the availability of the National Vaccine Injury Compensation Program.

The US Department of Health and Human Services has developed a pamphlet for this purpose (See Patient Resources). Other patient educational materials may be used if they provide the information required by the National Childhood Vaccine Injury Act. For additional information about this requirement, contact the Training Coordinator, National Immunization Program, Centers for Disease Control and Prevention; (404)639-8226.

8. Vaccine Storage and Handling

Store vaccine at 2 to 8°C (36 to 46°F); do not freeze. Do not use vaccine that has been frozen. Handle all vaccine preparations according to manufacturers' instructions.

Basics of Tetanus Prophylaxis

1. Indications

Patients who may have been exposed to tetanus because of wounds may need prophylaxis via immediate passive immunization with tetanus immune globulin (TIG), active immunization with tetanus toxoid (preferably Td), or both. See Table 12.3 for guidelines on passive and active immunization according to the nature of the wound and the patient's immunization status.

2. Dose and Administration

The recommended dose of TIG is 250 units. This should be given intramuscularly in a different site and with a different syringe than that used for concurrent administration of DTP, DTaP, or Td.

The recommended dose of Td is 0.5 mL. This should be given intramuscularly, in a different site and with a different syringe than that used for concurrent administration of TIG.

Table 12.3. Summary Guide to Tetanus Prophylaxis in Routine Wound Management

Number of previous tetanus vaccinations	Clean, minor wounds		All other wounds[1]	
	Give Td[2]	Give TIG	Give Td[2]	Give TIG
Unknown, uncertain or fewer than 3	Yes	No	Yes	Yes
3 or more [3]	No[4]	No	No[5]	No

1. Such as, but not limited to: wounds contaminated with dirt, feces, and saliva; puncture wounds; avulsions; and wounds resulting from missiles, crushing, burns, and frostbite

2. For children < 7 years of age DTaP or DTP (DT if pertussis vaccine is contraindicated) is preferred to tetanus toxoid alone. For persons ≥ 7 years of age, Td (tetanus-diphtheria toxoid for adult use) is preferred to tetanus toxoid alone.

3. If only 3 doses of fluid toxoid have been received, then a fourth dose of toxoid, preferably an adsorbed toxoid should be given.

4. Administer a booster if more than 10 years have elapsed since the last dose.

5. Administer a booster if more than 5 years have elapsed since the last dose. More frequent boosters are not needed and can accentuate side effects.

Adapted from: Centers for Disease Control. Diphtheria, tetanus, and pertussis: Recommendations for vaccine use and other preventive measures. MMWR. 1991;40(RR-10):1-28.

3. Adverse Reactions

The side effects of TIG are relatively minor (site soreness and mild temperature elevation), but a few cases of more serious side effects (anaphylaxis, angioneurotic edema, nephrotic syndrome) have been reported.

Patient Resources

Childhood Vaccines: What They Are and Why Your Child Needs Them. American Academy of Family Physicians, 8880 Ward Parkway, Kansas City, MO 64114-2797; (800)944-0000. Internet address: http://www.aafp.org

Vaccine Information Statement—*Diphtheria, Tetanus, and Pertussis: What you need To know before your child gets the vaccines,* #I1923; *Tetanus and Diphtheria Vaccine: What you need to know before you or your child gets the vaccine,* #I1733. US Department of Health and Human Services. This information is available from the National Immunization Program, Information/Distribution Center, MS E-34, Centers for Disease Control and Prevention, 1600 Clifton Rd NE, Atlanta, GA 30333; (404)639-8225. Fax (404)639-8828. Other sources of this information are state and local health departments or the American Academy of

Pediatrics, Division of Publications, PO Box 927, Elk Grove Village, IL 60009-0927; (800)433-9016.

Protecting Your Child Against Diphtheria, Tetanus, and Pertussis; Immunization Protects Children. American Academy of Pediatrics, Division of Publications, 141 Northwest Point Blvd, PO Box 927, Elk Grove Village, IL 60009-0927; (800)433-9016. Internet address: http://www.aap.org

Parents Guide to Childhoood Immunization, #00-590. US Department of Health and Human Services. This material is available from the National Immunization Program, MS E-34, Centers for Disease Control and Prevention, 1600 Clifton Rd NE, Atlanta, GA 30333; (404)639-8225. Fax (404)629-8828.

Provider Resources

Diphtheria, Tetanus, and Pertussis: Recommendations for Vaccine Use and Other Preventive Measures, #I1413; *Recommended Childhood Immunization Schedule,* #I1743; *Six Common Misconceptions about Vaccination and How to Respond to Them,* #00-6561; *Guide to Contraindications in Childhood Vaccines,* #00-6562. These documents are available from the National Immunization Program, MS E-34, Centers for Disease Control and Prevention, 1600 Clifton Rd NE, Atlanta, GA 30333; (404)639-8225. Fax (404)639-8828.

Immunization Protects Children. American Academy of Pediatrics, Division of Publications, 141 Northwest Point Blvd, PO Box 927, Elk Grove Village, IL 60009-0927; (800)433-9016. Internet address: http://www.aap.org

Immunization Action Coalition. Internet address: http://www.immunize.org

Selected References

American Academy of Family Physicians. *Summary of Policy Recommendations for Periodic Health Examination.* Kansas City, Mo: American Academy of Family Physicians; 1997.

American Academy of Pediatrics, Committee on Infectious Diseases. Acellular pertussis vaccine: Recommendations for use as the fourth and fifth doses. *Pediatrics.* 1992;90:121-123.

American Academy of Pediatrics, Committee on Infectious Diseases. Acellular Pertussis Vaccine: Recommendations for use as the initial series in infants and children. *Pediatrics.* 1997;98(2):282-288.

American Academy of Pediatrics, Committee on Infectious Diseases. Haemophilus influenzae type b conjugate vaccines: Recommendations for immunization with recently and previously licensed vaccines. *AAP News.* 1993;9:17-19.

American Academy of Pediatrics, Committee on Infectious Disease. *1991 Report.* Elk Grove Village, Ill: American Academy of Pediatrics; 1991.

Canadian Task Force on the Periodic Health Examination. Childhood immunizations. In: *The Canadian Guide to Clinical Preventive Health Care.* Ottawa, Canada: Minister of Supply and Services; 1994: chap 24.

Centers for Disease Control and Prevention. FDA approval of use of a new Haemophilus b conjugate vaccine and a combined diphtheria-tetanus-pertussis and Haemophilus b conjugate vaccine for infants and children. *MMWR*. 1993;42:296-298.

Centers for Disease Control and Prevention. Recommended childhood immunization schedule—United States, 1997. *MMWR*. 1997;46:35-40.

Centers for Disease Control. Summary of notifiable diseases, United States, 1989. *MMWR*. 1990;38:51-59.

Centers for Disease Control and Prevention. Pertussis vaccination: use of acellular pertussis vaccines among infants and young children—recommendations of the Advisory Committee on Immunization Practices (ACIP). *MMWR*. 1997;46(No.RR-7):1-25.

Centers for Disease Control and Prevention. CDC Surveillance Summaries, February 21, 1997. *MMWR*. 1997;46(No.SS-2).

Centers for Disease Control. Vaccine Adverse Event Reporting System—United States. *MMWR*. 1990;39:730-733.

Edwards KM, Karzon DT. Pertussis vaccines. *Pediatr Clin North Am*. 1990;37:549-563.

Farizo KM, Cochi SL, Zell ER, Brink EW, Wassilak SG, Patriarca PA. Epidemiological features of pertussis in the United States, 1980-89. *Clin Infect Dis*. 1992;14:708-719.

Gergen PJ, McQuillan GM, Kiely M, Ezzati-Rice TM, Sutter RW, Virella G. A population-based serologic survey of immunity to tetanus in the United States. *N Engl J Med*. 1995; 332:761-766.

Isselbacher KJ, Braunwald E, Wilson JD, et al. *Harrison's Principles of Internal Medicine, Companion Handbook*. 13th ed. New York: MacGraw-Hill, 1995.

McAuliffe JSM, Wadland WC. Pertussis vaccination. *Am Fam Physician*. 1988;37(3):231-235.

National Vaccine Advisory Committee. *Standards for Pediatric Immunization Practices*. Atlanta, Ga: Centers for Disease Control and Prevention; 1993.

Patel R, Kinsinger L. Childhood immunizations: American College of Preventive Medicine Practice Policy Statement. *Am J Prev Med*. 1997;13(2):74-77.

US Preventive Services Task Force. Childhood immunizations. In: *Guide to Clinical Preventive Services*. 2nd ed. Washington, DC: US Department of Health and Human Services; 1996: chap 65.

13

HAEMOPHILUS INFLUENZAE **TYPE B**

Before the introduction of *Haemophilus influenzae* type b (Hib) conjugate vaccines, Hib was the leading cause of bacterial meningitis in children younger than age 5 years and one of the leading causes of invasive bacterial disease (such as pneumonia, epiglottitis, septic arthritis, and cellulitis) in this age group. Even with the use of antibiotics, mortality from meningitis was approximately 5%. Among meningitis survivors, 15% to 30% had permanent neurologic sequelae. The peak incidence of Hib invasive disease occurred in children aged 6 to 12 months; 75% of all illness occurred in children younger than 24 months of age.

Risk factors for Hib invasive disease included attendance at day care centers, exposure to a family member of elementary school age, asplenia, sickle cell disease, and antibody-deficiency syndromes. In 1990, Hib conjugate vaccines were introduced and recommended as a primary series in infants. These vaccines have high efficacy (over 90%) for preventing Hib invasive disease, and since their introduction, a significant decline in the incidence of invasive disease has been documented. The efficacy of Hib vaccination in older children with chronic conditions associated with increased risk of Hib disease has not been studied. Studies suggest, however, good immunogenicity in patients with sickle cell disease, leukemia, splenectomy, and HIV infection.

Under certain circumstances, rifampin is used prophylactically to prevent the transmission of Hib (See Recommendations of Major Authorities). Rifampin prophylaxis eradicates Hib carriage in at least 95% of the contacts of persons with primary disease and reduces the risk of secondary invasive disease in exposed household contacts. The efficacy of rifampin prophylaxis in day care settings is not well defined.

H. influenzae type b (invasive disease only) is currently designated as an infectious disease notifiable at the national level. Refer to Appendix C for further information on nationally notifiable diseases.

Recommendations of Major Authorities

Immunization

Advisory Committee on Immunization Practices, American Academy of Family Physicians, American Academy of Pediatrics, American College of Preventive Medicine, Bright Futures, and **US Preventive Services Task Force**—All children should receive a primary series of one of the conjugate vaccines licensed for infant use beginning at 2 months of age. See below for details and schedule.

Canadian Task Force on the Periodic Health Examination—Recommends immunization with Hib conjugate vaccine at 2, 4, 6, and 18 months of age.

Prophylaxis

Advisory Committee on Immunization Practices and **American Academy of Pediatrics**—Rifampin prophylaxis is indicated for all household contacts of a person with Hib invasive disease if the household contains at least one child younger than 12 months old (regardless of immunization status). Prophylaxis is also indicated for all household contacts of a person with Hib invasive disease if the household contains children younger than 4 years of age who are not fully vaccinated against Hib disease. A household contact is defined as an individual residing with the patient, or a nonresident who spent 4 hours or more with the patient for at least 5 of the 7 days preceding the day of hospital admission of the patient. A child is considered fully immunized following (a) at least one dose of conjugate vaccine at 15 months of age or older, or (b) two doses of conjugate vaccine at 12 to 14 months of age, or (c) two or more doses of conjugate vaccine at less than 12 months of age, followed by a booster dose at 12 months of age or later.

Basics of *H. influenzae* Type b Immunization

1. Vaccine Types

Conjugate Vaccines

Four types of conjugate vaccines currently are licensed for use in the United States: HbOC (HibTITER®, Lederle-Praxis), PRP-OMP (PedvaxHIB®, Merck, Inc.), PRP-D (ProHIBIT®, Connaught Laboratories), and PRP-T (ActHIB®, Connaught Laboratories and OmniHIB®, Smith Kline Beecham). PRP-D is not licensed for use in primary immunization of children younger than 15 months of age; it may, however, be used as a booster dose beginning at 12 months of age. Ideally, use the same type of conjugate vaccine throughout the entire primary vaccination series. To facilitate this, note the vaccine type on the parent-held record and in the patient chart. If the type of vaccine used for previous immunization is not known, ensure that the 2- to 6-month-old patient receives a total of at least three doses of conjugate vaccine. Any type of conjugate Hib vaccine can be used for booster doses.

Combined Vaccines

A combined whole-cell DTP and Hib (HbOC) vaccine (TETRAMUNE®, Lederle-Praxis) is licensed for use in children aged 2 months to 5 years when indications for vaccination with DTP vaccine and Hib conjugate vaccine coincide.

The Food and Drug Administration has approved reconstituting the following *H. influenzae* type b conjugate vaccines: ActHIB® (Connaught Laboratories) or OmniHIB® (Smith Kline Beecham) with DTP vaccine (Connaught Laboratories) for use in the first four doses of the DTP series. Similarly, DTaP (Tripedia®, Connaught Laboratories) can be combined with either ActHIB® or OmniHIB® for the fourth dose in children who previously received three doses of DTP and three doses of Hib vaccine.

When both Hib and Hepatitis B vaccines are indicated, Comvax™ (Merck, Inc.), composed of the antigenic components used in PedvaxHIB® (Merck, Inc.), and RECOMBIVAX HB® (Merck, Inc.) can be used.

2. Schedule

The Advisory Committee on Immunization Practices, the American Academy of Pediatrics, and the American Academy of Family Physicians currently recommend the following schedule for *H. influenzae* type b (Hib) vaccination:

Table 13.1 Immunization Schedule for *Haemophilus influenzae* Type b (Hib)

Dose	Age	Notes
1*	2 months	If HbOC or PRP-T is used, the primary series consists of three vaccinations given at 2, 4, and 6 months of age with a booster vaccination given at 12-15 months.
		If PRP-OMP is used, the primary series consists of two vaccinations given at 2 and 4 months with a booster vaccination given at 12-15 months.
2	4 months	
3	6 months	
4	12-15 months	

*First vaccination may be given as early as 6 weeks of age.

3. Dose and Administration

The recommended dose of Hib vaccines (including DTP-HbOC) is 0.5 mL, given intramuscularly.

For infants younger than 12 months of age, the preferred site is the anterolateral thigh (although the deltoid may be used if necessary). Bunch the thigh muscle, using the free hand, and direct the needle (22- to 25-gauge, 7/8" to 1" in length) inferiorly at an angle to reach the muscle but avoid contact with neurovascular structures or bone.

For toddlers and older children, vaccination may be given in the deltoid (if muscle mass appears adequate), using a 22- to 25-gauge needle that is 5/8" to 1-1/4" in length.

NOTE: Hib vaccines and Hib combination vaccines may be given simultaneously with other childhood vaccinations but must be administered at different sites.

4. Contraindications/Precautions

There are few, true contraindications to administering vaccinations. See Appendix B, Table B.3 for a listing of valid contraindicaitons.

There are no known specific contraindications to Hib vaccination. Use in pregnant women is not recommended.

5. Adverse Reactions

The side effects of Hib vaccination are minor and are limited to mild fever and redness and/or swelling at the injection site.

All adverse side effects should be reported to the Vaccine Adverse Event Reporting System (VAERS). Refer to Table B.4 for a detailed listing of adverse events. VAERS forms and instructions are available in the FDA Drug Bulletin (Food and Drug Administration) and the Physician's Desk Reference or by calling the 24-hour VAERS information recording, (800)822-7967. Refer to Appendix B for details.

6. Special Cases

If the first vaccination is delayed beyond 6 months of age, the schedule for vaccination of previously unimmunized children should be followed (Table 13.2).

Hib vaccination is not recommended for healthy persons over the age of 5 years. However, one dose of Hib conjugate vaccine can be considered in persons older than 5 years who are vulnerable to Hib invasive disease (eg, persons with asplenia, sickle cell anemia, HIV infection, and leukemia).

Table 13.2. Schedule for Hib Conjugate Vaccine Administration Among Previously Unimmunized Children

Vaccine	Age at first vaccination (Months)	Primary series	Booster
HbOC/PRP-T	2-6	3 doses, 2 mos apart	12-15 mos
	7-11	2 doses, 2 mos apart	12-18 mos
	12-14	1 dose	2 mos later
	15-59	1 dose	not applicable
PRP-OMP	2-6	2 doses, 2 mos apart	12-15 mos
	7-11	2 doses, 2 mos apart	12-18 mos
	12-14	1 dose	2 mos later
	15-59	1 dose	not applicable
PRP-D	15-59	1 dose	not applicable

Source: Centers for Disease Control and Prevention. Recommendations for use of Haemophilus b conjugate vaccines and a combined diphtheria, tetanus, pertussis and Haemophilus b vaccine: Recommendation of the Advisory Committee on Immunization Practices (ACIP). MMWR. 1993;42(RR-13):1-15.

7. Patient Education

The US Department of Health and Human Services has developed vaccine information statements about *H. influenza* type b vaccination (see Patient Resources). Copies of these statements must be available to patients in facilities where federally purchased vaccines are used, and their availability in other settings is encouraged.

8. Vaccine Storage and Handling

Store vaccine at 2° to 8°C (36° to 46°F); do not freeze. Do not use vaccine that has been frozen. Handle all vaccine preparations according to manufacturers' instructions.

Basics of Rifampin Prophylaxis

1. Schedule

Begin rifampin prophylaxis as soon as possible, because most cases of secondary disease occur within the first week after occurrence of the index case. The efficacy of chemoprophylaxis is questionable if it is given 2 weeks after occurrence of the index case.

2. Dosage and Administration

The recommended prophylactic dosage of rifampin is 20 mg/kg (maximum, 600 mg), given orally once daily for 4 days. The recommended dosage for infants younger than age 1 month is 10 mg/kg. If a child is unable to swallow capsules, prescribe a rifampin suspension or rifampin powder, which may be mixed with several teaspoons of applesauce.

3. Contraindications

Do not administer rifampin to pregnant women; consult an infectious disease specialist for alternative therapies.

4. Adverse Reactions

Side effects of rifampin chemoprophylaxis include orange discoloration of urine and other bodily fluids, discoloration of soft contact lenses, decreased effectiveness of oral contraceptives, nausea, vomiting, diarrhea, headache, and dizziness.

All adverse side effects should be reported to the Vaccine Adverse Event Reporting System (VAERS). Refer to Table B.4 for a detailed listing of adverse events. VAERS forms and instructions are available in the FDA Drug Bulletin (Food and Drug Administration) and the Physician's Desk Reference or by calling the 24-hour VAERS information recording, (800)822-7967. Refer to Appendix B for details.

Patient Resources

Childhood Vaccines: What They Are and Why Your Child Needs Them. American Academy of Family Physicians, 8880 Ward Parkway, Kansas City, MO 64114-2797; (800)944-0000. Internet address: http://www.aafp.org

Vaccine Information Statement—*Haemophilus Influenzae Type B: What You Need to Know Before Your Child Gets the Vaccine,* #I1905. US Department of Health and Human Services. This material is available from the National Immunization Program, Information/Distribution Center, M/S E-34, Centers for Disease Control and Prevention, 1600 Clifton Rd, NE, Atlanta, GA 30333; (404)639-8225. Fax (404)639-8828; state and local health departments; and the American Academy of Pediatrics, Division of Publications, PO Box 927, Elk Grove Village, IL 60009-0927; (800)433-9016. Internet address: http://www.aap.org

Immunization Action Coalition. Internet address: http://www.immunize.org

Immunization Protects Children. American Academy of Pediatrics, Division of Publications, PO Box 927, Elk Grove Village, IL 60009-0927; (800)433-9016. Internet address: http://www.aap.org

Parents Guide to Childhood Immunizations, #00-590. US Department of Health and Human Services. This material is available from the National Immunization Program, M/S E-34, Centers for Disease Control and Prevention, 1600 Clifton Rd, NE, Atlanta, GA 30333; (404)639-8225; fax (404)639-8828.

Provider Resources

Recommended Childhood Immunization Schedule, #I1743; *Six Common Misconceptions about Vaccination and How to Respond to Them,* #00-6561; *Guide to Contraindications in Childhood Vaccine,* #00-6562; *Recommendations for Use of Haemophilus B Conjugate Vaccines and a Combined Diphtheria, Tetanus, Pertussis and Haemophilus B Vaccine,* #I1706; *Haemophilus b Conjugate Vaccines for Prevention of Haemophilus Influenzae Type B Disease among Infants and Children Two Months of Age and Older,* #I1417. These documents are available from the National Immunization Program, M/S E-34, Centers for Disease Control and Prevention, 1600 Clifton Road, NE, Atlanta, GA 30333; (404)639-8225, fax (404)639-8828.

Selected References

American Academy of Family Physicians, Commission on Public Health and Scientific Affairs. AAFP recommendations: new Haemophilus influenzae type b immunization schedule. *Am Fam Physician.* 1991;43(4):1473-1474.

Adams WG, Deaver KA, Cochi SL, et al. Decline of childhood Haemophilus influenzae type b (Hib) disease in the Hib vaccine era. *JAMA.* 1993;269:221-226.

American Academy of Pediatrics, Committee on Infectious Diseases. Haemophilus influenzae type b conjugate vaccines: recommendations for immunization with recently and previously licensed vaccines. *AAP News.* 1993;9:17-19.

American Academy of Pediatrics, Committee on Infectious Diseases. *1994 Red Book: Report of the Committee on Infectious Diseases.* Elk Grove Village, Ill: American Academy of Pediatrics; 1994;203-216.

Canadian Task Force on the Periodic Health Examination. Childhood immunizations. In: *The Canadian Guide to Clinical Preventive Health Care.* Ottawa, Canada: Minister of Supply and Services; 1994: chap 33.

Centers for Disease Control and Prevention. FDA approval of use of a new Haemophilus b conjugate vaccine and a combined diphtheria-tetanus-pertussis and Haemophilus b conjugate vaccine for infants and children. *MMWR.* 1993;42:296-298.

Centers for Disease Control. Haemophilus b conjugate vaccines for prevention of Haemophilus influenzae type b disease among infants and children two months of age and older: recommendations of the Advisory Committee on Immunization Practices (ACIP). *MMWR.* 1991;40(RR-1):1-6.

Centers for Disease Control and Prevention. Recommended childhood immunization schedule—United States, 1997. *MMWR.* 1997;46:35-40.

Centers for Disease Control and Prevention. Recommendations for use of Haemophilus b conjugate vaccines and a combined diphtheria, tetanus, pertussis and Haemophilus b vaccine: recommendations of the Advisory Committee on Immunization Practices (ACIP). *MMWR.* 1993;42(RR-13):1-15.

Patel R, Kinsinger L. Childhood immunizations: American College of Preventive Medicine Practice Policy Statement. *Am J Prev Med.* 1997;13(2):74-77.

Pomeroy SL, Holmes SJ, Dodge PR, Feigin RD. Seizures and other neurologic sequelae of bacterial meningitis in children. *N Engl J Med.* 1990;323:1651-1657.

Wilfert CM. Epidemiology of Haemophilus influenzae type b infections. *Pediatrics.* 1990;85(suppl 4):631-635.

US Preventive Services Task Force. Childhood immunizations. In: *Guide to Clinical Preventive Services.* (2nd ed). Washington, DC: US Department of Health and Human Services; 1996: chap 65.

14

HEPATITIS B

Infection with hepatitis B virus (HBV) is a major health problem in the United States. About 200,000 new cases are reported annually. Every year, approximately 4000 to 5000 people die of chronic liver disease caused by HBV infection, and persons with chronic infection are also at increased risk of death from hepatocellular cancer. See Table 14.1 for a list of groups at high risk for HBV infection.

In the United States, most HBV infections are acquired during adolescence or adulthood, largely as a result of sexual contact, injection drug use, or occupational/household contact. Rates of infection are also high in certain populations, including Alaska Natives, Pacific Islanders, and immigrants from HBV-endemic areas (particularly East Asia and Africa). Efforts to control HBV infection through vaccination and education of high-risk individuals, testing of pregnant women, and vaccination of the offspring of carrier women have been only partially successful. Children of HBV-infected mothers are at high risk for developing infection during the perinatal period and the first 5 years of life. Perinatal infection leads to a 90% risk of chronic infection and a 25% risk of death from chronic liver disease as an adult. Vaccination later in life (ie, adolescence) misses this vulnerable population and requires the use of more vaccine with a subsequent higher cost per dose.

Vaccination is highly effective (up to 95%) in preventing HBV infection in susceptible patients. Because hepatitis B vaccine was developed relatively recently, its length of effectiveness is unknown; it is thought to be 10 years, but much longer-lasting immunity is likely. The combination of hepatitis B vaccination and hepatitis B immune globulin (HBIG) is 80% to 95% effective for preventing perinatal HBV infection after acute exposure.

See chapter 48 for information on hepatitis immunization and prophylaxis for adults.

Hepatitis B is currently designated as an infectious disease notifiable at the national level. Refer to Appendix C for further information on nationally notifiable diseases.

Table 14.1. Groups at High Risk for Hepatitis B (HBV) Virus Infection

Heterosexual individuals who have had more than one sex partner in the previous 6 months and/or those with a recent episode of a sexually transmitted disease

Sexually active homosexual or bisexual males

Household contacts and sex partners of hepatitis B surface antigen (HBsAg)-positive persons

Injection drug users

Health care workers and others at occupational risk

Clients and staff of institutions for the developmentally disabled, including nonresidential day-care programs if attended by known HBV carriers

Hemodialysis patients

Hemophiliacs and other recipients of certain blood products

Household contacts of adoptees from HBV-endemic, high-risk countries who are HBsAg-positive

International travelers who spend more than 6 months in areas with high HBV infection rates and who have close contact with the local population; also short-term travelers who have contact with blood or sexual contact with residents in high- or intermediate-risk areas

Inmates of long-term correctional institutions

Adapted from: Advisory Committee on Immunization Practices (ACIP). Hepatitis B virus: a comprehensive strategy for eliminating transmission in the United States through universal childhood vaccination. MMWR. 1991;40(No. RR-13):1-25.

Recommendations of Major Authorities

Immunization

All major authorities, including **Advisory Committee on Immunization Practices, American Academy of Family Physicians (AAFP), American Academy of Pediatrics, American College of Preventive Medicine, American Medical Association, Canadian Task Force on the Periodic Health Examination (CTFPHE),** and **US Preventive Services Task Force**—All children should receive a complete series of hepatitis B immunizations during the first 18 months of life. Infants born to hepatitis B suface antigen (HBsAg) positive mothers should begin receiving these immunizations at birth. All adolescents should also be fully immunized. In addition, all major authorities recommend immunization of adolescents and young adults not previously immunized, particularly those at increased risk of infection. **AAFP** recommends offering immunization to persons aged 12 to 24 years. According to the **CTFPHE**, the optimal dose schedules and target populations for universal childhood immunization have not yet been determined, and vaccination of high-risk groups should continue to receive high priority. See below for details of schedule.

Prophylaxis

All major authorities—HBIG should be used as prophylaxis for nonimmunized or inadequately immunized individuals exposed to active hepatitis B infection. Prophylactic treatment may be needed in the following situations: percutaneous or mucosal exposure to HBsAg-positive blood, sexual exposure to a hepatitis B surface antigen (HBsAg) positive person, perinatal exposure of an infant to an HBsAg-positive mother, or household exposure of an infant younger than 12 months of age to a primary care-giver who has acute HBV infection. The **CTFPHE** indicates the prophylactic use of HBIG only in situations where there is perinatal exposure of an infant to an HBsAg positive mother.

Basics of Hepatitis B Immunization

1. Vaccine Types

Two licensed hepatitis B vaccines currently are produced in the United States: Engerix-B® and Recombivax HB® (available in three preparations for different age groups). Both vaccines are produced by recombinant DNA technology, and they may be used interchangeably at any point in the vaccination schedule, although the dosage may vary. A plasma-derived vaccine (Heptavax™) is also licensed, but it is no longer produced in the United States.

2. Schedule

According to the Advisory Committee on Immunization Practices, the schedule for administering hepatitis B vaccine to infants of hepatitis B surface antigen (HBsAg) negative mothers should be flexible and integrated into the routine childhood immunization schedule. Administer the first dose between birth and 2 months of age. Give the second dose between 1 and 4 months of age and at least 1 month after delivery of the first dose. Give the third dose between 6 and 18 months of age, with a minimum of 4 months between the second and third doses. Because of possible decreased seroconversion rates, premature infants of HBsAg-negative mothers with birth weights less than 2000 g should receive the first dose at the time of hospital discharge if the infant then weighs at least 2000 g, or when routine childhood immunizations are initiated at 2 months of age.

For infants (even if premature) born to HBsAg-positive mothers, initiate immunization within 12 hours of birth. Give subsequent doses at 1 and 6 months of age. A four-dose schedule (at birth, 1, 2, and 12 months) for post-exposure immunization has been licensed by Engerix-B®. This schedule may slightly increase the likelihood of development of immunity, but it has not been demonstrated to offer clinical advantage over the three-dose regimens. For information on perinatal prophylaxis see Table 14.3. For information on immunization for postexposure prophylaxis, see Table 48.2.

Adolescents not immunized as infants should receive a complete series of three immunizations by 11 to 12 years of age, with the second and third doses administered at least 1 and 4 months, respectively, after the first dose.

Long-term studies of healthy adults and children indicate that immunologic memory remains intact for at least 10 years, although antibody levels may become low or undetectable. Therefore, booster doses of vaccine are not recommended for children and adults whose immune status is normal, and serologic testing to assess antibody levels is not necessary. The possible need for booster doses will be assessed as additional information becomes available.

3. Dose and Administration

The recommended dose of hepatitis B vaccine varies according to the vaccine type and the age of the child (Table 14.2). Administer the vaccine as an intramuscular injection. In infants younger than 12 months of age, the preferred site is the anterolateral thigh (although, if necessary, the deltoid may be used). Bunch the thigh muscle, using the free hand, and direct the needle (22- to 25-gauge, 7/8" to 1" in length) inferiorly at an angle to reach the muscle but avoid contact with neurovascular structures or bone. In toddlers and older children, the vaccination may be given in the deltoid (if muscle mass appears adequate), using a 22- to 25-gauge needle that is 5/8" to 1-1/4" in length. Hepatitis B vaccines may be given simultaneously with other childhood vaccinations but at different sites.

4. Contraindications/Precautions

There are few, true contraindications to administering vaccinations. See Appendix B, Table B.3 for a listing of valid contraindications.

A history of an anaphylactic reaction to common baker's yeast is a specific contraindication to hepatitis B vaccination. The only other contraindication is a known serious adverse reaction to the vaccine. Pregnancy and lactation are not contraindications.

Table 14.2. Recommended Doses for Children of Currently Licensed Recombinant Hepatitis B Vaccines

Group	Vaccines			
	Recombivax HB®		Engerix-B®	
	µg	mL	µg	mL
Infants of HBsAg-negative mothers and children <11 years of age	2.5	0.25	10	0.5
Infants of HBsAg-positive mothers; prevention of perinatal infection	5	0.5	10	0.5
Children and adolescents 11-19 years of age	5	0.5	20	1.0

Adapted from: Advisory Committee on Immunization Practices (ACIP). Hepatitis B virus: a comprehensive strategy for eliminating transmission in the United States through universal childhood vaccination. MMWR. 1991;40(No. RR-13):1-25.

5. Adverse Reactions

The side effects of hepatitis B vaccination are relatively minor in children. These include pain at the injection site (3% to 29%) and temperature higher than 38°C (100.4°F) (0.5% in infants and 1% to 6% in other children). Based on surveillance for adverse reactions in adults in the United States, a possible association between Guillain-Barré syndrome (GBS) and receipt of plasma-derived hepatitis B vaccine has been suggested; however, available data do not indicate an association between receipt of recombinant hepatitis B vaccine and GBS. Although systematic surveillance for adverse events following administration of recombinant hepatitis B vaccine to infants and children has been limited, no association has been found between vaccination and the occurrence of severe adverse events, including seizures and GBS.

Any adverse side effects should be reported to the Vaccine Adverse Event Reporting System (VAERS). Refer to Table B.4 for a detailed listing of adverse events. VAERS forms and instructions are available in the FDA Drug Bulletin (Food and Drug Administration) and the Physician's Desk Reference or by calling the 24-hour VAERS information recording at (800)822-7967. Refer to Appendix B for details.

6. Patient Education

The US Department of Health and Human Services has developed vaccine information statements about hepatitis B vaccination (see Patient Resources). These statements must be available to patients in facilities where federally purchased vaccines are used, and their availability in other settings is encouraged.

7. Vaccine Storage and Handling

Store vaccine at 2° to 8°C (36° to 46°F). Do not freeze. Do not use vaccine that has been frozen. Handle all vaccine preparations according to manufacturers' instructions.

Basics of Postexposure Prophylaxis

1. Schedule

See Table 14.3 for the recommended schedule of HBV immunoprophylaxis to prevent perinatal transmission. See Table 48.2 for the recommended schedule

---

Table 14.3. Recommended Schedule of Hepatitis B Immunoprophylaxis to Prevent Perinatal Transmissizon

---

Infant Born to Mother Known to be HBsAg[1] Positive

Intervention	Age of Infant
First hepatitis B	Birth (within 12 hours)
HBIG[2]	Birth (within 12 hours)
Second hepatitis B	1 month
Third hepatitis B	6 months

Infant Born to Mother Not Screened for HBsAg

Intervention	Age of Infant
First hepatitis B[3]	Birth (within 12 hours)
HBIG	If mother is found to be HBsAg-positive, administer a dose to infant as soon as possible, but not later than 1 week after birth
Second hepatitis B[4]	1-2 months[5]
Third hepatitis B[4]	6 months

---

[1] Hepatitis B surface antigen   [2] Hepatitis B immune globulin

[3] Give same dose as for infants born to HBsAg-positive mothers.

[4] Give additional doses based on mother's HBsAg status (see Table 14.2).

[5] Infants of women who are HBsAg-positive and who have not received HBIG should be vaccinated at 1 month of age; infants of women who are HBsAg-negative may be vaccinated at 2 months of age.

Adapted from: Advisory Committee on Immunization Practices (ACIP). Hepatitis B virus: a comprehensive strategy for eliminating transmission in the United States through universal childhood vaccination. MMWR. 1991;40(No. RR-13);1-25.

of HBV immunoprophylaxis for percutaneous and mucosal exposure in children and adults.

2. Dose and Administration

The recommended dose of HBIG for infants 12 months of age or younger is 0.5 mL. The dose for children older than 12 months of age is 0.06 mL/kg. Administer HBIG as an intramuscular injection. The recommended site is the anterolateral thigh muscle for infants and the deltoid muscle for children and adolescents. HBIG may be given at the same time as hepatitis B vaccine but must be given at a different site. The recommended dose of hepatitis B vaccine for perinatal exposure varies according to vaccine type (Table 14.2).

3. Contraindications/Precautions

The only contraindication to HBIG injection is a history of hypersensitivity to HBIG.

4. Adverse Reactions

The main side effects of HBIG are pain and swelling at the injection site. Urticaria, angioedema, and, very rarely, anaphylaxis can occur. HIV is not known to be transmitted by HBIG injection.

Patient Resources

Childhood Vaccines: What They Are and Why Your Child Needs Them. American Academy of Family Physicians, 8880 Ward Parkway, Kansas City, MO 64114-2797; (800)944-0000.

Vaccine Information Statement—*Hepatitis B Vaccine & Hepatitis B Immune Globulin: What you need to know before you or your child gets the vaccine,* #I1906. US Department of Health and Human Services. This material is available from the National Immunization Program, M/S E-34, Centers for Disease Control and Prevention, 1600 Clifton Rd NE, Atlanta, GA 30333, (404)639-8225, fax (404)639-8828; state and local health departments; and the American Academy of Pediatrics, Division of Publications, PO Box 927, Elk Grove Village, IL 60009-0927; (800)433-9016. Internet address: http://www.aap.org

Your Baby: Protecting Your Baby Against Hepatitis B (videotape), #00-6320; *Protect Your Baby With Hepatitis B Shots,* #00-6550; *Why Does My Baby Need Hepatitis B Vaccine?,* #00-6230; *Parents Guide to Childhood Immunizations,* #00-590. US Department of Health and Human Services. These and other materials are available from the National Immunization Program, M/S E-34, Centers for Disease Control and Prevention, 1600 Clifton Rd NE, Atlanta, GA 30333; (404)639-8225. fax (404)639-8828.

Provider Resources

Recommended childhood immunization schedule, #I1743; Six common misconceptions about vaccination and how to respond to them, #00-6561; Guide to contraindications in childhood vaccines, #00-6562; Hepatitis B Virus Infection—From Mother to Child: A Cycle of Tragedy (videotape), #99-4149. These documents are available from the National Immunization Program, M/S E-34, Centers for Disease Control and Prevention, 1600 Clifton Rd NE, Atlanta, GA 30333; (404)639-8225. fax (404)639-8828.

Selected References

Centers for Disease Control and Prevention. Recommended childhood immunization schedule—United States, 1997. *MMWR.* 1997;46:35-40.

Centers for Disease Control. Hepatitis B virus: a comprehensive strategy for eliminating transmission in the United States through universal childhood vaccination: recommendations of the Advisory Committee on Immunization Practices (ACIP). *MMWR.* 1991;40(No. RR-13):1-25.

Centers for Disease Control. Protection against viral hepatitis: recommendatoins of the Advisory Committee on Immunization Practices. *MMWR.* 1990;39(No. RR-2):1-26.

American Academy of Pediatrics, Committee on Infectious Diseases. *1994 Red Book: Report of the Committee on Infectious Diseases.* Elk Grove Village, Ill: American Academy of Pediatrics; 1994:224-237.

American Academy of Family Physicians. *Recommendations for Hepatitis B Preexposure Vaccination and Postexposure Prophylaxis.* Kansas City, Mo: American Academy of Family Physicians; 1992.

American Academy of Pediatrics. Universal hepatitis B immunization. *AAP News.* February 1992:13-15, 22.

American Medical Association. Rationale and recommendations: infectious diseases. In: *AMA Guidelines for Adolescent Preventive Services (GAPS): Recommendations and Rationale.* Chicago, Ill: American Medical Association; 1994: chap 15.

Canadian Task Force on the Periodic Health Examination. Hepatitis B immunization in childhood. In: *The Canadian Guide to Clinical Preventive Health Care.* Ottawa, Canada: Minister of Supply and Services; 1994: chap 35.

National Vaccine Advisory Committee. *Standards for Pediatric Immunization Practices.* Atlanta, Ga: Centers for Disease Control and Prevention; 1993.

Patel R, Kinsinger L. Childhood immunizations: American College of Preventive Medicine Practice Policy Statement. *Am J Prev Med.* 1997;13(2):74-77.

US Preventive Services Task Force. Childhood immunizations. In: *Guide to Clinical Preventive Services.* 2nd ed. Washington, DC: US Department of Health and Human Services; 1996: chap 65.

US Preventive Services Task Force. Postexposure prophylaxis for selected infectious diseases. In: *Guide to Clinical Preventive Services.* 2nd ed. Washington, DC: US Department of Health and Human Services; 1996: chap 67.

15

MEASLES, MUMPS, AND RUBELLA

The incidence of measles (rubeola), mumps, and rubella is now at record low levels following outbreaks that occurred in the late 1980s and early 1990s. The predominant cause of these outbreaks was failure to immunize children on time. An outbreak that occurred in the mid 1980s among school- and college-aged students was attributed to lack of vaccination and vaccine failure. Since 1989, administration of a second dose of vaccine has been recommended either in primary, middle, or junior high school to ameliorate the problem of vaccine failure.

Measles outbreaks in the United States principally affect four groups: unvaccinated preschool-aged children, persons opposed to vaccination, unvaccinated young adults, and school-aged children who receive only a single dose of measles-containing vaccine. Genetic studies of measles viruses isolated from outbreak-related cases suggest that importation of measles virus from countries with less developed measles control programs is the source of most and maybe all outbreaks of measles. The annual number of reported cases of measles was 312 in 1993, 963 in 1994, and 309 in 1995, the three lowest annual totals ever. Death, usually caused by pneumonia or encephalitis, occurs in one to two patients per every 1000 reported cases; however, no deaths have been reported since 1992.

In the early 1990s, 4264 mumps cases were reported in the United States; the number of reported cases fell steadily, to a record low of 906 cases in 1995. Orchitis occurs in up to 38% of postpubertal males with mumps. Five of every 1000 reported cases are complicated by encephalitis.

In 1995, 128 cases of rubella were reported; this is the lowest number of cases ever reported. Use of rubella vaccine has led to a significant decrease in the overall incidence of both rubella and congenital rubella syndrome (CRS), which develops in an estimated 85% of infants born to women who acquire rubella during the first trimester of pregnancy. Only six cases of CRS were reported in 1995. The most frequently occurring clinical manifestations of CRS are deafness, low birth weight, hepatomegaly, splenomegaly, ocular lesions, psychomotor retardation, congenital heart disease, and petechiae. Half of noncongenital rubella infections are subclinical, with occasional serious complications such as thrombocytopenia (1 per 3000 cases) and encephalitis (1 per 6000 cases).

See chapter 51 for information about rubella immunization of adults.

Measles, mumps, and rubella are currently designated as infectious diseases notifiable at the national level. Refer to Appendix C for further information on nationally notifiable diseases.

Recommendations of Major Authorities

Normal-Risk Children

All major authorities, including **Advisory Committee on Immunization Practices (ACIP), American Academy of Family Physicians (AAFP), American Academy of Pediatrics (AAP), American College of Preventive Medicine, Bright Futures, Canadian Task Force on the Periodic Health Examination (CTFPHE), and US Preventive Services Task Force (USPSTF)**—A primary measles-mumps-rubella (MMR) immunization should be given at 12 to 15 months of age. The **AAFP, AAP, and ACIP** recommend that the booster dose be given either at 4 to 6 years or 11 to 12 years of age, consistent with state school immunization requirements. The **AAFP** recommends increased attention to adolescents and young adults from congregate settings (eg, schools) who might lack a second dose. The **USPSTF** and **CTFPHE** recommend that the booster dose be given at 4 to 6 years of age. The **USPSTF** recommends immunization of older children who present for care so that all children have had two doses of measles or MMR vaccine by age 11 to 12 years. The **AAP** has recommended that colleges and other institutions require all entering students to have documentation of physician-diagnosed measles, serologic evidence of immunity, birth before 1957, or receipt of two doses of measles-containing vaccines. Students without documentation of any measles vaccination or immunity should receive a dose on entry, followed by a repeat dose 1 or more months later.

High-Risk Children

Advisory Committee on Immunization Practices and **American Academy of Pediatrics**—Although MMR is recommended routinely at 12 to 15 months of age, the first vaccination should be given at 12 months of age in areas at high risk for recurrent measles transmission. A high-risk area is: a county with more than five cases among preschool-aged children during each of the last 5 years; a county with a recent outbreak among nonimmunized preschool-aged children; or a county with a large inner-city population. In order to control outbreaks of measles among preschool-aged children, the first immunization (either as monovalent measles vaccine or MMR) may be given as early as 6 months of age if cases are occurring in children younger than 1 year of age. Children immunized before 12 months of age should be revaccinated at 12 to 15 months of age and at 4 to 6 years or 11 to 12 years of age, according to state school immunization requirements.

Postexposure

Advisory Committee on Immunization Practices (ACIP) and **American Academy of Pediatrics**—Exposure to measles is not a contraindication to vaccination. If live measles vaccine is given within 72 hours of measles exposure, it may provide some protection. **ACIP** states that use of vaccine is preferable to the use of immunoglobulin (IG) for children 12 months of age or older. The use of IG within 6 days of exposure can prevent or modify measles in susceptible individuals. IG may be particularly indicated for susceptible household contacts of measles patients, particularly contacts younger than 1 year of age, pregnant women, or immunocompromised individuals.

Basics of Measles, Mumps, and Rubella Immunization

1. Vaccine Types

Measles, mumps, and rubella are live attenuated virus vaccines. They are available as single-antigen preparations and as combination preparations: measles-rubella, mumps-rubella, and measles-mumps-rubella (MMR). Unless a specific antigen is contraindicated, use MMR.

2. Schedule

Give primary immunization at 12 to 15 months of age. Some high-risk children may benefit from receiving this immunization earlier. Revaccinate children who received MMR before their first birthdays at 12 to 15 months of age. The Advisory Committee on Immunization Practices, the American Academy of Pediatrics, and the American Academy of Family Physicians recommend giving a second dose either at age 4 to 6 years (before school entry) or at age 11 to 12 years (before middle school or junior high school entry). Administer doses of MMR or other measles-containing vaccines at least 1 month apart. MMR may be given simultaneously with other childhood immunizations.

3. Assessing Immunity

Children and adolescents are considered susceptible to measles unless there is documentation of physician-diagnosed measles, serologic evidence of measles immunity, or documentation of receipt of adequate immunization. Patient or parental reports of measles illness or measles immunization are not adequate documentation.

Children and adolescents are considered susceptible to mumps unless there is documentation of physician-diagnosed mumps, laboratory evidence of immunity, or documentation of immunization with live mumps vaccine on or after the first birthday. Vaccinate children whose immunization status is uncertain. Susceptibility testing of adolescents before vaccination is not necessary.

Children and adolescents are considered susceptible to rubella unless there is documentation of immunity by laboratory testing or documentation of immunization on or after the first birthday. Patient or parental reports or clinician diagnosis are not adequate evidence of immunity. See chapter 51 for more information about indications for rubella immunization in adults.

4. Dose and Administration

The recommended dose of MMR and the single-antigen preparations is 0.5 mL. Give the injection subcutaneously into the thigh in infants and the deltoid area in children, using a 5/8" to 3/4", 23- to 25-gauge needle.

5. Contraindications/Precautions

There are few, true contraindications to administering vaccinations. See Appendix B, Table B.3 for a listing of valid contraindications. See Table 15.1 for a list of contraindications specific to MMR vaccination.

6. Adverse Reactions

The measles component may cause a transient rash in 5% of vaccinees. Fever higher than 39.4°C (103°F) develops in 5% to 15% of individuals susceptible to measles, beginning 5 to 12 days after immunization and usually lasting 1 to 2 days, but can persist for up to 5 days. Because of the late onset of fever, acetaminophen prophylaxis may not be practical in preventing febrile seizures.

The rubella component is associated with development of a mild rash lasting 1 to 2 days and mild pain and stiffness in the joints 1 to 2 weeks after immunization, usually lasting up to 3 days. Rarely, pain or stiffness can last for months or longer and can recur. Joint swelling (arthritis) lasting a few days to a week develops in 1% of children. Damage to joints is a very rare occurrence.

Both the rubella and mumps components can cause swollen anterior cervical, posterior auricular, or mandibular lymph nodes 1 to 2 weeks after immunization. This happens rarely with the mumps component but may affect one in seven children receiving the rubella component. Development of encephalitis is temporally related to receipt of MMR in about one of every 1 million persons immunized.

Table 15.1. Contraindications and Precautions for MMR Vaccination

True Contraindications and Precautions‡	NOT Contraindications (vaccine may be given)
Anaphylactic reactions to egg ingestion and to neomycin*	Tuberculosis or positive PPD
	Simultaneous TB skin testing†
Pregnancy	Breast feeding
Known altered immune function (hematologic and solid tumors, congenital immunodeficiency, and long-term immunosuppressive therapy)	Pregnancy of mother of recipient
	Immunodeficient family member or household contact
Recent IG administration (within 3-11 months)	
	Infection with HIV
	Nonanaphylactic reactions to eggs or neomycin

*Persons with a history of anaphylactic reactions following egg ingestion should be vaccinated only with caution. Protocols have been developed for vaccinating such persons and should be consulted (Herman et al, 1983; Greenberg and Birx, 1988; Lavi et al, 1990).

†Measles vaccination may temporarily suppress tuberculin reactivity. If testing cannot be done the day of MMR vaccination, the test should be postponed for 4-6 weeks.

‡Precautions should be carefully reviewed. The benefits and risks of administering a specific vaccine to an individual under these circumstances should be considered. If the risks are believed to outweigh the benefits, the immunization should be withheld; if the benefits are believed to outweigh the risks (eg, during an outbreak or foreign travel), it should be given. It is prudent on theoretical grounds to avoid vaccinating pregnant women. (See also MMWR. 1994;43[RR-1]:1-38.)

Adapted from: National Vaccine Advisory Committee. Standards for Pediatric Immunization Practices. Atlanta, Ga: Centers for Disease Control and Prevention; 1993, and CDC General Recommendations on Immunization: Recommendations of the Advisory Committee on Immunization Practices (ACIP). MMWR. 1994:43(RR-1).

Any adverse side effects should be reported to the Vaccine Adverse Event Reporting System (VAERS). Refer to Table B.4 for a detailed listing of adverse events. VAERS forms and instructions are available in the FDA Drug Bulletin (Food and Drug Administration) and the Physician's Desk Reference or by calling the 24-hour VAERS information recording at (800)822-7967. Refer to Appendix B for details.

7. Special cases

Do not administer MMR vaccine to patients who have received high doses of a systemically administered corticosteroid (2 mg/kg or 20 mg per day of prednisone or equivalent) until at least 3 months after discontinuation of the corticosteroid.

Immune globulin-containing preparations, such as immune globulin (IG), tetanus immune globulin (TIG), hepatitis B immune globulin (HBIG), varicella zoster immune globulin (VZIG), rabies immune globulin (HRIG), and packed red blood cells, whole blood, and plasma or platelet products may interfere with the immune response to MMR vaccination. Do not administer MMR vaccine 2 weeks before or until 3 to 11 months after such preparations are given (depending on the immune globulin content). Repeat vaccination after the window of immune globulin interference has expired, or perform antibody testing to determine the patient's immunity status. See Advisory Committee on Immunization Practices (MMWR. 1994;43[RR-1]:1-38) for more detailed information regarding this issue.

8. Patient Education

The National Childhood Vaccine Injury Act requires health care providers to provide the following information to patients prior to administering MMR: (1) a concise description of the benefits of the vaccine, (2) a concise description of the risks associated with the vaccine, and (3) notice of the availability of the National Vaccine Injury Compensation Program.

The US Department of Health and Human Services has developed a pamphlet for this purpose (see Patient Resources). Other patient educational materials may be used if they provide the information required by the National Childhood Vaccine Injury Act. For additional information about this requirement, contact the Training Coordinator, National Immunization Program, Centers for Disease Control and Prevention; (404)639-8226.

9. Vaccine Storage and Handling

Measles, mumps, rubella, and MMR vaccines must be shipped at temperatures lower than 10°C (50°F) and stored at 2° to 8°C (36° to 46°F) or colder and must be protected from light exposure at all times. After vaccine is reconstituted, keep it refrigerated at 2° to 8°C (36° to 46°F), protect it from light, and discard any that is not used within 8 hours. Do not freeze reconstituted vaccine and the diluent. Handle all vaccine preparations according to manufacturers' instructions.

Basics of Postexposure Prophylaxis (Measles)

1. Dose and Administration

The recommended dose of IG for immunocompetent individuals is 0.25 mL/kg of body weight (maximum dose, 15 mL) given intramuscularly. The recommended dose for immunocompromised patients is 0.5 mL/kg of body weight (maximum dose, 15 mL).

Administer IG deep into a large muscle mass such as the anterolateral thigh. If the gluteal region must be used, limit injection to the ventrogluteal site or the upper outer quadrant. Divide large volumes of IG, and administer it in different sites for patient comfort. Administer no more than 5 mL in one site to an adult or large child; give smaller amounts (1 to 3 mL) to smaller children and infants.

2. Precautions

Do not give IG to patients with severe thrombocytopenia or any coagulation disorder that would preclude IM injection. Although such instances are rare, persons with selective serum IgA deficiency can develop anti-IgA antibodies from the receipt of IG and react to a subsequent dose of IG, whole blood, or plasma with systemic symptoms. Use IG with caution in patients with a history of past allergic reactions after injections of IG.

3. Adverse Reactions

Local pain and swelling (often mistaken for an allergic reaction) are the most common adverse effects of IG injection. Urticaria, angioedema, and (rarely) anaphylaxis may occur.

Patient Resources

Childhood Vaccines: What They Are and Why Your Child Needs Them. American Academy of Family Physicians, 8880 Ward Parkway, Kansas City, MO 64114-2797; (800)944-0000. Internet address: http:/www.aafp.org

Vaccine Information Statement—*Measles, Mumps, and Rubella: What You Need to Know Before You or Your Child Gets the Vaccine,* #I1730. US Department of Health and Human Services. This material is available from the National Immunization Program, M/S E-34, Centers for Disease Control and Prevention, 1600 Clifton Rd NE, Atlanta, GA 30333; (404)639-8225; fax (404)639-8828. Other sources include state and local health departments and the American Academy of Pediatrics, Division of Publications, PO Box 927, Elk Grove Village, IL 60009-0927, (800)433-9016; Internet address: http://www.aap.org

Parents Guide to Childhood Immunizations, #00-590. US Department of Health and Human Services. This material is available from the National Immunization Program, M/S E-34, Centers for Disease Control and Prevention, 1600 Clifton Rd NE, Atlanta, GA 30333; (404)639-8225; fax (404)639-8828.

Protecting Your Child Against Diphtheria, Tetanus, and Pertussis; Immunization Protects Children. American Academy of Pediatrics, PO Box 927, Elk Grove Village, IL 60009-0927; (800)433-9016. Internet address: http://www.aap.org

Provider Resources

Immunization Protects Children. American Academy of Pediatrics, Division of Publications, 141 Northwest Point Blvd, PO Box 927, Elk Grove Village, IL 60009-0927; (800)433-9016. Internet address: http:/www.aap.org

Rubella Prevention, #I1428; *Measles Prevention,* #I1418; *Recommended Childhood Immunization Schedule,* #I1743; *Six Common Misconceptions About Vaccination and How to Respond to Them,* #00-6561; *Guide to Contraindications in Childhood Vaccines,* #00-6562. These and other documents are available from the National Immunization Program, M/S E-34, Centers for Disease Control and Prevention, 1600 Clifton Road NE, Atlanta, GA 30333; (404)639-8225. Fax (404)639-8828.

Selected References

American Academy of Family Physicians. *Summary of Policy Recommendations for Periodic Health Examination.* Kansas City, Mo: American Academy of Family Physicians; 1997.

American Academy of Pediatrics, Committee on Infectious Diseases. *1994 Red Book: Report of the Committee on Infectious Diseases.* Elk Grove Village, Ill: American Academy of Pediatrics; 1994:308-322, 329-333, 406-412.

Canadian Task Force on the Periodic Health Examination. Childhood immunizations. In: *The Canadian Guide to Clinical Preventive Health Care.* Ottawa, Canada: Minister of Supply and Services; 1994: chap 33.

Centers for Disease Control and Prevention. General recommendations on immunization: recommendations of the Advisory Committee on Immunization Practices (ACIP). *MMWR.* 1994;43(No. RR-1):1-38.

Centers for Disease Control and Prevention. Recommended childhood immunization schedule—United States, January 1995. *MMWR.* 1995;43:959-960.

Centers for Disease Control. Measles prevention: recommendations of the Advisory Committee on Immunization Practices (ACIP). *MMWR.* 1989;38(No. S-9):1-13.

Centers for Disease Control. Mumps prevention. *MMWR.* 1989;38:388-392.

Centers for Disease Control. Rubella prevention: recommendations of the Advisory Committee on Immunization Practices (ACIP). *MMWR.* 1990;39(No. RR-15):1-13.

Centers for Disease Control. Vaccine Adverse Event Reporting System—United States. *MMWR.* 1990;39:730-733.

Centers for Disease Control and Prevention. Recommended childhood immunization schedule—United States, 1997. *MMWR.* 1997;4635-4640.

Greenberg MA, Birx DL. Safe administration of mumps-measles-rubella vaccine in egg-allergic children. *J Pediatr.* 1988;113:504-506.

Herman JJ, Radin R, Schneiderman R. Allergic reactions to measles (rubeola) vaccine in patients hypersensitive to egg protein. *J Pediatr.* 1983;102:196-199.

Lavi S, Zimmerman B, Koren G, Gold R. Administration of measles, mumps, and rubella vaccine (live) to egg-allergic children. *JAMA.* 1990;263:269-271.

National Vaccine Advisory Committee. *Standards for Pediatric Immunization Practices.* Atlanta, Ga: Centers for Disease Control and Prevention; 1993.

National Vaccine Advisory Committee. The measles epidemic: the problems, barriers and recommendations. *JAMA.* 1991;166(11):1547-52.

Patel R, Kinsinger L. Childhood immunizations: American College of Preventive Medicine Practice Policy Statement. *Am J Prev Med.* 1997;13(2):74-77.

US Preventive Services Task Force. Childhood immunizations. In: *Guide to Clinical Preventive Services.* 2nd ed. Washington, DC: US Department of Health and Human Services; 1996: chap 65.

Watson JC, Pearson JA, Markowitz LE, et al. An evaluation of measles revaccination among school-entry-age children. *Pediatrics.* In press

16

POLIOMYELITIS

In 1994, the Western Hemisphere was certified as being free of indigenous wild-type (not vaccine-related) poliovirus, the enterovirus that causes paralytic poliomyelitis. The last cases of wild, indigenously acquired poliomyelitis in the United States were reported in 1979. The current risk of exposure to wild poliovirus in the United States is very low and continues to diminish as global eradication continues. In comparison, the risk of vaccine-associated poliomyelitis (VAPP) from oral polio vaccine (OPV), for both vaccine recipients and their susceptible contacts, is greater than the risk of paralytic poliomyelitis from wild-type virus. The risk of VAPP is approximately one per 750,000 first doses of OPV administered

Between 1980 and 1994, only six imported cases and two indeterminate cases of polio occurred in the United States, while there were 125 cases of VAPP. Although the successful elimination of indigenous wild-type polio is primarily attributable to the wide use of OPV, these recent changes in the epidemiological patterns of poliomyelitis in the United States prompted a re-examination and subsequent change in many of the recommendations regarding the routine use of OPV and inactive polio vaccine (IPV) beginning in the 1997 calendar year.

Paralytic poliomyelitis is currently designated as an infectious disease notifiable at the national level. Refer to Appendix C for further information on nationally notifiable diseases.

Recommendations of Major Authorities

In 1997, the **Advisory Committee on Immunization Practices (ACIP), American Academy of Family Physicians (AAFP),** and **American Academy of Pediatrics (AAP)** changed their recommendations for routine poliovirus vaccination, and now recommend expanded use of IPV for routine poliovirus vaccination. The **American College of Preventive Medicine** and **Bright Futures** have also adopted these guidelines. The revised recommendations include three acceptable options (sequential IPV-OPV; all IPV; and all OPV), and parents and providers may choose among them. Parents and other care-givers should be informed of the poliovirus vaccines available, alternative immunization schedules, and the basis for poliovirus vaccination recommendations. The benefits and risks of the vaccines and the advantages and disadvantages of the three vaccination options, for individuals and the community, should be discussed.

Sequential: IPV at 2 and 4 months; OPV at 12 to 18 months and 4 to 6 years
All-IPV: IPV at 2, 4, 12 to 18 months, and 4 to 6 years
All-OPV: OPV at 2, 4, 6-18 months, and 4 to 6 years

Advisory Committee on Immunization Practices recommends a sequential IPV-OPV schedule for greatest overall public health benefit by decreasing the incidence of VAPP while maintaining high levels of population immunity to poliovirus to prevent outbreaks should wild poliovirus be reintroduced in the United States.

American Academy of Pediatrics and **American Academy of Family Physicians** recommend parent and provider choice in the selection of the vaccination schedule most suitable for the child.

Canadian Task Force on the Periodic Health Examination recommends either IPV or OPV. The IPV vaccination schedule is at 2, 4, 6 and 18 months and 4 to 6 years. The OPV schedule is at 2, 4, and 18 months and 4 to 6 years.

US Preventive Services Task Force acknowledged the potential benefits of incorporating IPV into the childhood immunization schedule, but has not updated its recommendations since the change in the **ACIP** guidelines.

Basics of Poliomyelitis Immunization

1. Vaccine Types

Two types of trivalent vaccine are available for use in the United States: live oral poliovirus vaccine (OPV) and enhanced-potency inactivated poliovirus vaccine (IPV). Both vaccines contain antigens to poliovirus types I, II, and III and are highly effective. OPV, through its induction of intestinal immunity against poliovirus, is effective in controlling circulation of the wild virus. IPV also induces mucosal immunity, but to a lesser extent.

2. Schedule

a. Primary:

IPV at 2 and 4 months; OPV at 12 to 18 months and 4 to 6 years
OR
IPV at 2, 4, and 12 to 18 months and 4 to 6 years
OR
OPV at 2, 4, and 12 to 18 months and 4 to 6 years

Parents of children who are to be vaccinated should be informed of the poliovirus vaccines available, the three alternative vaccination schedules, and the basis for the vaccination recommendations. The benefits and risks of the vaccines as well as the advantages and disadvantages of the three vaccination options for individuals and for the community should be discussed (Table 16.1).

Table 16.1. Advantages and Disadvantages of Three Poliovirus Vaccination Options

Attribute	OPV	IPV	IPV-OPV
Occurrence of VAPP	8-9 cases/yr	None	2-5 cases/yr*
Other serious adverse events	None known	None known	None known
Systemic Immunity	High	High	High
Immunity of GI mucosa	High	Low	High
Secondary transmission of vaccine virus	Yes	No	Some
Extra injections or visits needed	No	Yes	Yes
Compliance with immunization schedule	High	Possibly reduced	Possibly reduced
Future combination vaccines	Unlikely	Likely	Likely (IPV)
Current cost	Low	Higher	Intermediate

*Estimated

Adapted from: Centers for Disease Control and Prevention. Poliomyelitis prevention in the United States: introduction of a sequential vaccination schedule of inactivated poliovirus vaccine followed by oral poliovirus vaccine: recommendations of the Advisory Committee on Immunization Practices (ACIP). MMWR. 1997;46(No. RR-3):12.

b. Late or Accelerated Schedule for Children:

An all-OPV schedule is preferred for infants and children starting vaccination late (ie, after 6 months of age) or when accelerated protection against poliomyelitis is required. Three doses of OPV constitute a primary series and are required to assure seroconversion to all three serotypes of poliovirus. Under such circumstances, the minimum time interval between doses of OPV is 4 weeks. Administer a supplemental dose of OPV between 4 and 6 years of age. For infants and children for whom IPV is indicated and accelerated protection is needed, the minimum interval between doses of IPV is 4 weeks, although the preferred interval between the second and third dose is six months. Administer an additional dose of IPV between ages 4 and 6 years.

c. Late or Accelerated Schedule for Adults:

Routine poliovirus vaccination of adults (generally those aged 18 years and older) residing in the United States is not necessary. Immunization is recommended for certain adults who are at risk of exposure to poliovirus, including travelers, laboratory and health-care workers, and unvaccinated adults residing in households of children receiving OPV. For unvaccinated adults, primary vaccination with IPV is recommended because the risk for VAPP after receiving OPV is higher among adults than among children. Two doses of IPV should be administered at intervals of 4 to 8 weeks; a third dose should be administered 6 to 12 months after the second. If three doses of IPV cannot be administered within the recommended intervals before protection is needed, the following alternatives are recommended:

If 8 or more weeks are available, three doses of IPV should be administered at least 4 weeks apart.

If less than 8 but more than 4 weeks are available, two doses of IPV should be administered at least 4 weeks apart.

If less than 4 weeks are available, a single dose of OPV or IPV is recommended.

The remaining doses of vaccine should be administered later, at the recommended intervals, if the person remains at increased risk.

Adults who previously completed a primary series of either OPV or IPV who are at increased risk of exposure to poliovirus may be given another dose of either OPV or IPV. These adults are not at increased risk for VAPP.

3. Dose and Administration

OPV is supplied in a disposable pipette containing a single dose of 0.5 mL or in 10-dose vials. The vaccine should be dropped on the back of the tongue. If a substantial amount of OPV is regurgitated or spit out within 5 to 10 minutes of administration, it may be readministered. If the repeat dose is also lost, attempt readministration at the next visit.

The recommended dose of IPV is 0.5 mL, given subcutaneously or intramuscularly in the thigh of infants and in the deltoid area of older children and adults with a 5/8" to 3/4", 23- to 25-gauge needle.

4. Contraindications/Precautions

There are few, true contraindications to administering vaccinations. See Appendix B, Table B.3 for a listing of valid contraindications. See Table 16.2 for a list of contraindications specific to polio immunization.

Because of the increased risk for VAPP, OPV should not be administered to persons with immunodeficiency disorders or malignant diseases or to persons whose immune systems have been compromised by therapy (corticosteroids,

Table 16.2. True Contraindications and Precautions* for OPV/IPV Vaccination

Vaccine	True Contraindications and Precautions	NOT Contraindications (vaccines may be given)
OPV	Infection with HIV or a household contact with HIV	Breast feeding
		Current antimicrobial therapy
	Known altered immunodeficiency	Diarrhea
	Immunodeficient household contact	
	Pregnancy	
IPV	Anaphylactic reaction following a previous dose of IPV or anaphylactic reaction to neomycin, polymyxin B or streptomycin	Breast feeding
		Current antimicrobial therapy
	Pregnancy	Diarrhea

*Precautions should be carefully reviewed. Consider the benefits and risks of administering a specific vaccine to a child under the circumstances. If the risks are believed to outweigh the benefits, withhold the immunization; if the benefits are believed to outweigh the risks (eg, during an outbreak or foreign travel), administer the vaccine. It is prudent on theoretical grounds to avoid vaccinating pregnant women. However, if immediate protection against poliomyelitis is needed, OPV is preferred, although IPV may be considered if full immunization can be completed before the anticipated imminent exposure. Pregnancy of a mother is not a contraindication to giving polio vaccine to her child.

Adapted from: Centers for Disease Control and Prevention. General recommendations on immunization: recommendations of the Advisory Committee on Immunization Practices (ACIP). MMWR. 1994; 43(RR-1): 24–25, and Centers for Disease Control and Prevention. Poliomyelitis prevention in the United States: introduction of a sequential vaccination schedule of inactivated poliovirus vaccine followed by oral poliovirus vaccine: recommendations of the Advisory Committee on Immunization Practices (ACIP). MMWR. 1997; 46 (No. RR-3): 1–25.

alkylating drugs, antimetabolites or radiation) (see Adverse Reactions). Use IPV for these patients and their household contacts. Do not administer OPV to hospitalized infants until after discharge, because of the theoretical risk of poliovirus transmission in the hospital.

5. Adverse Reactions

The risk of paralysis in recipients of OPV and their close contacts is extremely low. The rate of VAPP after the first dose of OPV is approximately one case per 750,000 doses. All adults who are not immunized or inadequately immunized against polio should be informed of the very low risk of developing paralytic poliomyelitis after a child with whom they have close contact has been immunized with the OPV vaccine. Advise them to wash their hands well after diaper changes and avoid contact with feces. Nonimmunized and partially immunized adults may be offered immunization with IPV. Because of the overriding importance of ensuring prompt and complete immunization, sequential IPV-OPV vaccination of children should begin regardless of the polio vaccination status of adult contacts.

IPV does not induce paralysis, and its side effects are minor (eg, local pain and swelling at the injection site).

Any adverse effects should be reported to the Vaccine Adverse Event Reporting System (VAERS). Refer to Table B.4 for a detailed listing of adverse events. VAERS forms and instructions are available in the FDA Drug Bulletin (Food and Drug Administration) and the Physician's Desk Reference or by calling the 24-hour VAERS information recording at (800)822-7967. Refer to Appendix B for details.

6. Patient Education

The National Childhood Vaccine Injury Act requires health care providers to provide the following information to patients prior to administering a polio vaccination: (1) a concise description of the benefits of the vaccine, (2) a concise description of the risks associated with the vaccine, and (3) notice of the availability of the National Vaccine Injury Compensation Program.

The US Department of Health and Human Services has developed a pamphlet for this purpose (see Patient Resources). Other patient educational materials may be used if they provide the information required by the National Childhood Vaccine Injury Act. For additional information about this requirement, contact the Training Coordinator, National Immunization Program, Centers for Disease Control and Prevention; (404)639-8226.

7. Vaccine Storage and Handling

Store OPV at temperatures low enough to keep it solidly frozen. Temperatures below -14°C (+7°F) may be required. Completely thaw the vaccine before use. A container of vaccine may be subjected to a maximum of 10 cycles of thawing and refreezing as long as the temperature of the vaccine does not exceed 8°C (46°F) and the total cumulative time thawed is not more than 24 hours. If the vaccine is thawed for more than 24 hours, it should not be refrozen but should be stored at 2 to 8°C (36 to 46°F) and used within 30 days. Store IPV at 2 to 8°C (36 to 46°F); do not freeze it. Do not use IPV vaccine that has been frozen. Handle all vaccine preparations according to manufacturers' instructions.

Patient Resources

Childhood Vaccines: What They Are and Why Your Child Needs Them. American Academy of Family Physicians, 8880 Ward Parkway, Kansas City, MO 64114-2797; (800)944-0000; Internet address: http://www.aafp.org.

Vaccine Information Statement—*Polio Vaccines: What You Need to Know,* #I1921. US Department of Health and Human Services. This material is available from the National Immunization Program, M/S E-34, Centers for Disease Control and Prevention, 1600 Clifton Rd NE, Atlanta, GA 30333; (404)639-8225, fax (404)639-8828; state and local health departments, or the American Academy of Pediatrics, PO Box 927, Elk Grove Village, IL 60009-0927; (800)433-9016. Internet address: http://www.aap.org

Immunization Protects Children. American Academy of Pediatrics, PO Box 927, Elk Grove Village, IL 60009-0927; (800)433-9016.
Internet address: http://www.aap.org

Parents Guide to Childhood Immunizations, #00-590. US Department of Health and Human Services. This material is available from the National Immunization Program, M/S E-34, Centers for Disease Control and Prevention, 1600 Clifton Rd NE, Atlanta, GA 30333; (404)639-8225; fax (404)639-8828.

Provider Resources

Poliomyelitis prevention: enhanced potency inactivated poliomyelitis vaccine-supplementary statement, #I1925; *Recommended childhood immunization schedule,* #I1743; *Six common misconceptions about vaccination and how to respond to them,* #00-6561; *Guide to contraindications in childhood vaccines,* #00-6562. These and other documents are available from the National Immunization Program, Centers for Disease Control and Prevention, M/S E-34, 1600 Clifton Rd NE, Atlanta, GA 30333; (404)639-8225; fax (404)639-8828.

Selected References

American Academy of Family Physicians. *Summary of Policy Recommendations for Periodic Health Examination.* Kansas City, Mo: American Academy of Family Physicians; 1997.

American Academy of Pediatrics, Committee on Infectious Diseases. Poliomyelitis prevention: recommendations for use of inactivated poliovirus vaccine and live oral poliovirus vaccine. *Pediatrics.* 1997;99(2):300-305.

Canadian Task Force on the Periodic Health Examination. Childhood immunizations. In: *The Canadian Guide to Clinical Preventive Health Care.* Ottawa, Canada: Minister of Supply and Services; 1994: chap 33.

Centers for Disease Control. Paralytic poliomyelitis—Senegal, 1986-1987: update on the N-IPV efficacy study. *MMWR.* 1988;37:257-259.

Centers for Disease Control. Vaccine Adverse Event Reporting System—United States. *MMWR.* 1990;39:730-733.

Centers for Disease Control and Prevention. General recommendations on immunization: recommendations of the Advisory Committee on Immunization Practices (ACIP). *MMWR.* 1994;43 (RR-1): 24-25.

Centers for Disease Control and Prevention. Poliomyelitis prevention in the United States: introduction of a sequential vaccination schedule of inactivated poliovirus vaccine followed by oral Poliovirus vaccine: recommendations of the Advisory Committee on Immunization Practices (ACIP). *MMWR.* 1997;46(No. RR-3):1-25.

Centers for Disease Control and Prevention. Recommended childhood immunization schedule-United States. 1997. *MMWR.* 1997;46:35-40.

Kimpen JL, Ogra PL. Poliovirus vaccines: a continuing challenge. *Pediatr Clin North Am.* 1990;37(3):627-649.

LaForce FM. Poliomyelitis vaccines: success and controversy. *Infect Dis Clin North Am.* 1990;4:75-83.

National Center for Health Statistics. *Health, United States, 1995.* Hyattsville, Md: Public Health Service. 1996.

Patel R, Kinsinger L. Childhood immunizations: American College of Preventive Medicine Practice Policy Statement. *Am J Prev Med.* 1997;13(2):74-77.

Physician's Desk Reference. 51st ed. Montvale, NJ: Medical Economics Co: 1997:3005-3007.

Strebel PM, Sutter RW, Coohi SL, et al. Epidemiology of poliomyelitis in the United States one decade after the last reported case of indigenous wild virus-associated disease. *Clin Infect Dis.* 1992;14:568-579.

US Preventive Services Task Force. Childhood immunizations. In: *Guide to Clinical Preventive Services.* 2nd ed. Washington, DC: US Department of Health and Human Services; 1996: chap 65.

17

VARICELLA (Including Adult Immunization)

Approximately 3.9 million cases of primary varicella-zoster virus (VZV) disease (chickenpox) occur annually in the United States. Chickenpox is typically a mild disease but may be severe in newborn infants, immunocompromised persons, and susceptible adults. Approximately 90 fatal cases of chickenpox are reported annually. Infants born to women who contract varicella in the first or second trimester of pregnancy may be afflicted with congenital varicella syndrome, with abnormalities in the skin, limbs, eyes, and central nervous system. In approximately 15% of chickenpox cases, subsequent reactivation in the form of zoster (shingles) occurs; shingles is particularly prevalent and severe in persons who are elderly or immunocompromised.

A varicella vaccine was licensed for use in the United States in 1995. A similar vaccine has been widely used in Japan and Korea. The varicella vaccine has been shown to be highly efficacious in children (70% to 90% effective at preventing all clinical disease, 95% effective at preventing severe disease). Clinical disease that does occur in vaccinated children tends to be less severe than that experienced by nonimmunized children. Varicella vaccine has not been as well studied in adults. Because adults tend to have a poorer immune response to the vaccine, two doses are required to achieve optimal conversion rates. Chickenpox results in considerable costs to society in the form of hospitalizations, lost days of schooling, and lost days of work. Cost-benefit analysis has indicated that routine use of varicella vaccine in children at 1 year of age would result in savings of $384 million per year in the United States.

Recommendations of Major Authorities

Children/Adolescents

Advisory Committee on Immunization Practices (ACIP), American Academy of Family Physicians, American Academy of Pediatrics (AAP), and **US Preventive Services Task Force**—Clinicians should routinely vaccinate children between the ages of 12 and 18 months. Children within this age range who have a prior history of chickenpox do not need to be immunized, although the **ACIP** has stated that it is acceptable to do so. Immunization is also recommended for children 19 months to 12 years of age who lack a prior history of immunization or clinical disease. Serologic testing of children before vaccination is not warranted, because most children aged 12 months to 12 years who do not have a history of chickenpox are susceptible, and the vaccine is well tolerated in seropositive persons. The **AAP** states that clinicians may decide to offer serologic testing to healthy adolescents who may be susceptible to VZV.

Adults

Advisory Committee on Immunization Practices (ACIP) and **US Preventive Services Task Force**—Given the high prevalence of immunity in adults who have no history of chickenpox and the results of cost-effectiveness analysis, clinicians may wish to offer serologic testing for varicella susceptibility in lieu of routine immunization to history-negative adults who are likely to comply with return visits. **ACIP** and **Centers for Disease Control and Prevention (CDC)** recommend vaccination for susceptible persons aged 13 years and over who have close contact with persons at high risk for serious complications (eg, health-care workers and family contacts of immunocompromised persons). **ACIP** and **CDC** further state that vaccination should be considered for susceptible persons aged 13 years and over who: (1) live or work in environments in which transmission of VZV is likely (eg, teachers of young children, day-care workers, residents and staff in institutional settings); (2) live or work in environments in which transmission may occur (eg, college students, military personnel); (3) are women of childbearing age (if not pregnant and willing to avoid pregnancy for 1 month); and/or (4) travel internationally (especially if the traveler expects to have close personal contact with local populations).

Basics of Varicella Vaccination

1. Vaccine Types

The single vaccine available in the United States (Varivax®, Merck and Co, Inc) is a live, cell-free preparation. A multiple-antigen, measles-mumps-rubella-varicella (MMR) vaccine is currently being tested.

2. Schedule

Children should receive a single vaccination between 12 and 18 months of age. Older children, up to 12 years of age, should also receive a single vaccination at the earliest convenient date. Children and healthy adults who are immunized after age 13 years should receive two doses of varicella vaccine delivered 4 to 8 weeks apart. Do not administer varicella vaccine until at least 5 months after a patient has received any form of immune globulin or other blood product.

Varicella vaccine and other childhood vaccines may be given simultaneously but at different sites. If varicella vaccine and MMR are not given concurrently, these vaccines should be given at least 1 month apart.

Booster doses are currently not recommended. The duration of immunity provided by varicella vaccine has not been established, and research is needed to determine whether booster doses will be necessary to maintain protection throughout adulthood.

3. Dose and Administration

The recommended dose of varicella vaccine for children and adults is 0.5 mL. Administer the vaccine subcutaneously into the thigh of infants and the deltoid area of older children and adults using a 5/8" to 3/4", 23- to 25-gauge needle.

4. Contraindications/Precautions

There are few, true contraindications to administering vaccinations. See Appendix B, Table B.3 for a listing of valid contraindicaitons.

Varicella vaccine is specifically contraindicated in persons with a history of an anaphylactic reaction to neomycin. VZV should be used with caution in any immunocompromised individual, including individuals taking steroids and recent recipients of blood or blood products (including immunoglobulin). Varicella vaccine should not be given to any pregnant women or women who intend to become pregnant within 1 month of vaccination. Individuals suffering from a severe illness should not be vaccinated until full recovery.

Advise parents to avoid administering salicylates to their children for 6 weeks following vaccination, because of the theoretical risk of developing Reye's syndrome.

5. Adverse Reactions

The vaccine is well tolerated. Transient pain and redness at the injection site are reported by approximately 25% of vaccinees. Fewer than 10% of vaccinees report a mild maculopapular or varicelliform rash, either local or generalized. Because of the small potential for transmission of the vaccine virus, vaccinees in whom a rash develops should avoid contact with immunocompromised susceptible persons. Inadvertent administration of varicella vaccine to individuals who are immune to varicella has not resulted in an increased number of adverse reactions.

Any adverse side effects should be reported to the Vaccine Adverse Event Reporting System (VAERS). Refer to Table B.4 for a detailed listing of adverse events. VAERS forms and instructions are available in the FDA Drug Bulletin

(Food and Drug Administration) and the *Physician's Desk Reference* or by calling the 24-hour VAERS information recording at (800)822-7967. Refer to Appendix B for details.

6. Patient Education

The US Department of Public Health has developed vaccine information statements about varicella vaccination (see Patient Resources). Copies of these statements must be available to patients in facilities where federally purchased vaccines are used, and their availability in other settings is encouraged.

7. Vaccine Storage and Handling

The lyophilized vaccine must be stored frozen at an average temperature of -15°C (8°F) or colder. Store the diluent separately at room temperature or in the refrigerator. Use the vaccine within 30 minutes of reconstitution with the supplied diluent. Discard any reconstituted vaccine that is not used within 30 minutes. Handle all vaccine preparations according to manufacturers' instructions.

Patient Resources

Childhood Vaccines: What They Are and Why Your Child Needs Them. American Academy of Family Physicians, 8880 Ward Pkwy, Kansas City, MO 64114-2797; (800)944-0000. Internet address: http://www.aafp.org

Vaccine Information Statement—*Chickenpox Vaccine: What you need to know before you or your child gets the vaccine*, #I1894. US Department of Health and Human Services. This information is available from the National Immunization Program, Information/Distribution Center, M/S E-34, Centers for Disease Control and Prevention, 1600 Clifton Rd NE, Atlanta, GA 30333, (404)639-8225, Fax (404)639-8828; or the American Academy of Pediatrics, PO Box 927, Elk Grove Village, IL 60009-0927; (800)433-9016.
Internet address: http://www.aap.org

Immunization Protects Children. American Academy of Pediatrics, PO Box 927, Elk Grove Village, IL 60009-0927; (800)433-9016. Internet address: http://www.aap.org

Parents Guide to Childhood Immunizations, #00-590; *Immunization of Adults: A Call to Action,* #00-6040. US Department of Health and Human Services. This material is available from the National Immunization Program, Information/Distribution Center, M/S E-34, Centers for Disease Control and Prevention, 1600 Clifton Rd NE, Atlanta, GA 30333; (404)639-8225; fax (404)639-8828.

Provider Resources

Rules of Childhood Immunization. Immunization Action Coalition, 1573 Selby Ave, Suite 229, St. Paul, MN 55104; (612)647-9009. Internet address: http://www.immunize.org

Recommended Childhood Immunization Schedule, #I1743; *Six Common Misconceptions About Vaccination and How to Respond to Them,* #00-6561; *Guide to Contraindications in Childhood Vaccines,* #00-6562. These and other documents are available from the National Immunization Program, M/S E-34, Centers for Disease Control and Prevention, 1600 Clifton Rd NE, Atlanta, GA 30333; (404)639-8225; fax (404)639-8828.

Selected References

American Academy of Family Physicians. *Summary of Policy Recommendations for Periodic Health Examination.* Kansas City, Mo: American Academy of Family Physicians; 1997.

American Academy of Pediatrics, Committee on Infectious Diseases. Recommendation for use of live attenuated varicella vaccine. *Pediatrics.* 1995;95:791-796.

Centers for Disease Control and Prevention. Prevention of varicella: recommendations of the Advisory Committee on Immunization Practices (ACIP). *MMWR.* 1996;45:(No. RR-11) 1-36.

Centers for Disease Control and Prevention. Recommended childhood immunization schedule-United States. 1997. *MMWR.* 1997;46:35-40.

Lieu T, Cochi SL, Black SB, et al. Cost-effectiveness of a routine varicella vaccination program for US children. *JAMA.* 1994;271:375-381.

Patel R, Kinsinger L. Childhood immunizations: American College of Preventive Medicine Practice Policy Statement. *Am J Prev Med.* 1997;13(2):74-77.

US Preventive Services Task Force. Adult immunizations. In: *Guide to Clinical Preventive Services.* 2nd ed. Washington, DC: US Department of Health and Human Services; 1996: chap 66.

US Preventive Services Task Force. Childhood immunizations. In: *Guide to Clinical Preventive Services.* 2nd ed. Washington, DC: US Department of Health and Human Services; 1996: chap 65.

18

ALCOHOL AND OTHER DRUG ABUSE

Abuse of alcohol and other drugs is a major health problem for older children and adolescents. Accidental injuries are the leading cause of death for adolescents, and approximately 40% of such injuries are related to alcohol use. Alcohol use has also been implicated in a significant percentage of adolescent homicides and suicides—the second and third leading causes of death in this age group. Cocaine use leads to increased cardiovascular morbidity and mortality in adolescents and young adults and indirectly contributes to the number of violent deaths of young people that are related to illegal drug activities. Use of illegal drugs is also related to poor school performance, social withdrawal, and family dysfunction.

Drug abuse affects children in all cultural and socioeconomic groups, not only minorities, the poor, and the undereducated. A 1990 survey of high school seniors found that the percentage of white youths reporting use of alcohol, marijuana, and cocaine in the month prior to the survey was higher than that of African-American youths (alcohol: 62.2% versus 32.9%; marijuana: 15.6% versus 5.2%; cocaine: 1.8% versus 0.5%). In this same study, alcohol and marijuana use were found to be directly related to parental educational levels. Higher parental educational levels were associated with greater drug use by the child. In general, the prevalence of alcohol and other drug abuse among females is lower than that among males.

See chapter 53 for information on counseling adults about abuse of alcohol and other drugs. See chapters 24 and 60 for information on counseling about tobacco use and smoking cessation.

Recommendations of Major Authorities

American Academy of Family Physicians—Recommends counseling about accidental injury prevention with regard to impaired driving.

American Academy of Pediatrics—Clinicians should condemn the nontherapeutic use of all psychoactive drugs, including alcohol and nicotine, by children and adolescents. All providers of adolescent health care should discuss the hazards of alcohol and other drug use with their patients as a routine part of risk behavior assessment. Providers should reinforce abstinent behaviors and assess current use with a nonjudgmental approach. Special attention should be paid to the discussion of this issue when risk factors for problem drinking, such as family history of alcoholism, are present. Preventive child health care visits provide an opportunity to inquire about a family history of alcoholism and parental attitudes about alcohol use.

American Medical Association—Clinicians should counsel all adolescents on the dangers of substance use and strategies to refrain from use. This approach should be complemented by counseling parents to monitor adolescents' social behaviors. Clinicians should screen adolescents for use of alcohol and other drugs. Previsit questionnaires may be used to determine risk for substance abuse, with direct questioning about actual use during a clinical interview. Once use is identified, a positive response to any of the following questions should alert the health care provider to possible abuse and prompt a referral:

1. Does the adolescent ever use drugs when alone?

2. Does the adolescent ever use alcohol when alone?

3. Does the adolescent ever get drunk or high at social events or have friends who do?

4. Does the adolescent ever consume alcohol on school grounds?

5. Does the adolescent ever miss school because of drinking or hangovers?

6. When truant, does the adolescent ever go drinking or get high on drugs?

All adolescent males who participate in high school athletic programs should be asked about their knowledge and use of anabolic steroids. Particular attention should be given to those who participate in sports that require weight and strength, such as football, track and field, and weightlifting.

Bright Futures—Child and adolescent health supervision visits should include interview questions, developmental surveillance questions, and anticipatory guidance that address alcohol and other drug abuse, as well as tobacco use.

Canadian Task Force on the Periodic Health Examination—
Routine active case-finding of problem drinking among patients in medi-

cal practices is highly recommended on the basis of the high prevalence of this problem, its association with adverse consequences before the stage of dependency is reached, and its amenability to a counseling intervention by clinicians. Active case-finding should be performed through structured interviews and questionnaires. Clinicians should be sensitive to the possibility of alcohol-related stressors in offspring of alcoholic or alcohol-abusing parents and in some high-risk groups, particularly children hospitalized for injury. Primary health care providers are in an excellent position to prevent children's injuries by identifying, evaluating, and assisting families in recovery from the effects of family alcoholism.

US Preventive Services Task Force—Screening to detect problem drinking is recommended for all adult and adolescent patients. Screening should involve a careful history of alcohol use and /or the use of standardized screening questionnaires. Routine measurement of biochemical markers is not recommended in asymptomatic persons. Pregnant women should be advised to limit or cease drinking during pregnancy. Although there is insufficient evidence to prove or disprove harms from light drinking in pregnancy, recommendations that women abstain from alcohol during pregnancy may be made on other grounds. All persons who use alcohol should be counseled about the dangers of operating a motor vehicle or performing other potentially dangerous activities after drinking alcohol.

There is insufficient evidence to recommend for or against routine screening for drug abuse with standardized questionnaires or biologic assays. Including questions about drug use and drug-related problems when taking a history from all adolescents and adult patients may be recommended on other grounds, including the prevalence of drug use and the serious consequences of drug abuse and dependence. All pregnant women should be advised of the potential adverse effects of drug use on the development of the fetus. Clinicians should be alert to the signs and symptoms of drug abuse in patients and refer drug-abusing patients to specialized treatment facilities where available.

Basics of Alcohol and Other Drug Abuse Counseling

1. Begin educational discussions with children and parents during the preteen years. Sample questions for discussing drug use with children in this age group are listed in Table 18.1. Similar questions can be used to discuss alcohol use. Inform all children and adolescents of the dangers of alcohol and drug use. Emphasize the dangers of operating a motor vehicle while under the influence of alcohol or drugs. Explain the potential risk for exposure to hepatitis B, HIV, and other STDs and the risk of unintended pregnancies from sexual encounters while under the influence of alcohol or other drugs.

Table 18.1. Sample Questions Concerning Drugs for School-aged Children

What have you learned about drugs at school?

Have you and your friends ever talked about drugs?

Have you ever wondered why some people use drugs?

Has anyone ever tried to sell you drugs or tried to force you to take drugs?

Adapted from: Schonberg KS, ed. Substance Abuse: A Guide for Health Professionals. Elk Grove Village, Ill: American Academy of Pediatrics; 1988. Used with permission of the American Academy of Pediatrics; copyright 1988.

2. Ask parents about their own use of alcohol and other drugs and whether they discuss the use of alcohol and other drugs with their children. Assess whether a family history of alcoholism or other drug use exists and whether family stress places the child at increased risk. See chapter 53 for information on counseling adults about abuse of alcohol and other drugs.

3. Establish a caring and confidential relationship with adolescent patients. Inform both the parents and the adolescent of the limits of this confidentiality. Such limits can be summarized as follows: absolute confidentiality is not possible if the provider judges the adolescent's actions to be of immediate and serious danger to him/herself or to others. There is a duty to disclose to protect the adolescent from him/herself (eg, suicidality), a duty to warn others of imminent or likely harm (eg, homicidality), and also a duty to report (eg, sexually transmitted diseases and abuse or neglect). Discussions about confidentiality should assure the teen that in all other situations, information will not be shared with parents or others without the teen's permission. Clinicians should reinforce the limits of confidentiality at each visit. Using one or more examples as illustration is also helpful.

4. Begin by asking children and adolescents about alcohol and drug use in their environment—at home, school (including use of drugs to enhance athletic ability), or work. This may be less threatening than first asking about their personal use. A set of questions using this indirect approach is listed in Table 18.2.

5. If a history of alcohol or other drug use is elicited, ask the adolescent in a nonjudgmental manner about the type of drugs used, the quantity and frequency of use, and the setting of use.

6. Evaluate the extent to which alcohol or other drug use is adversely affecting important aspects of the patient's life, such as school performance,

Table 18.2. Sample Questions Concerning Drug Use for Adolescents

Do most of your friends drink alcohol or smoke marijuana at parties?

Do any of your friends use drugs other than alcohol or marijuana?

Do you smoke cigarettes? How many per day?

Have you ever tried alcohol? Marijuana? Other drugs?

Have you ever been ill as a result of using drugs or drinking? In what way?

Have you ever been in trouble with the law as a result of drugs or alcohol?

Do your parents know that you've used _____ ?

What would (did) they say?

Have you ever worried about your _____ use?

Have you ever been drunk or stoned and driven a car (or motorcycle)?

Adapted from: Schonberg KS, ed. Substance Abuse: A Guide for Health Professionals. Elk Grove Village, Ill: American Academy of Pediatrics; 1988. Used with permission of the American Academy of Pediatrics; copyright 1988.

peer relationships, family relationships, work performance, and sexual relationships. "Drinking and You," in The Adolescent Drinking Index, is an evaluation tool designed and tested with adolescents (see Provider Resources).

7. Counsel patients at increased risk for hepatitis B, HIV, and other STDs about the importance of screening for these conditions and receiving hepatitis B vaccination.

8. Remain alert for signs and symptoms of physiologic dependence or withdrawal, such as craving, compulsive alcohol- or drug-seeking behavior, tremulousness, agitation, weight loss, headaches, and changes in mental status.

9. The presence of significant psychosocial impairment or physiological dependence attributable to alcohol or other drug abuse suggests the need for early referral of the patient for comprehensive evaluation and possible inpatient, outpatient, or day treatment. Be familiar with the range of referral and treatment options in your community. Examples of types of community resources may include behavioral health centers, community mental health centers, alcohol and drug treatment centers specializing in adoles-

cent care, child and adolescent guidance centers (in some states these are part of local public health clinics), and school health centers. The primary care provider may counsel patients who are not seriously impaired.

10. Chapter 53 discusses basic principles of substance abuse counseling, including:

- Establishing a therapeutic relationship

- Making the medical office or clinic off-limits for substance abuse

- Presenting information about negative health consequences

- Involving family and other support

- Setting goals

- Becoming familiar with community treatment services

- Providing follow-up

Patient Resources

Anabolic Steroids and Athletes. American College of Sports Medicine, PO Box 1440, Indianapolis, IN 46206-1440; (317)637-9200. Internet address: http://www.acsm.org/sportsmed

Alcohol: What to Do If It's a Problem for You. American Academy of Family Physicians, 8880 Ward Parkway, Kansas City, MO 64114-2797; (800)944-0000. Internet address: http://www.aafp.org

Alcohol: Your Child and Drugs; Cocaine: Your Child and Drugs; Marijuana: Your Child and Drugs; Teens Who Drink and Drive: Reducing the Death Toll; Inhalent Abuse: Your Child and Drugs. American Academy of Pediatrics, PO Box 927, Elk Grove Village, IL 60009-0927; (800)433-9016. Internet address: http://www.aap.org

Let's Talk Facts about Substance Abuse. American Psychiatric Association, 1400 K Street, NW, Washington, DC 20005; (800)368-5777. Internet address: http://www.psych.org

National Clearinghouse for Alcohol and Drug Information. Information about numerous publications available in both English and Spanish. (800)729-6686.

Provider Resources:

The Adolescent Drinking Index. Manual and 25 test booklets (cost $55). Available from Psychological Assessment Resources, Inc, PO Box 998, Odessa, FL 33556; (800)331-TEST.

Bright Futures: Guidelines for Health Supervision of Infants, Children and Adolescents; Bright Futures Pocket Guide; Bright Futures Anticipatory Guidance Cards. Available from the National Center for Education in Maternal and Child Health, 2000 15th Street North, Suite 701, Arlington, VA 22201-2617; (703)524-7802. Internet address: http://www.brightfutures.org

Selected References

American Academy of Family Physicians. *Summary of Policy Recommendations for Periodic Health Examination.* Kansas City, Mo: American Academy of Family Physicians; 1997.

American Academy of Pediatrics, American Academy of Family Physicians, American College of Obstetricians and Gynecologists, NAACOG—The Organization for Obstetric, Gynecologic, and Neonatal Nurses, National Medical Association (joint policy statement). Confidentiality in adolescent health care. In: *Policy Reference Guide: A Comprehensive Guide to AAP Policy Statements Published through December 1996.* Elk Grove Village, Ill: American Academy of Pediatrics; 1997:129.

American Academy of Pediatrics, Committee on Adolescence, Committee on Substance Abuse. Marijuana: A continuing concern for pediatricians. *Pediatrics.* 1991;88:1070-1072.

American Academy of Pediatrics. Committee on Substance Abuse and Committee on Native American Child Health. Inhalent Abuse. *Pediatrics.* 1996;97:420-423.

American Academy of Pediatrics, Committee on Substance Abuse. Alcohol use and abuse: a pediatric concern. *Pediatrics.* 1995;95:439-442.

American Academy of Pediatrics, Committee on Substance Abuse. Role of pediatricians in prevention and management of substance abuse. *Pediatrics.* 1993;91:1010-1013.

American Academy of Pediatrics, Committee on Substance Abuse. The role of schools in combating substance abuse. *Pediatrics.* 1995;95:784-785.

American Medical Association. Use of alcohol, drugs, and steroids. In: *AMA Guidelines for Adolescent Preventive Services (GAPS): Recommendations and Rationale.* Chicago, Ill: American Medical Association; 1994.

Canadian Task Force on the Periodic Health Examination. Children of alcoholics. In: *The Canadian Guide to Clinical Preventive Health Care.* Ottawa, Canada: Minister of Supply and Services; 1994: chap 41.

Canadian Task Force on the Periodic Health Examination. Early detection and counseling of problem drinking. In: *The Canadian Guide to Clinical Preventive Health Care.* Ottawa, Canada: Minister of Supply and Services; 1994: chap 42.

Green M, ed. Bright Futures: *Guidelines for Health Supervision of Infants, Children, and Adolescents.* Arlington, Va: National Center for Education in Maternal and Child Health; 1994.

National Center for Health Statistics. *Health, United States, 1991 Prevention Profile.* Hyattsville, Md: Public Health Service; 1992. US Department of Health and Human Services publication PHS 92-1232.

Schonberg KS, ed. *Substance Abuse: A Guide for Health Professionals.* Elk Grove Village, Ill: American Academy of Pediatrics; 1988.

US Preventive Services Task Force. Screening for drug abuse. In: *Guide to Clinical Preventive Services.* 2nd ed. Washington, DC: US Department of Health and Human Services; 1996: chap 53.

US Preventive Services Task Force. Screening for problem drinking. In: *Guide to Clinical Preventive Services.* 2nd ed. Washington, DC: US Department of Health and Human Services; 1996: chap 52.

19

DENTAL AND ORAL HEALTH

Dental and oral health problems are common in children. Caries and peri-odontal diseases are the most frequent, but other significant problems include malocclusion, trauma, congenital anomalies, and oral malignancies. Widespread use of fluoride and other preventive dental health practices have led to a significant decrease in the incidence of dental caries. Nonetheless, two thirds of 12- to 17-year-old children have decayed or filled permanent teeth, and among teens aged 13 to 17 years, 73% have some gingival bleeding. In most cases, these problems are preventable, and the dental and oral health status of adults is largely determined by the quality of preventive and treatment services received during childhood.

See chapter 54 for information on dental and oral health counseling for adults. See chapters 24 and 60 for information on counseling on tobacco and smoking cessation.

Recommendations of Major Authorities

Primary Care

All major dental and medical authorities—Dental and oral health counseling for children and parents should be provided routinely by primary care clinicians.

Dental and Oral Care

American Academy of Pediatrics—Referral for the first dental visit should occur at 3 years of age, with frequency of subsequent visits determined by the dentist. Earlier referrals may be appropriate for some children.

American Academy of Pediatric Dentistry, American Society of Dentistry for Children, American Dental Association, and **Bright Futures**—A child's first dental visit should occur at 6 months of age or when the first tooth erupts, whichever comes later, but no later than 1 year of age. Frequency of subsequent visits should be determined by the dentist.

US Preventive Services Task Force—All patients should be encouraged to visit a dental-care provider on a regular basis, with the optimal frequency determined by the patient's dental-care provider.

Basics of Dental and Oral Health Counseling

1. Begin oral health education and care at an infant's first visit, and continue education and care throughout childhood and adolescence.

2. Assess an infant's need for fluoride supplementation. Only 62% of Americans live in areas with fluoridated community water supplies. If a child lives in an area without an optimally fluoridated community water supply, the water supply should be tested and other sources of fluoride identified before recommending supplementation. Information about fluoride content of community water supplies can be obtained from the local water department.

   See Table 19.1 for the recommended dosages for fluoride supplementation. Fluoride supplementation may begin as early as 6 months of age and continue until approximately 16 years of age, if necessary. Fluoride supplements are available as drops (for infants and young children) and as chewable tablets. Prescribe the recommended dose once daily. When chewable tablets are used, encourage children to chew and swish the resultant fluid in the mouth for 30 seconds before swallowing.

Table 19.1. Daily Fluoride Dosage (mg) According to Age and Water Supply Content

Age	Fluoride Concentration in Local Water Supply (ppm)		
	<0.3	0.3-0.6	>0.6
Birth-6 mo	0	0	0
6 mo-3 y	0.25	0	0
3-6 y	0.50	0.25	0
6-16 y	1.00	0.50	0

From: American Academy of Pediatrics, Committee on Nutrition. Fluoride supplementation for children: interim policy recommendations. Pediatrics. 1995;95:777. Reproduced by permission of Pediatrics; copyright 1995.

3. Instruct parents to wipe their infant's gums and teeth after each feeding, using a moist washcloth or gauze pad. As multiple teeth appear, parents should begin brushing the infant's teeth daily with a small toothbrush and a very small (pea-sized) amount of fluoride-containing toothpaste. Swallowing large amounts of toothpaste by infants and children may lead later to enamel discoloration of permanent teeth because of fluorosis. To avoid gum tissue injury, use a brush with soft end-rounded or polished bristles, and replace it when bristles are bent or worn. Although children should actively participate in their dental care, they should continue to receive assistance from parents or other care givers until they are 7 or 8 years old.

4. Parents can sooth irritability caused by teething by allowing the infant to chew on a cold teething ring, by gently massaging the infant's gums with a finger, or by administering acetaminophen. Advise parents that fever is not a symptom of teething; if fever is present, parents should contact their child's primary care provider.

5. Address strategies to prevent tooth decay from breast- or bottle-feeding. Infants should not be permitted to nurse throughout the night or fall asleep with a bottle containing anything other than water. If a bottle is required to quiet or comfort the infant before sleep, instruct parents to use only water. Also, a child should not be allowed to keep a bottle during the day for extended periods for *ad libitum* drinking with anything other than water. Parents should encourage infants to begin using a cup instead of a bottle at 1 year of age.

6. Advise parents to talk with their dentist or dental hygienist about when their child should begin using dental floss.

7. Thumb-sucking or use of a pacifier generally does not cause permanent dental problems for children younger than 4 years of age. Children who thumb-suck beyond age 5 years, however, may develop alignment problems of their permanent teeth. These children may need to be referred to a dentist for assessment.

8. Counsel parents about the impact of dietary habits on oral health: Avoid foods that are high in simple sugars or starches or those that are particularly sticky. If snacks are eaten, select them carefully; encourage consumption of raw fruits and vegetables, nuts, and low-sugar drinks. Limit ingestion of sweets to once or twice a day, preferably with a meal.

9. If a child has a permanent tooth knocked out that is intact and whole, rinse it gently without removing any attached tissue, and immediately reinsert it into the socket. If this is not possible, place it in cool water or milk. The child should see a dentist as soon as possible for emergency treatment. Replacement of the tooth within the first hour is critical for long-term retention. Primary teeth should not be reinserted.

10. Advise parents that children between the ages of 5 and 13 years should be evaluated by their dentist regarding the need for dental sealants on newly erupted permanent molars. First molars usually erupt at about 6 years of age and second molars at about 12 years of age. The sealant is most effective if applied soon after eruption, before the decay process has had time to begin.

11. Give children and adolescents special counseling about dental and oral health problems, such as dental injuries and tobacco-related illnesses, for which they are at increased risk. Advise those involved in contact sports to use appropriate mouth protectors and helmets. Advise adolescents of the cosmetic (yellowed teeth, bad breath) and health (lung cancer, heart disease, leukoplakia, and oral and pharyngeal cancers) problems caused by tobacco use. Smokeless tobacco (snuff and chewing tobacco) is a particular problem among adolescents, and its use should be seriously discouraged (chapter 24).

12. When examining the oral cavity, remain alert for signs of oral diseases, such as caries and inflamed or cyanotic gingiva, mucosal changes such as white patches or wrinkling characteristic of spit tobacco, malalignment or crowding of teeth, and mismatching upper and lower dental arches.

13. Transient bacteremia is common during dental procedures, including cleaning. Give antibiotic prophylaxis to children before a dental cleaning or procedure if they have underlying great vessel or heart disease (Tables 54.2 and 54.3).

Patient Resources

A Guide to Children's Dental Health; Baby Bottle Tooth Decay: How to Prevent It. American Academy of Pediatrics, PO Box 927, Elk Grove Village, IL 60009-0927; (800)433-9016. Internet address: http://www.aap.org

Dental Emergency Procedures; Seal Out Decay; Your Child's Teeth; Smokeless Tobacco: Think Before You Chew; Diet and Dental Health; Smoking Can Really Do a Number on Your Health; Oral Health Guidelines for Special Patients. American Dental Association, Department of Salable Materials, 211 E Chicago Ave, Chicago, IL 60611; (800)947-4746.

For a Lifetime of Smiles.... American Dental Hygienists' Association, 444 N Michigan Ave, Suite 3400, Chicago, IL 60611; (312)440-8900. Internet address: http://www.adha.org

Baby's Bright Smile. American Society of Dentistry for Children, 875 N Michigan Ave, Suite 4040, Chicago, IL 60611; (312)943-1244.

A Healthy Mouth for Your Baby; Prevent Baby Bottle Tooth Decay; Rx for Sound Teeth (Spanish and English); Seal Out Dental Decay (English and Spanish); Kids-Snack Smart for Healthy Teeth, Fever Blisters and Canker Sores, Sealants and Fluorides (bookmark). National Institute of Dental Research, Building 31 Room 2C35, 31 Center Dr MSC 2290, Bethesda, MD 20890-2290; (301)496-4261. Internet address: http://www.nidr.nih.gov

Provider Resources

Bright Futures: Guidelines for Health Supervision of Infants, Children and Adolescents; Bright Futures Pocket Guide; Bright Futures in Practice: Oral Health; Bright Futures in Practice: Oral Health Quick Reference Cards. National Center for Education in Maternal and Child Health, 2000 15th Street North, Suite 701, Arlington VA 22201-2617; (703)524-7802. Internet address: http://www.bright-futures.org

Detection and Prevention of Periodontal Disease: A Guide for Health Care Providers. National Institute of Dental Research, Building 31 Room 2C35, 31 Center Dr MSC 2290, Bethesda, MD 20890-2290; (301)496-4261. Internet address: http://www.nidr.nih.gov

Getting the Picture on Dental X Rays. FDA Office of Consumer Affairs. HFE 88 Room 1675, 5600 Fishers Lane, Rockville, MD 20857. (800)532-4440.

Selected References

American Academy of Pediatrics, Committee on Nutrition. Fluoride supplementation. *Pediatrics.* 1986;77:758-761.

American Academy of Pediatrics, Committee on Practice and Ambulatory Medicine. Recommendations for pediatric preventive health care. *Pediatrics.* 1995;96:373-374.

American Academy of Pediatrics. Committee on Nutrition. Fluoride supplementation for children: interim policy recommendations. *Pediatrics.* 1995;95:777.

American Academy of Pediatric Dentistry. *Reference Manual 1991-1992.* Chicago, Ill: American Academy of Pediatric Dentistry; 1991.

American Dental Association. *Baby Bottle Tooth Decay.* Chicago, Ill: American Dental Association; 1989.

American Dental Association. Fluoride compounds. In: *Accepted Dental Therapeutics.* 40th ed. Chicago, Ill: American Dental Association; 1984.

Brunelle JA, Bhat M, Lipton JA. Prevalence and distribution of selected occlusal characteristics. *Journal of Dental Research.* 1996;75:706-713.

Green M, ed. *Bright Futures: Guidelines for Health Supervision of Infants, Children, and Adolescents.* Arlington, Va: National Center for Education in Maternal and Child Health; 1994.

Greene JC, Louie R, Wycoff SJ. US Preventive Services Task Force: Preventive dentistry: I. Dental caries. *JAMA.* 1989;262:3459-3563.

Greene JC, Louie R, Wycoff SJ. US Preventive Services Task Force: Preventive dentistry: II. Periodontal diseases, malocclusion, trauma, and oral cancer. *JAMA.* 1990;263:421-423.

Helfetz SB. Amounts of fluoride in self-administered dental products: safety considerations for children. *Pediatrics.* 1986;77:876-882.

Kaste LM, Selwitz RH, Oldakowski RJ, et. al. Coronal caries in the primary and permanent dentition of children and adolescents 1-17 years of age: United States, 1988-1991. *Journal of Dental Research.* 1996;75:631-641.

Kaste LM, Gift HC, Bhat M, Swango PA. Prevalence of incisor trauma in persons 6 to 50 years of age: United States, 1988-1991. *Journal of Dental Research.* 1996;75:696-705.

Selwitz RH, Albertini TF, Brown LJ, et al. The prevalence of dental sealants in the US population: Findings from NHANES III, 1988-1991. *Journal of Dental Research.* 1996;75:652-660.

US Preventive Services Task Force. Counseling to prevent dental and periodontal disease. In: *Guide to Clinical Preventive Services.* 2nd ed. Washington, DC: US Department of Health and Human Services; 1996: chap 61.

20

NUTRITION

Proper nutrition during childhood is essential for normal growth and development. Inadequate intake of nutrients is reflected in slow growth rates, inadequate mineralization of bones, and low body reserves of micronutrients. The nutrients most commonly deficient in children's diets are iron and calcium. Excessive caloric intake is a greater problem for children in United States than is inadequate caloric intake. Many children are substantially overweight, physically inactive, and have high dietary intakes of total fat and saturated fat. These factors may lead to obesity and poor nutritional habits as adults, resulting in an increased risk of heart disease, type 2 diabetes, high blood pressure, certain types of cancer, and other chronic diseases. Primary care clinicians face the challenge of helping children develop dietary habits that promote growth and development and reduce the risk of chronic diseases later in life.

Recommendations of Major Authorities

Most major authorities, including the **American Academy of Family Physicians, American Academy of Pediatrics, American Dietetic Association, American Medical Association, Bright Futures,** and **US Preventive Services Task Force (USPSTF)**—Primary care providers should counsel children and adolescents and their parents about proper nutrition. The USPSTF has reported that there is insufficient evidence that nutritional counseling by physicians has an advantage over dietitian counseling or community interventions in changing the dietary habits of patients.

American Academy of Family Physicians—Counseling should be provided to promote breast-feeding through at least 6 months of age.

American Academy of Pediatrics, American Medical Association, Bright Futures, Canadian Task Force on the Periodic Health Examination, and **US Preventive Services Task Force**—Parents should be counseled about the benefits and techniques of breast-feeding for infants.

American College of Obstetricians and Gynecologists, US Preventive Services Task Force, and **Canadian Task Force on the Periodic Health Examination** — Women of childbearing age who are capable of becoming pregnant should consume 0.4 mg of folic acid per day.

Basics of Nutrition Counseling

Younger than 2 Years of Age

1. Breast milk is the best choice for feeding almost all infants. Encourage mothers to breast-feed for 6 to 12 months, if possible, but even a few weeks is desirable. Breast-feeding is contraindicated in a few situations, such as certain maternal infections or use of certain drugs or medications by the mother. Educate parents about the benefits of breast-feeding and techniques for successfully initiating and maintaining breast-feeding.

2. Counsel parents to begin introducing single-ingredient foods when infants are developmentally ready, usually at 4 to 6 months of age. A child should be able to sit up with some help, maintain good head and neck control, and accept soft food from a spoon. Infant cereal mixed with breast milk or formula is often a good first choice. Introduce new foods one at a time, at 3- to 5-day intervals, to permit detection of food intolerances.

3. Encourage use of iron-rich foods, such as iron-fortified infant formula and iron-fortified cereal. Infants who are exclusively breast-fed may need iron supplementation beginning at 6 months of age. Many authorities recommend hemoglobin/hematocrit testing to detect iron deficiency anemia before 1 year of age (chapter 1).

4. Advise parents not to feed cow's milk to children younger than 1 year of age, because its nutrient composition is inadequate to meet the needs of younger children. Do not use reduced-fat milk until the child is at least 2 years of age.

5. Advise parents not to limit fat in children's diets during the first 2 years of life.

6. Counsel parents not to feed honey to infants during the first year of life because of the risk of infant botulism.

7. Counsel parents that vitamin supplements have not been proven to be necessary in healthy children who have balanced diets that include a variety of foods. Infants who are exclusively breast-fed, particularly if they are dark-skinned or are not regularly exposed to sunlight, may need vitamin D supplementation.

8. Children 6 months of age and older who live in areas with low fluoride content in the drinking water may need fluoride supplementation for prevention of dental caries (chapter 19).

Over 2 Years of Age

1. Counsel parents that children, like adults, need a balanced diet that includes a wide variety of foods. The US Departments of Agriculture and Health and Human Services have published the *Dietary Guidelines for Americans* and the Food Guide Pyramid (Figure 56.1) to assist the public in planning a healthful diet.

2. Help parents and children choose a diet that is low in total fat (30% or less of total calories), saturated fat (less than 10% of total calories), and cholesterol. Encourage inclusion of poultry (without skin), fish, lean meat, low-fat and skim milk products, cooked dry peas and beans, whole-grain breads and cereals, and fruits and vegetables.

3. Encourage parents and children to use sugar and salt only in moderation and to choose foods with low or reduced sugar and salt content.

4. Advise children, particularly adolescent girls, and their families to eat foods rich in calcium (such as milk and milk products) and iron (such as lean meats, dry legumes, fortified cereals, and whole-grain products).

5. Counsel parents and children about the importance of maintaining a healthy weight. A child's weight should be related to height, age, body build, and other factors that may influence weight. The limits of "healthy" weight are not well defined for children. As a rule of thumb, however, weight-for-height values from the 5th through the 95th percentiles (chapter 3) can be considered "healthy." However, for individuals with a family history of obesity-related diseases or conditions, such as high blood pressure or abnormal lipid patterns, a weight lower than the 85th percentile is desirable.

6. Weight reduction through dieting or other means is not advisable for children and adolescents, because they are still growing. Counsel overweight children and their parents to strive to maintain the child's weight at a constant level as the child continues to grow, while increasing physical activity to improve fitness and to avoid gaining weight. Ask patients about their dietary habits and determine if they try to limit their food intake for any reason. Pay special attention to individuals who participate in sports requiring stringent weight standards or those who perceive their weight to be too high.

7. Discuss the use of dietary supplements. Advise patients that vitamin supplements have not been proven to be necessary in normal children and adolescents with balanced diets. Those who live in areas with low fluoride content in the drinking water may need fluoride supplements to prevent dental caries until approximately 16 years of age (chapter 19).

8. Advise adolescent females of the following options for comsuming adequate amounts of folic acid:

- Consumption of a diet consistent with the Dietary Guidelines for Americans (chapter 56) and the Food Guide Pyramid (Figure 56.1) is likely to provide the proper amount of folic acid. Dry beans, leafy green vegetables, and citrus fruits are good sources of folic acid.

- Consumption of fortified foods, such as breakfast cereals, may help patients consume enough folic acid.

- Folic acid supplement pills and multivitamin preparations containing 0.4 mg folic acid are available.

- Caution patients against consuming more than 1 mg of folic acid daily, because the effects of excess folic acid are not well known. Such effects may include a delay in the detection of vitamin B12 deficiency, thus allowing neurologic damage to progress. However, women who have had a previous neural tube defect-affected pregnancy should consult with their clinicians several months before they plan to become pregnant about consuming a higher dose of folic acid. Public health measures to fortify the US food supply with folic acid are currently being implemented.

Patient Resources

The Gift of Love; Feeding Kids Right Isn't Always Easy: Tips for Preventing Food Hassles; Growing Up Healthy: Fat, Cholesterol and More; Right from the Start: ABC's of Good Nutrition for Young Children; What's to Eat? Healthy Foods for Hungry Children. American Academy of Pediatrics, PO Box 927, Elk Grove Village, IL 60009-0927; (800)433-9016. Internet address: http://www.aap.org

Nutrition and Sports Performance: A Guide for High School Athletes. American College of Sports Medicine, PO Box 1440, Indianapolis, IN 46202-1440; (317)634-7817.

Nutrition and Your Health: Dietary Guidelines for Americans; The Food Guide Pyramid. These booklets are available through the Cooperative Extension System, or contact the Superintendent of Documents, US Government Printing Office, Washington, DC 20402; (202)783-3238.

The Food Guide Pyramid: Beyond the Basic 4. Food Marketing Institute, 800 Connecticut Ave NW, Washington, DC 20006.

Provider Resources:

Bright Futures: Guidelines for Health Supervision of Infants, Children and Adolescents; Bright Futures Pocket Guide; Bright Futures Anticipatory Guidance Cards. Available from the National Center for Education in Maternal and Child Health, 2000 15th Street North, Suite 701, Arlington, VA 22201-2617; (703)524-7802. Internet address: http://www.brightfutures.org

Selected References

American Academy of Family Physicians. *Summary of Policy Recommendations for Periodic Health Examination.* Kansas City, Mo: American Academy of Family Physicians; 1997.

American Academy of Pediatrics, Committee on Nutrition. *Pediatric Nutrition Handbook.* 3rd ed. Elk Grove Village, Ill: American Academy of Pediatrics; 1993.

American Academy of Pediatrics, Committee on Nutrition. The promotion of breast-feeding. *Pediatrics.* 1982;69:654-661.

American Academy of Pediatrics, Committee on Nutrition. The use of whole cow's milk in infancy. *Pediatrics.* 1992;89:1105-1109.

American Medical Association. *Guidelines for Adolescent Preventive Services (GAPS).* Chicago, Ill: American Medical Association; 1992.

Canadian Task Force on the Periodic Health Examination. The periodic health examination: 2. 1984 update. *Can Med Assoc J.* 1984;130:1278-1285.

Cunningham AS. Morbidity in breast-fed and artificially fed infants. *J Pediatr.* 1977;90:726.

Freed GL, Landers S, Schanler RJ. A practical guide to successful breast-feeding management. *Am J Dis Child.* 1991;145:917-921.

Green M, ed. *Bright Futures: Guidelines for Health Supervision of Infants, Children, and Adolescents.* Arlington, Va: National Center for Education in Maternal and Child Health; 1994.

Mallick MJ. Health hazards of obesity and weight control in children: a review of the literature. *Am J Public Health.* 1983;73:78-82.

National Cholesterol Education Program. Report of the Expert Panel on Blood Cholesterol Levels for Children and Adolescents. *Pediatrics.* 1992;89(suppl 3):525-584.

US Department of Agriculture, US Department of Health and Human Services. *Nutrition and Your Health: Dietary Guidelines for Americans.* Washington, DC: US Goverment Printing Office; 1995. Home and Garden Bulletin 232.

US Preventive Services Task Force. Counseling to promote a healthy diet. In: *Guide to Clinical Preventive Services.* 2nd ed. Washington, DC: US Department of Health and Human Services; 1996: chap 56.

US Public Health Service. Recommendations for the use of folic acid to reduce the number of cases of spina bifida and other neural tube defects. *MMWR.* 1992;41:1-7.

US Public Health Service. *The Surgeon General's Report on Nutrition and Health.* Washington DC: US Department of Health and Human Services; 1988. DHHSPHS publication 88-50210.

21

PHYSICAL ACTIVITY

Most Americans, including American children and adolescents, are not physically active. Although the health consequences of physical inactivity usually become apparent in adulthood, the early changes that lead to their development may begin in childhood and adolescence. Physical activity, even moderate levels, confers significant health benefits including: building and maintaining healthy bones, muscles, and joints; controlling weight; reducing body fat; and preventing or delaying the development of hypertension and diabetes. Further, physical activity patterns developed in childhood and adolescence are believed to influence adult activity patterns.

According to the 1996 Report of the Surgeon General on Physical Activity and Health, only about half of young persons in the United States aged 12 to 21 years regularly participate in vigorous physical activity. The level of participation in all types of physical activity declines strikingly as age or grade in school increases. Physical education requirements in schools vary widely in terms of days per week and total physical education requirements. During the first half of the 1990s, total enrollment of high school students in physical education remained unchanged, although daily attendance in physical education classes decreased from 42% to 25%. A corollary of escalating physical inactivity among children and adolescents is the increase of obesity among this age group. A 55-year follow-up study by Must, Jacques, Dallai, Bajema, and Dietz (Selected References) that controlled for adult weight found that being overweight in adolescence was a more powerful predictor of premature mortality than was being overweight as an adult.

See chapter 57 for information about physical activity counseling for adults. See chapters 20 and 56 for information on nutrition counseling for children and adolescents and adults, respectively.

Recommendations of Major Authorities

American Academy of Family Physicians and **US Preventive Services Task Force**—Counseling to promote regular physical exercise is recommended for all children and adults.

American Academy of Pediatrics—Clinicians should assess the frequency, type, and duration of physical activities during any health supervision visit for a child 3 years of age or older. They should teach the importance of regular moderate-to-vigorous physical activity as a way to prevent illness in adult life. Parents should be encouraged to serve as role models by participating in regular physical activity, ideally with their child or as a family. Clinicians should also serve as role models by participating in regular physical activity themselves, work with schools to promote daily physical education, encourage measurements of physical fitness in physical education classes, and develop the ability to perform or refer children for body composition analysis, such as skinfold measurement.

American College of Sports Medicine—The health-care professions need to become more actively involved in promoting physical fitness for children and youth. Health-care professionals can make a major impact by promoting and supporting physical fitness programs for children and youth.

American Medical Association—Adolescents should receive annual counseling about the benefits of exercise and should be encouraged to engage in safe exercise on a regular basis.

Bright Futures—Parents, children, and teenagers should be counseled regarding physical activity using open-ended trigger questions, developmental surveillance questions, and anticipatory guidance.

National Institutes of Health Consensus Panel on Physical Activity and Cardiovascular Health—All Americans should engage in regular physical activity at a level appropriate to their capacity, needs, and interest. Children and adults should set a goal of accumulating at least 30 minutes of moderate-intensity physical activity on most, and preferably, all days of the week.

US Preventive Services Task Force—Clinicians should encourage regular physical activity, encouraging a variety of self-directed, moderate-level physical activities that can be incorporated in an individual's daily routine. The effectiveness of physician counseling to change patients' physical activity behaviors is not proven.

Basics of Physical Activity Counseling

1. Use every office visit as an opportunity to inquire about the physical activity habits of both children and parents. The physical activity levels of parents and parental encouragement of physical activity can strongly influence children.

2. Preschool children generally do not need structured activities to achieve physical fitness; they need only a safe environment in which to express their innate curiosity and natural propensity for active exploration. School-aged children may benefit from participating in more structured activities.

3. Encourage involvement in physical activities for enjoyment, not only for competition. Unpleasant experiences with competition in sports can discourage children from involvement in physical activity.

4. Encourage involvement in physical activities that can be enjoyed into adulthood, such as walking, running, swimming, basketball, tennis, golf, dancing, or bicycle riding.

5. Encourage activities that can easily be incorporated into a child's daily routine and enjoyed all year. Activity levels tend to decrease significantly in the winter months.

6. Counsel children and parents about the importance of engaging in a variety of activities that help develop a range of abilities.

7. Stress the appropriate use of safety equipment, such as helmets and pads.

8. Counsel that the use of cigarettes, alcohol, and other drugs impairs performance and may increase the risk for injuries.

9. Encourage children with functional limitations to participate fully in appropriate physical activities. The American Academy of Pediatrics has issued sports guidelines for children with certain medical conditions (Table 21.1).

10. Advise children and adolescents that they can reduce the risk of musculoskeletal injuries by following proper training techniques, avoiding sudden changes or increases in activity, and having current or prior injuries properly addressed before playing.

11. Advise all adolescents of the dangers of anabolic steroids and other performance-enhancing drugs.

12. Establish an office or clinic environment that conveys the message that physical activity is valued, using posters, pamphlets, and other means.

Table 21.1. Sports Guidelines for Children with Certain Medical Conditions

Condition	May Participate?
Atlantoaxial instability Explanation: Athlete needs evaluation* to assess risk of spinal cord injury during sports participation.	Qualified Yes
Bleeding Disorder Explanation: Athlete needs evaluation*.	Qualified Yes
Cardiovascular diseases Carditis Explanation: Carditis may result in sudden death with exertion.	No
Hypertension Explanation: Those with significant essential hypertension should avoid weight lifting, body building, and strength training. Those with secondary hypertension or severe essential hypertension need evaluation*.	Qualified Yes
Congenital heart disease Explanation: Those with mild forms may participate fully; those with moderate or severe forms, or who have undergone surgery, need evaluation*.	Qualified Yes
Dysrhythmia Explanation: Athlete needs evaluation* because some types require therapy or make certain sports dangerous.	Qualified Yes
Mitral valve prolapse Explanation: Those with symptoms or evidence of mitral regurgitation on physical examination need evaluation*. All others may participate fully.	Qualified Yes
Heart Murmur Explanation: If the murmur is innocent, full participation is permitted. Otherwise the athlete needs evaluation*. (See congenital heart disease and mitral valve prolapse, above.)	Qualified Yes
Cerebral palsy Explanation: Athlete needs evaluation*.	Qualified Yes
Diabetes mellitus Explanation: All sports can be played with proper attention to diet, hydration, and insulin therapy. Particular attention is needed for activities that last 30 minutes or more.	Yes

continued

Table 21.1. Sports Guidelines for Children with Certain Medical Conditions —*Continued*

Condition	May Participate?
Diarrhea	Qualified No

Explanation: Unless disease is mild, no participation is permitted, because diarrhea may increase the risk of dehydration and heat illness. (See Fever, below.)

Eating disorders	
Anorexia nervosa / Bulimia nervosa	Qualified Yes

Explanation: These patients need both medical and psychiatric assessment before participation.

Eyes	
Functionally one-eyed athlete	Qualified Yes
Loss of an eye	
Detached retina	
Previous eye surgery or serious eye injury	

Explanation: A functionally one-eyed athlete has a best corrected visual acuity of <20/40 in the worse eye. These athletes would suffer significant disability if the better eye was seriously injured, as would those with loss of an eye. Some athletes who have previously undergone eye surgery or had a serious eye injury may have an increased risk of injury because of weakened eye tissue. Availability of eye guards approved by the American Society for Testing Materials (ASTM) and other protective equipment may allow participation in most sports, but this must be judged on an individual basis (needs evaluation*).

Fever	No

Explanation: Fever can increase cardiopulmonary effort, reduce maximum exercise capacity, make heat illness more likely, and increase orthostatic hypotension during exercise. Fever may rarely accompany myocarditis or other infections that may make exercise dangerous.

Heat illness, history of	Qualified Yes

Explanation: Because of the increased likelihood of recurrence, the athlete needs evaluation* to determine the presence of predisposing conditions and to arrange a prevention strategy.

HIV Infection	Yes

Explanation: Because of the apparent minimal risk to others, all sports may be played that the state of health allows. In all athletes, skin lesions should be properly covered, and athletic personnel should use universal precautions when handling blood or body fluids.

continued

Table 21.1. Sports Guidelines for Children with Certain Medical Conditions —*Continued*

Condition	May Participate?
Kidney: absence of one	Qualified Yes
Explanation: Athlete needs evaluation* for contact/collision and limited-contact sports.	
Liver: enlarged	Qualified Yes
Explanation: If the liver is acutely enlarged, participation should be avoided because of risk of rupture. If the liver is chronically enlarged, the athlete needs evaluation* before collision/contact or limited-contact sports are played.	
Malignancy	Qualified Yes
Explanation: Athlete needs evaluation*.	
Musculoskeletal disorder	Qualified Yes
Explanation: Athlete needs evaluation*.	
Neurologic	
History of serious head or spine trauma, severe or repeated concussions, or craniotomy.	Qualified Yes
Explanation: Athlete needs evaluation* for collision/contact or limited-contact sports, and also for noncontact sports, if there are deficits in judgement or cognition. Recent research supports a conservative approach to management of concussion.	
Convulsive disorder, well controlled	Yes
Explanation: Risk of convulsion during participation is minimal	
Convulsive disorder, poorly controlled	Qualified Yes
Explanation: Athlete needs evaluation* for collision/contact or limited-contact sports. Avoid the following noncontact sports: archery, riflery, swimming, weight or power lifting, strength training, or sports involving heights. In these sports, occurrence of a convulsion may be a risk to self or others.	
Obesity	Qualified Yes
Explanation: Because of the risk of heat illness, obese persons need careful acclimatization and hydration.	
Organ transplant recipient	Qualified Yes
Explanation: Athlete needs evaluation*.	
Ovary: absence of one	Yes
Explanation: Risk of severe injury to the remaining ovary is minimal.	

continued

Table 21.1. Sports Guidelines for Children with Certain Medical Conditions —Continued

Condition	May Participate?
Respiratory	
Pulmonary compromise, including cystic fibrosis Explanation: Athlete needs evaluation*, but generally all sports may be played if oxygenation remains satisfactory during a graded exercise test. Patients with cystic fibrosis need acclimatization and good hydration to reduce the risk of heat illness.	Qualified Yes
Asthma Explanation: With proper medication and education, only athletes with the most severe asthma will have to modify their participation.	Yes
Acute upper respiratory infection Explanation: Upper respiratory obstruction may affect pulmonary function. Athlete needs evaluation* for all but mild disease. (See Fever, above.)	Qualified Yes
Sickle cell disease Explanation: Athlete needs evaluation*. In general, if status of the illness permits, all but high-exertion, collision/contact sports may be played. Overheating, dehydration, and chilling must be avoided.	Qualified Yes
Sickle cell trait Explanation: It is unlikely that individuals with sickle cell trait have an increased risk of sudden death or other medical problems during athletic participation except under the most extreme conditions of heat, humidity, and possibly increased altitude. These individuals, like all athletes, should be carefully conditioned, acclimatized, and hydrated to reduce any possible risk.	Yes
Skin	
Boils, herpes simplex, impetigo, scabies, molluscum contagiosum Explanation: While the patient is contagious, participation in gymnastics with mats, martial arts, wrestling, or other collision/contact or limited-contact sports is not allowed. Herpes simplex virus probably is not transmitted via mats.	Qualified Yes
Spleen, enlarged Explanation: Patients with acutely enlarged spleens should avoid all sports because of risk of rupture. Those with chronically enlarged spleens need evaluation* before playing collision/contact or limited-contact sports.	Qualified Yes

continued

Table 21.1. Sports Guidelines for Children with Certain Medical Conditions —Continued

Condition	May Participate?
Testicle, absent or undescended	Yes
Explanation: Certain sports may require a protective cup.	

* "Needs evaluation" indicates that a clinician with appropriate medical knowledge and experience should assess the safety of a given sport for an athlete with the listed medical condition. Unless otherwise noted, this is due to either the variability of the severity of the disease or the risk of injury among different sports.

Adapted from: American Academy of Pediatrics, Committee on Sports Medicine and Fitness. Medical Conditions Affecting Sports Participation. Pediatrics. 1994; 94:757-760. Used with permission of the American Academy of Pediatrics, copyright 1994.

Patient Resources

Better Health and Fitness Through Physical Activity; Sports and Your Child. American Academy of Pediatrics, PO Box 927, Elk Grove Village, IL 60009-0927; (800)433-9016. Internet address: http://www.aap.org

Get Fit: A Handbook for Youth Ages 6-17; Kids in Action: Fitness for Children Ages 2-17; Presidential Sports Awards: 4-Month Qualifications for Anyone Ages 6 and Up; The Physician's Rx: Exercise. The President's Council on Physical Fitness and Sports, 701 Pennsylvania Ave, SW, Suite 250, Washington, DC 20004; (202)272-3421.

Anabolic Steroids and Athletes; Nutrition and Sports Performance: A Guide for High School Athletes; Weight Loss and Wrestlers; Youth Fitness. American College of Sports Medicine, Public Information Department, PO Box 1440, Indianapolis, IN 46206-1440; (317)637-9200. Internet address: http://www.acsm.org/sportsmed

Provider Resources

Bright Futures: Guidelines for Health Supervision of Infants, Children and Adolescents; Bright Futures Pocket Guide; Bright Futures Anticipatory Guidance Cards. Available from the National Center for Education in Maternal and Child Health, 2000 15th Street North, Suite 701, Arlington VA, 22201-2617; (703)524-7802. Internet address: http://www.brightfutures.org

Physician-based Assessment and Counseling for Exercise. Project PACE, San Diego State University, San Diego, CA 92182-0567; (619)594-5949.

Sports Medicine: Health Care for Young Athletes, 2nd ed; *Pre-Participation Physical Evaluation,* 2nd ed; *A Self Appraisal Checklist for Health Supervision in Scholastic Athletic Programs.* American Academy of Pediatrics. PO Box 927, Elk Grove Village, IL 60009-0927; (800)433-9016. Internet address: http://www.aap.org

Selected References

American Academy of Family Physicians, *Summary of Policy Recommendations for Periodic Health Examination*. Kansas City, Mo: American Academy of Family Physicians; 1997.

American Academy of Pediatrics, Committee on Psychosocial Aspects of Child and Family Health. *Guidelines for Health Supervision*. 3rd ed. Elk Grove Village, Ill: American Academy of Pediatrics; 1997.

American Academy of Pediatrics, Committee on Sports Medicine and Fitness. Assessing physical activity and fitness in the office setting. *Pediatrics*. 1994;93:686-689.

American Academy of Pediatrics, Committee on Sports Medicine and Fitness. Fitness, activity, and sports participation in the pre-school child. *Pediatrics*. 1992;89:1002-1004.

American Academy of Pediatrics, Committee on Sports Medicine and Fitness. Medical conditions affecting sports participation. *Pediatrics*. 1994;94:757-760.

American Academy of Pediatrics, Committee on Sports Medicine and Fitness. Strength training, weight and power lifting, and body building by children and adolescents. *Pediatrics*. 1990;86:801-803.

American Academy of Pediatrics, Committee on Sports Medicine. Counseling families. In: *Sports Medicine: Health Care for Young Athletes*. Elk Grove Village, Ill: American Academy of Pediatrics; 1983: chap 2.

American College of Sports Medicine. Physical fitness in children and youth. *Med Sci Sports Exerc*. 1988;20:422-423.

American Medical Association. Rationale and recommendation: physical fitness. In: *AMA Guidelines for Adolescent Preventive Services (GAPS): Recommendations and Rationale*. Chicago, Ill: American Medical Association; 1994: chap 6.

Baranowski T, Bouchard C, Bar-Or O, et al. Assessment, prevalence, and cardiovascular benefits of physical activity and fitness in youth. *Med Sci Sports Exerc*. 1992;24(suppl):S237-S247.

Canadian Task Force on the Periodic Health Examination. Physical activity counseling. In: *The Canadian Guide to Clinical Preventive Health Care*. Ottawa, Canada: Minister of Supply and Services; 1994: chap 47.

Green M, ed. *Bright Futures: Guidelines for Health Supervision of Infants, Children, and Adolescents*. Arlington, Va: National Center for Education in Maternal and Child Health; 1994.

Must A, Jacques PF, Dallai GE, Bajema CJ, Dietz WH. Long-term morbidity and mortality of overweight adolescents: a follow-up of the Harvard Growth Study of 1922 to 1935. *N Engl J Med*. 1992;327:1350-1355.

Pate RR, Small ML, Ross JG, Young JC, Flint KH, Warren CW. School Physical Education. *J School Health*. 1995;65(8):312-317.

Physical Activity and Cardiovascular Health. NIH Consensus Statement. Bethesda, Md: National Institutes of Health. 1995:13(3):1-33.

Sallis JF, Simons-Morton BG, Stone EJ, et al. Determinants of physical activity and interventions in youth. *Med Sci Sports Exerc*. 1992;24(suppl):S248-S257.

US Department of Health and Human Services. *Physical Activity and Health: A Report of the Surgeon General*. Atlanta, Ga: US Department of Health and Human Services, Centers for Disease Control and Prevention, National Center for Chronic Disease Prevention and Health Promotion; 1996.

US Preventive Services Task Force. Counseling to promote physical activity. In: *Guide to Clinical Preventive Services*. 2nd ed. Washington, DC: US Department of Health and Human Services; 1996: chap 55.

22

SAFETY

Injuries are the number one cause of death for children in the United States. Each year childhood injuries result in 20,000 deaths, 600,000 hospitalizations, and 16 million visits to emergency rooms, with an associated cost of approximately $165 billion.

Almost half of the injury-related deaths of children involve motor vehicles. Other causes of unintentional childhood injuries are drowning, burns and scalds, choking, firearms, falls, poisoning, and sports.

The vast majority of unintentional childhood injuries are preventable. Children at a higher risk of injury include males, children with previous serious injuries, children in families with low income, and children in families with young mothers. Among adolescents, alcohol and drug use are significant risk factors.

For additional information on safety, refer to chapter 26, which deals with counseling children and adolescents on violent behavior and firearms, and to chapter 55 for information about counseling adults about injury prevention.

Recommendations of Major Authorities

All major authorities, including **American Academy of Pediatrics (AAP), Bright Futures, Canadian Task Force on the Periodic Health Examination,** and **US Preventive Services Task Force**— Age-specific safety counseling should be provided as a part of routine well-child care. **American Academy of Family Physicians** specifies counseling for accidental injury prevention, including (as appropriate) child safety seats, lap and shoulder belt use, bicycle safety, motorcycle helmet use, poison control center numbers, and driving while intoxicated. **AAP** specifies unintentional injury counseling as appropriate for traffic safety, burn prevention, fall prevention, poisoning prevention, drowning, water safety, sports safety, and firearm safety.

American Academy of Pediatrics and **Bright Futures**—Healthy, sleeping infants should be positioned on the back, instead of prone, to decrease the risk of sudden infant death syndrome (SIDS).

Basics of Safety Counseling

Encourage parents to learn basic life-saving skills, including cardiopulmonary resuscitation (CPR).

Counsel parents to teach their children to dial 911 or other local emergency numbers.

Encourage parents to teach their children self-esteem and how to handle peer pressure that might result in risk-taking behavior that may interfere with making good safety decisions.

Encourage parents to be good role models for safe behavior. In particular, counsel parents to avoid drinking alcohol before or while driving, to always wear a seat belt and bicycle helmet, and to drive within the posted speed limit.

Be attentive to issues involving limited parental and community access to resources for child safety. Be aware of programs in your practice community offering affordable, reliable equipment, devices, and assistance for parents of limited means, and have referrals to these sources available at the time of counseling.

Specific Safety Topics

Choking and Suffocation

Advise parents to keep objects that can cause suffocation (such as plastic bags) and choking (such as coins, small toy parts, and certain foods, including whole grapes, gum, peanuts, popcorn kernels and pieces of raw carrots, and hot dogs) away from small children.

Drowning

Inform parents that children can drown in small depths of water such as may be contained in buckets, toilets, bathtubs, and wading pools. Empty and store buckets after use. Never leave infants in the bathtub without supervision.

- Do not allow children to swim alone.

- Advise parents to protect their children from drowning by installing fences around swimming pools/spas; fences should be at least 4 ft (1.2 m) high with completely self-closing gates.

Electrical Safety

Advise parents to keep unused electrical outlets covered with plastic guards or to install breaker outlets. Ground fault interrupter circuits (GFIC) should be used in bathrooms and other areas where water is likely to touch bare skin.

Fall Prevention

- Safety gates: Advise parents to use safety gates (preferably not the accordion type) across stairways (both top and bottom), to install window guards above the first floor, and to move furniture away from upper-story windows so children cannot use the furniture to climb onto the window sill.

- Baby Walkers: Baby walkers are associated with more injuries each year than any other baby product. If they are used, strict supervision must be maintained to avoid falls down stairwells.

Fire and Burn Prevention

- Water heaters: Counsel parents to protect their children from scald burns by reducing the temperature setting of their water heater to 49° C (120° F), if possible, or install anti-scald devices on bathroom and kitchen faucets.

- Smoke detectors : Counsel parents about the importance of using smoke alarms to prevent residential fire injuries. Emphasize proper installation, semiannual battery changes, and monthly checks to make sure they work. Discuss the use of a family fire drill and escape plan.

Firearms

Advise parents about the dangers of keeping a firearm in the home. If a gun is kept in the home, counsel parents to keep it unloaded and locked up separately from the ammunition.

Motor Vehicle Safety

- Car seats: Use of child safety seats is required by law in all 50 states. Counsel parents to install child safety seats in the rear seat of the car, preferably in the middle, and to use them every time children ride. Safety seats should be used until children weigh at least 40 lbs (18 kg). Safety seats should face backward until children weigh at least 20 lbs (9 kg) or reach 1 year of age. Failure to properly secure either the child in the seat or the seat in the car is common; therefore, urge parents to take particular care when securing both.

- Booster seats/Seat belts: Advise parents to have their children sit in the rear seat of cars and to use safety belts every time they ride. Until children grow tall enough so that the lap belt stays low on their hips and the shoulder belt crosses their shoulders or until children's ears come above the top of the vehicle seat back, they should use properly secured booster seats. Remind parents that children should not ride in the cargo areas of pickup trucks, vans, or station wagons.

- Air bags: Infants riding in rear-facing safety seats should never be placed in the front seat of a vehicle equipped with a passenger-side air bag. Children should ride in a car's rear seat. If a vehicle does not have a rear seat, children riding in the front seat should be positioned as far back as possible from an air bag.

- Impaired driving: Advise children and adolescents to avoid riding in a vehicle driven by anyone who has been or is drinking. Counsel adolescents not to drink and drive.

Poison Ingestion

Remind parents to keep medicines and other dangerous substances locked up and in child-resistant containers, to have the local poison control center telephone number posted in a prominent place near the telephone, and to keep a 1-oz bottle of syrup of ipecac at home and to replace it when it reaches its expiration date. Advise parents not to administer syrup of ipecac without first consulting with a poison control center or health care professional.

Pedestrian Safety

Encourage parents to teach and demonstrate pedestrian safety to their children. Remind them that children younger than aged 9 to 12 years need supervision when crossing streets, depending on the density and speed of traffic.

Recreational Safety

- A safety helmet approved by the American National Standards Institute (ANSI), Snell Memorial Foundation, or the American Society for Testing Materials (ASTM) should be worn by all persons every time they ride or are a passenger on a bicycle. Helmets should also be worn while using roller skates, in-line skates, and skateboards.

- Wrist guards, elbow pads, and knee pads should be worn by all children of all ages using roller skates, in-line skates, and skateboards.

- Personal flotation devices should be worn by every child engaged in any boating activity.

Sudden Infant Death Syndrome (SIDS)

Advise parents that positioning sleeping infants on their backs, rather than prone, may decrease the risk of SIDS.

Patient Resources

Auto Safety Hot Line. National Highway Traffic Safety Administration: (800)424-9393.

Child Safety: How to Keep Your Home Safe for Your Baby. American Academy of Family Physicians, 8880 Ward Parkway, Kansas City, MO 64114-2797; (800)944-0000. Internet address: http://www.aafp.org

Fun in the Sun: Keep Your Baby Safe; 1995 Family Shopping Guide To Car Seats: Guidelines for Parents. American Academy of Pediatrics, PO Box 927, Elk Grove Village, IL 60009-0927; (800)433-9016. Internet address: http://www.aap.org

Reduce The Risk of Sudden Infant Death Syndrome (SIDS). Brochures available in English and Spanish. Back to Sleep, PO Box 29111, Washington, DC 20040; (800)505-2742.

Safe Kids Gear Up Guide; How to Protect Your Child From Injury. These and other injury-prevention magazines, brochures, posters, videos, and other materials are available from the National SAFE KIDS Campaign, 1301 Pennsylvania Ave NW, Suite 1000, Washington, DC 20004; (202)662-0600.

US Consumer Product Safety Commission, Publication Requests, Washington, DC 20207. Brochures about preventing injuries from toys, household goods, and other common items. Available in English and Spanish; (800)638-2772.

Provider Resources

Bright Futures: Guidelines for Health Supervision of Infants, Children and Adolescents; Bright Futures Pocket Guide. Available from the National Center for Education in Maternal and Child Health, 2000 15th Street North, Suite 701, Arlington, VA 22201-2617; (703)524-7802. Internet address: http://www.brightfutures.org

Centers for Disease Control and Prevention: National Center for Injury Prevention and Control; Internet address: http://www.cdc.gov/ncipc

The Injury Prevention Program (TIPP). American Academy of Pediatrics, PO Box 927, Elk Grove Village, IL 60009-0927; (800)433-9016. Internet address: http://www.aap.org

A Guide to Safety Counseling in Office Practice; Physician's Resource Guide for Bicycle Safety Education; Injury Prevention for Children and Youth. American

Academy of Pediatrics, PO Box 927, Elk Grove Village, IL 60009-0927; (800)433-9016. Internet address: http://www.aap.org

National Highway Traffic Safety Administration, Office of Occupant Protection, NTS-13, 400 7th St SW, Washington, DC 20590; (202)366-2727.

US Consumer Product Safety Commission, Washington, DC 20207. Recorded messages, in both English and Spanish, (800)638-2772.

Injury Control News. Association for the Advancement of Injury Control, 888 17th St NW, Suite 1000, Washington, DC 20006; (202)296-6161.

Selected References

American Academy of Family Physicians, *Summary of Policy Recommendations for Periodic Health Examination.* Kansas City, Mo: American Academy of Family Physicians; 1997.

American Academy of Pediatrics, Committee on Accident and Poison Prevention. Office-based Counseling for Injury Prevention. *Pediatrics.* 1994;94:566-567.

American Academy of Pediatrics, Committee on Accident and Poison Prevention. Injury prevention. Selecting and using the most appropriate car seats for growing children: Guidelines for counseling parents. *Pediatrics.* 1996;97:761-763.

American Academy of Pediatrics, Committee on Practice and Ambulatory Medicine. Recommendations for pediatric preventive health care. *Pediatrics.* 1995;96:373-374.

American Academy of Pediatrics. *The Injury Prevention Program (TIPP).* Elk Grove Village, Ill: American Academy of Pediatrics; 1989.

American College of Obstetricians and Gynecologists. *Automobile Passenger Restraints for Children and Pregnant Women.* Washington, DC: American College of Obstetricians and Gynecologists; 1991. ACOG Technical Bulletin 151.

American Medical Association. Rationale and recommendation: intentional and unintentional injuries. In: *AMA Guidelines for Adolescent Preventive Services (GAPS): Recommendations and Rationale.* Chicago, Ill: American Medical Association; 1994: chap 4.

Baker SP, O'Neill B, Ginsberg, Li G. *The Injury Fact Book.* New York, NY: Oxford University Press; 1995.

Canadian Task Force on the Periodic Health Examination. Prevention of household and recreational injuries in children (<15 years of age). In: *The Canadian Guide to Clinical Preventive Health Care.* Ottawa, Canada: Minister of Supply and Services; 1994: chap 28.

Canadian Task Force on the Periodic Health Examination. Prevention of motor vehicle accidents. In: *The Canadian Guide to Clinical Preventive Health Care.* Ottawa, Canada: Minister of Supply and Services; 1994: chap 44.

Centers for Disease Control and Prevention. Airbag-associated fatal injuries to infants and children riding in front passenger seats—United States. *MMWR.* 1995;44(45):845-847.

Centers for Disease Control. Childhood injuries in the United States. *Am J Dis Child.* 1990;144:627–646.

Green M, ed. *Bright Futures: Guidelines for Health Supervision of Infants, Children, and Adolescents.* Arlington, Va: National Center for Education in Maternal and Child Health, 1994.

National Committee for Injury Prevention and Control. Injury prevention: meeting the challenge. *Am J Prev Med.* 1989;5(3)(suppl).

US Preventive Services Task Force. Counseling to prevent household and recreational injuries. In: *Guide to Clinical Preventive Services.* Washington, DC: US Department of Health and Human Services; 1996: chap 58.

23

SEXUALLY TRANSMITTED DISEASES AND HIV INFECTION

Sexually transmitted diseases (STDs), including infection with human immunodeficiency virus (HIV), represent a major health problem for adolescents. Approximately 3 million American teenagers acquire an STD annually. According to national surveys of male and female high school students taken in 1990, 1991, 1993, and 1995, the proportion of students who reported being sexually experienced (having ever had sexual intercourse) has remained stable, ranging from 53.0% to 54.2%. In contrast, the percentage of those who reported condom use at last sexual intercourse increased significantly, from 46.2% in 1991 to 54.4% in 1995. Despite the increase in condom use, many adolescents continue to be at risk for STDs, including HIV infection, because they engage in unprotected sexual intercourse.

The consequences of sexually transmitted diseases can be very serious for teenagers. Female adolescents are more susceptible to certain STDs than older adult women because of the histology of their cervix. Gonorrhea and chlamydial infection lead to pelvic inflammatory disease and potential sterility. Although the primary phase of syphilis is relatively asymptomatic, the later stages of this disease may cause great damage to multiple organ systems. Human papilloma virus (HPV) infection, which may be the most prevalent sexually transmitted disease in adolescents, can lead to cervical cancer. Transmission of HIV may be facilitated by the presence of other STDs. During pregnancy, STDs, if left untreated, can lead to serious consequences for the fetus or newborn child, including congenital infection and malformations, prematurity, low birth weight, and increased mortality.

Adolescents at high risk for HIV infection and other STDs include those who: (1) have unprotected intercourse; (2) are homosexual or bisexual males; (3) have been sexually abused by or have had sexual contact with individuals with documented STDs/HIV infection or injection drug use; (4) have a past history of STDs; (5) trade sex for money or drugs; and/or (6) use drugs, particularly if injected, or alcohol.

Refer to chapter 40 for information on screening for STDs and HIV infection. See chapter 59 for information on counseling adults about STDs and HIV infection. See chapters 25 and 61 for related information on counseling adolescents and adults to prevent unintended pregnancy. See chapters 14 and 48 for information about hepatitis B in children and adults, respectively.

Recommendations of Major Authorities

American Academy of Family Physicians—Adolescents should be counseled about the risks for sexually transmitted diseases and how to prevent them.

American Academy of Pediatrics—As a routine part of health supervision, adolescents should be asked about sexual behavior and provided with counseling about responsible sexual behavior, including contraception and prevention of STDs and HIV. Clinicians should encourage abstaining from intercourse as the surest way to prevent STDs, including HIV infection, and pregnancy in adolescents. Adolescents who have been sexually active previously should be counseled regarding the benefits of postponing future sexual relationships. Clinicians should actively support and encourage the use of reliable contraception and condoms by adolescents who are sexually active or contemplating sexual activity. The responsibility of male as well as female adolescents in preventing unintended pregnancies and STDs should be emphasized. Clinicians need to be actively involved in community programs directed toward this goal.

American College of Obstetricians and Gynecologists—Adolescents should be routinely counseled about sexual practices and sexually transmitted diseases, including partner selection and use of barrier protection.

American Medical Association—All adolescents should be asked annually about involvement in sexual behaviors that may result in unintended pregnancy and STDs, including HIV infection. This should include their use of and motivation to use condoms. All sexually active adolescents should be screened for gonorrhea and chlamydia; high-risk adolescents should be screened for syphilis; and HIV testing should be offered to high-risk adolescents.

American Nurses Association—Education about the risks of HIV infection, basic sex information, including the option of abstinence, and the essential features of safer sex practices should be a major priority within community health practice, with a special emphasis in school health settings and school-based clinics.

Canadian Task Force on the Periodic Health Examination—Adolescents should be counseled on sexual activity, and sexually active adolescents should be advised about the correct use of condoms.

US Preventive Services Task Force (USPSTF)—All adolescent and adult patients should be advised about risk factors for sexually transmitted diseases and HIV infection and counseled appropriately about effective measures to reduce risk of infection. This recommendation is based on the proven efficacy of risk reduction, although the effectiveness of clinician counseling in the primary care setting is uncertain. Counseling should be tailored to the individual risk factors, needs, and abilities of each patient. Assessment of risk should be based on a careful sexual and drug use history and consideration of the local epidemiology of STDs and HIV infection. Patients at risk of STDs and HIV infection should receive information on their risk and be advised about measures to reduce their risk. Effective measures include abstaining from sex, maintaining a mutually faithful monogamous sexual relationship with a partner known to be uninfected, regular use of latex condoms, and avoiding sexual contact with high-risk individuals (eg, injection drug users, commercial sex workers, and persons with numerous sex partners). Women at risk of STDs should be advised of options to reduce their risk in situations when their male partner does not use a condom, including the female condom. Warnings should be provided that using alcohol and drugs can increase high-risk sexual behavior. Persons who inject drugs should be referred to available drug treatment facilities, warned against sharing drug equipment and, when possible, referred to sources for uncontaminated injection equipment and condoms. All patients at risk for STDs should be offered testing in accordance with USPSTF recommendations for screening for syphilis, gonorrhea, chlamydia, genital herpes, hepatitis B, and HIV infection (chapter 40).

Basics of STD and HIV Counseling

1. Establish a trusting, caring relationship with both patients and parents. Sensitivity to the cultural and personal needs of patients and families is essential.

2. Counsel parents about the role of emerging sexuality in teenagers' lives and the importance of preventing STDs and HIV infection. Foster effective communication between adolescents and parents regarding responsible, safe sexual behavior.

3. Provide an atmosphere in which adolescents feel comfortable discussing their sexual behaviors. Conduct interviews without parents being present. Explain to both patients and parents the importance and limits of confidentiality in the clinician's relationship with patients.

4. Begin discussing sexual behavior and drug use indirectly by asking patients about the behavior of their friends and peers before moving to an explicit discussion of the patient's own knowledge, attitudes, behaviors, and beliefs. See Tables 18.2 and 59.1 for examples of questions used to take clinical histories about sexual behavior and drug use.

5. Counsel all adolescents that abstinence is the most effective way to prevent STDs and HIV infection. Offer support to adolescents who wish to abstain from sexual activity.

6. Provide explicit education to adolescents about which sexual practices and drug use behaviors will put them and their partners at high risk for STDs and HIV infection and about measures that will minimize risk (eg, use of condoms). Provide explicit education about the long- and short-term consequences of STDs and HIV infections. Provide this education, as appropriate, to preadolescents as well.

7. Ensure that adolescents understand that their partners' sexual and drug behaviors can put them at risk. A thorough drug use history is important not only because HIV and hepatitis B can be transmitted through injection drug use but also because of the "disinhibiting" effects of alcohol and other drug use, which can lead to unsafe behaviors responsible for transmission of STDs and HIV.

8. Contact the state or local health agency responsible for communicable disease reporting to determine the local prevalence of STDs and HIV infection. This agency also can provide information regarding state and local laws regulating testing, confidentiality, and reporting cases of infection. See Appendix C for information on notifiable diseases.

9. Counsel all adolescents about the importance of using condoms properly to prevent STDs and HIV infection (Table 23.1). Many adolescents, particularly those who are younger, are hesitant to purchase condoms on their own. Counsel adolescents about how to purchase condoms and about access to other sources of condoms. Some authorities advocate providing condoms at office visits.

10. Provide educational materials about prevention of STDs and HIV infection to patients and parents. (Patient Resources.)

Table 23.1. Guidelines for Proper Condom Use

Use condoms made of latex rather than natural membrane.

Do not use torn condoms, those in damaged packages, or those with signs of age (brittle, sticky, discolored, past expiration date).

Put the condom on the penis before it touches a partner's mouth, vagina, or anus.

Put the condom on the penis when it is erect. Make sure you have the rim side up so you can unroll it all the way down to the base of the penis, before the penis comes in contact with a body opening.

Leave a space at the tip of the condom to collect semen; remove air pockets in the space by pressing the air out towards the base.

Use only water-based lubricants. Lubricants such as petroleum jelly, mineral oil, cold cream, vegetable oil, or other oils may damage the condom.

Use of Nonoxynol 9 inside the condom or inside the vagina may increase protection against STDs and HIV infection. However, if spermicides cause local irritation, they may increase the risk of HIV infection. Nonoxynol 9 does not give added protection in anal intercourse.

Replace a broken condom immediately.

After ejaculation and while the penis is still erect, withdraw the penis while holding the condom carefully against the base of the penis so that the condom remains in place.

Do not reuse condoms.

Adapted from: Centers for Disease Control and Prevention. Update: barrier protection against HIV infection and other sexually transmitted diseases. *MMWR*. 1993;42:589-591, 597.

Patient Resources

Being a Teenager: You and Your Sexuality; Sexually Transmitted Diseases. American College of Obstetricians and Gynecologists, 409 12th St, SW, Washington, DC 20024-2188; (800)762-2264; Internet address: http://www.acog.com

Sex Education: A Bibliography of Educational Materials for Children, Adolescents, and Their Families. American Academy of Pediatrics, PO Box 927, Elk Grove Village, IL 60009-0927; (800)433-9016; Internet address: http://www.aap.org

The Correct Use of Condoms: A Message to Teens. American Academy of Pediatrics, PO Box 927, Elk Grove Village, IL 60009-0927, (800)433-9016; Internet address: http://www.aap.org

Know the Facts about HIV and AIDS. American Academy of Pediatrics, PO Box 927, Elk Grove Village, IL 60009-0927; (800)433-9016; Internet address: http://www.aap.org

Teenagers and HIV (#329 536); *Children, Parents, and HIV* (#329 540). American Red Cross. Contact your local chapter.

On the Teen Scene: Preventing STDs. Contact the FDA Office of Consumer Affairs. HFE 88 Room 1675, 5600 Fishers Lane, Rockville, MD 20857. (800)532-4440.

Jimmy and the Eggs Virus. To order this parent-information booklet and other materials on pediatric AIDS, contact the National Pediatric HIV Resource Center, 15 S Ninth St, Newark, NJ 07107; (201)268-8251; Internet address: http://www.wdcnet.com/peds.aids

Surgeon General's Report to the American Public on HIV Infection and AIDS; Condoms and Sexually Transmitted Diseases...Especially AIDS. CDC National AIDS Information Hot Line: (800)342-AIDS (English); (800)344-SIDA (Spanish); (800)AIDS-TTY (hearing impaired). All phone calls are confidential.

HIV in America: A Profile of the Challenges Facing Americans Living With HIV. National Association of People Living with AIDS, 1413 K St, NW, Washington, DC 20005; (202)898-0435.

National STD Hot Line: (800)227-8922 or (809)765-1010 (Spanish; call collect).

Provider Resources

Hemophilia and AIDS Network for the Dissemination of Information, 110 Green St, New York, NY 10012. For information on hemophilia and HIV, call: (800)424-2634.

HIV and AIDS in Children: Questions and Answers. National Pediatric HIV Resource Center, 15 S Ninth Street, Newark, NJ 07107; (201)268-8251. Internet address: http://www.wdcnet.com/peds.aids

National AIDS Information Clearinghouse, PO Box 6003, Rockville, MD 20850. To order brochures on STDs, HIV, AIDS, and AIDS-related diseases or a Fact Sheet packet, call: (800)458-5231 (English and Spanish).

Pediatric Human Immunodeficiency Virus (HIV) Infection. American Academy of Pediatrics, PO Box 927, Elk Grove Village, IL 60007-0927, (800)433-9016; Internet address: http://www.aap.org

Adolescent Sexuality: Guidelines to Professional Involvement. American Academy of Pediatrics, PO Box 927, Elk Grove Village, IL 60009-0927, (800)433-9016; Internet address: http://www.aap.org

Selected References

AIDS & Adolescents Network of New York. *HIV Antibody Counseling and Testing for Adolescents: Policy Recommendations and Practical Guidelines.* New York, NY: AIDS & Adolescents Network of New York; 1992.

American Academy of Family Physicians. *Summary of Policy Recommendations for Periodic Health Examination.* Kansas City, Mo: American Academy of Family Physicians; 1997.

American Academy of Pediatrics, Committee on Adolescence. Contraception and adolescents. *Pediatrics.* 1990;86:134-138.

American Academy of Pediatrics, Committee on Adolescence. Homosexuality and adolescence. *Pediatrics.* 1993;92(4);631-634.

American Academy of Pediatrics, Committee on Adolescence. Sexually transmitted diseases. *Pediatrics.* 1994;94(4):901-905.

American Academy of Pediatrics, Committee on Adolescence. Sexuality, contraception, and the media. *Pediatrics.* 1986;78:535-536.

American Academy of Pediatrics, Committee on Psychosocial Aspects of Child and Family Health. *Guidelines for Health Supervision III.* 2nd ed. Elk Grove Village, Ill: American Academy of Pediatrics; 1996.

American Academy of Pediatrics, Committee on School Health. Acquired immunodeficiency syndrome education in schools. *Pediatrics.* 1988;82:278-280.

American College of Obstetricians and Gynecologists. *The Adolescent Obstetric-Gynecologic Patient.* Washington, DC: American College of Obstetricians and Gynecologists; 1990. ACOG Technical Bulletin 145.

American College of Obstetricians and Gynecologists. *Guidelines for Women's Health Care.* Washington, DC: American College of Obstetricians and Gynecologists; 1996.

American Medical Association. *Guidelines for Adolescent Preventive Services (GAPS).* Chicago, Ill: American Medical Association; 1992.

Boekeloo BO, Schamus LA, Simmens SJ, Cheng TL. Tailoring STD/HIV prevention messages for young adolescents. *Academic Medicine.* 1996:71 October Suppl:S97-99.

Boekeloo BO, Schamus LA, Cheng TL, Simmens SJ. Young adolescents' comfort with discussion about sexual problems with their physician. *Archives of Pediatric and Adolescent Medicine.* 1996;150:1146-1152.

Brookman RR. Adolescent Sexual Behavior. In: Holmes KK, Mardh P, Sparling PF, Wiesner PJ, eds. *Sexually Transmitted Diseases.* New York, NY: McGraw-Hill Book Co; 1990: chap 8.

Cates W. The epidemiology and control of sexually transmitted diseases in adolescents. *Adolescent Medicine: State of the Art Reviews.* 1990;1:409-427.

Centers for Disease Control and Prevention. Trends in sexual risk behavior among high school students—United States, 1990, 1991, and 1993. *MMWR.* 1995;44:124-125; 131-132.

Centers for Disease Control and Prevention. CDC surveillance summaries: youth risk behavior surveillance—United States, 1995. *MMWR.* 1996;45 (No. SS-4).

Centers for Disease Control and Prevention. Update: barrier protection against HIV infection and other sexually transmitted diseases. *MMWR.* 1993;42:589–591,597.

Hatcher RA, Stewart F, Trussell J, et al. *Contraceptive Technology 1990-1992.* New York, NY: Irvington Publishers; 1990.

Institute of Medicine. *The Hidden Epidemic: Confronting Sexually Transmitted Diseases.* Eng TR, Butler WT, eds. Washington, DC: National Academy Press, 1997.

US Department of Health and Human Services. Sexually transmitted diseases. In: *Healthy People 2000: National Health Promotion and Disease Prevention Objectives.* Washington, DC: US Department of Health and Human Services, Public Health Service; 1991: chap 19. DHHS publication PHS 91-50212.

US Preventive Services Task Force. Counseling to prevent human immunodeficiency virus infection and other sexually transmitted diseases. In: *Guide to Clinical Preventive Services.* 2nd ed. Washington, DC: US Department of Health and Human Services; 1996: chap 62.

24

TOBACCO

Tobacco use continues to be the single largest cause of preventable illness and death in the United States. Cigarette use is related to heart disease, lung and esophageal cancer, and chronic lung disease. Smokeless tobacco use is associated with numerous cancers, including cancers of the gum, mouth, larynx, pharynx, and esophagus.

The decision to start smoking is often made during the teenage years. Approximately 22% of high school students now report smoking cigarettes daily. However, cigarette smoking is becoming increasingly common among younger children. Surveys indicate that 10% to 25% of children try cigarettes before or during sixth grade. Similarly, use of smokeless or chewing tobacco is increasing among children and adolescents. An estimated 11.4% of high school students use smokeless tobacco. The majority of smokeless tobacco users begin by 13 years of age, and some begin as early as 4 or 5 years of age. Nicotine addiction is rapidly established; therefore, initiation of tobacco use by youth perpetuates tobacco-related chronic health problems in our country. In 1993, smoking-related illnesses cost the nation $50 billion in direct health care costs.

Exposure to environmental tobacco smoke is a potential health hazard for infants and children. An estimated 31.2% of children aged 10 years and younger are exposed to tobacco smoke daily in their homes. Passive smoking can exacerbate the symptoms of asthma and allergies and decrease pulmonary function. The rates of lower respiratory tract infection and middle ear effusions are higher in children who are exposed to environmental tobacco smoke. Each year, an estimated 300,000 children suffer from lower respiratory tract infections attributable to environmental tobacco smoke.

Parental smoking is a risk factor for the initiation of smoking by youth. Children from families in which one or both parents smoke are twice as likely to smoke as are those whose parents do not smoke. See chapter 60 for information about smoking cessation.

Recommendations of Major Authorities

All major authorities, including **American Academy of Family Physicians, American Academy of Pediatrics, American Medical Association, Bright Futures, Canadian Task Force on the Periodic Health Examination, National Cancer Institute, Smoking Cessation Guideline Panel convened by the Agency for Health Care Policy and Research and the Centers for Disease Control and Prevention** and the **US Preventive Services Task Force**—Primary care clinicians should counsel both parents and children about the importance of abstaining from initiating tobacco use and of stopping tobacco use after initiation.

American Academy of Family Physicians—Children, adolescents, and young adults should be counseled on the risks of tobacco use. Parents who smoke while children are in the house should be counseled regarding the harmful effects of smoking on children's health. All tobacco users should be provided with tobacco cessation counseling on a regular basis. Clinicians should discuss nicotine replacement therapy as an adjunct for smoking cessation with patients desiring to quit smoking.

American Academy of Pediatrics and **Bright Futures**—Inquiry into tobacco use and smoke exposure should be a routine part of pediatric health supervision visits. Clinicians should inform parents of the dangers of environmental tobacco smoke and the implications and complications of exposing their children to tobacco smoke. Information about available smoking cessation assistance should be offered. Discussion and anticipatory guidance about smoking and tobacco use should begin well before the patient enters junior high school, with particular emphasis on the importance of resisting the influence of advertising and the peer group. Clinicians should obtain a history of environmental tobacco smoke exposure when encountering a child with a respiratory illness.

American Medical Association—Adolescents should receive annual screening and health guidance to promote avoidance of tobacco use. A cessation plan should be provided for adolescents who use tobacco products.

Canadian Task Force on the Periodic Health Examination— There is good evidence to support counseling for smoking cessation in the periodic health examination for individuals who smoke. There is fair evidence to support counseling to prevent smoking initiation for adolescents. Counseling by physicians has not been evaluated but given the burden of disease, the benefits of preventing addiction, the effectiveness of other smoking-related counseling, and the support of expert opinion, all children and adolescents should be counseled on avoiding tobacco use.

National Cancer Institute—Clinicians treating children should follow five principles that start with the letter A in counseling about smoking prevention/cessation:

1. Anticipate the risk for tobacco use at each developmental stage.

2. Ask about exposure to tobacco smoke and tobacco use at each visit.

3. Advise all smoking parents to stop and all children not to use tobacco products.

4. Assist children in resisting tobacco use; assist tobacco users in quitting.

5. Arrange follow-up visits as required.

US Preventive Services Task Force—Tobacco cessation counseling is recommended on a regular basis to all patients who use tobacco. Parents of children living at home should be counseled on the potential harmful effects of smoking on child health. Anti-tobacco messages should be included in health promotion counseling of children and adolescents based on the proven efficacy of risk reduction from avoiding tobacco use, although the evidence for the effectiveness of clinical counseling to prevent the initiation of tobacco use is less clear. Clinicians should support school-based programs to prevent initiation of tobacco use.

Basics of Tobacco Counseling: Preventing Initiation of Use

1. Maintain a smoke-free environment in the medical office or clinic. Do not permit smoking by staff, patients, or their parents. Post no-smoking signs, and provide literature about the importance of smoking cessation and avoiding tobacco use.

2. Obtain a history for all patients regarding tobacco use in the child's household and day-care or school settings. If parents or other family members smoke, stress the importance of stopping. Emphasizing the negative health consequences for the child can be an effective strategy in dealing with parents.

3. Advise all parents to quit smoking, and support parents who desire to quit smoking, with either counseling or referral (chapter 60). Discourage use of ineffective measures, such as blowing smoke away from a child, attempting to increase ventilation in a room, or smoking in another but contiguous room.

4. Begin in the early elementary school grades to discuss tobacco use and its negative effects. When discussing avoidance of tobacco use or smoking cessa-

tion with children or adolescents, emphasize the unattractive cosmetic (stained teeth and fingernails, oral sores, and foul-smelling breath and clothes) and athletic (decreased endurance, shortness of breath) consequences of tobacco use. Also emphasize the negative social consequences, such as disapproval by peers. Such strategies generally are more effective with children and adolescents than is discussing the long-term health consequences.

5. Elicit information in a nonthreatening manner. Having the parents leave the room is often helpful. Discussion during a physical examination is often well received by children and adolescents. Adolescents may be asked to complete a previsit questionnaire, which is a nonthreatening way to reveal information about tobacco use and other sensitive issues.

Patient Resources

Chew or Snuff Is Real Bad Stuff; Why Do You Smoke? National Cancer Institute. Superintendent of Documents, Consumer Information Center—3C, PO Box 100, Pueblo, CO 81002.

Stop Smoking Kit; Smoking: Steps To Help You Break the Habit. American Academy of Family Physicians, 8880 Ward Parkway, Kansas City, MO 64114-2797; (800)944-0000; Internet address: http://www.aafp.org

Through with Chew. American Academy of Otolaryngology, 1 Prince St, Alexandria, VA 22314; (703)836-4444.

Smoking: Guidelines for Teens; Tobacco Abuse—A Message to Parents and Teens; Straight Talk About Smokeless Tobacco; Smoking: Straight Talk for Teens; Environmental Tobacco Smoke: A Danger for Children. American Academy of Pediatrics, PO Box 927, Elk Grove Village, IL 60009-0927; (800)433-9016; Internet address: http://www.aap.org

Smoking and Reproductive Health; Smoking in Women. American College of Obstetricians and Gynecologists, 409 12th St SW, Washington, DC 20024; (800)762-2264; Internet address: http://www.acog.com

Smokeless Tobacco: Think Before You Chew; Smoking Can Really Do A Number on Your Health. American Dental Association, Department of Salable Materials, 211 E Chicago Ave, Chicago, IL 60611; (800)947-4746.

You Can Quit Smoking: Smoking Cessation Consumer Guide, Clinical Practice Guideline Number 18. Publication number 96-0695. Agency for Health Care Policy and Research, Publications Clearinghouse, PO Box 8547, Silver Spring Md 20907; (800)358-9295, Also available through InstantFAX at (301)594-2800 (push 1 and start, wait for directions); Internet address: http://www.ahcpr.gov

Provider Resources

Bright Futures: Guidelines for Health Supervision of Infants, Children and Adolescents; Bright Futures Pocket Guide; Bright Futures Anticipatory Guidance Cards. Available from the National Center for Education in Maternal and Child Health, 2000 15th Street North, Suite 701, Arlington VA, 22201-2617; (703)524-7802. Internet address: http://www.brightfutures.org

Centers for Disease Control and Prevention Information and Prevention Source Page: http://www.cdc.gov/tobacco

Clinical Interventions To Prevent Tobacco Use by Children and Adolescents. National Cancer Institute; (800)4-CANCER; Internet address: http://wwwicic.nci.nih.gov

Doctors Helping Smokers. For information about this office-based tobacco cessation program and video, contact: Doctors Helping Smokers at Blue Plus, PO Box 64179, R 3-11, St Paul, MN 55164; (800)382-2000, ext 1975.

How To Help Your Patients Stop Smoking: A National Cancer Institute Manual for Physicians; How To Help Your Patients Stop Using Tobacco: A National Cancer Institute Manual for the Oral Health Team. Office of Cancer Communications, National Cancer Institute, Bldg 31, Rm 10A16, Bethesda, MD 20892; (800)4-CANCER; Internet address: http://wwwicic.nci.nih.gov

Helping Smokers Quit: A Guide for Primary Care Clinicians, Clinical Practice Guideline No. 18, AHCPR Publication No. 96-0693. Agency for Health Care Policy and Research, Publications Clearinghouse, PO Box 8547, Silver Spring, MD 20907; (800)358-9295. Also available through InstantFAX at (301)594-2800 (push 1 and start, wait for directions). Internet address: http://www.ahcpr.gov

Nurses: Help Your Patients Stop Smoking. National Heart, Lung, and Blood Institute Smoking Education Program, PO Box 30105, Bethesda, MD 20824-0105; (301)251-1222; Available in both English and Spanish. Internet address:gopher://fido.nhlbi.nih.gov:70/11/nhlbi/health/lung/other/prof/nrsmk

On the Teen Scene: Young People Talk with FDA Commissioner About Smoking. FDA Office of Consumer Affairs, HFE 88 Room 1675, 5600 Fishers Ln, Rockville, MD 20857; (800)532-4440.

Selected References

American Academy of Family Physicians. *Summary of Policy Recommendations for Periodic Health Examination.* Kansas City, Mo: American Academy of Family Physicians; 1997.

American Academy of Pediatrics, Committee on Environmental Hazards. Involuntary smoking—a hazard to children. *Pediatrics.* 1986;77:755-757.

American Academy of Pediatrics, Committee on Environmental Hazards. Smokeless tobacco—a carcinogenic hazard to children. *Pediatrics.* 1985;75:1009-1011.

American Academy of Pediatrics, Committee on Substance Abuse. Tobacco-free environment: an imperative for the health of children and adolescents. *Pediatrics.* 1994;93:866-868.

American Medical Association. Rationale and recommendations: use of tobacco products. In: *AMA Guidelines for Adolescent Preventive Services (GAPS): Recommendations and Rationale.* Chicago, Ill: American Medical Association; 1994: chap. 10.

Canadian Task Force on the Periodic Health Examination. Prevention of tobacco-caused disease. In: *The Canadian Guide to Clinical Preventive Health Care.* Ottawa, Canada: Minister of Supply and Services; 1994: chap 43.

Centers for Disease Control and Prevention. Health-care provider advice on tobacco use to persons aged 10-22 years—United States, 1993. *MMWR.* 1995;44:826-830.

Centers for Disease Control and Prevention. United States, Youth Risk Behavior Survey, 1995. In: Tobacco use and usual source of cigarettes among high school students-United States, 1995. *MMWR.* 1996;45(20):413-418.

Epps RP, Manley MW. *Clinical Interventions to Prevent Tobacco Use by Children and Adolescents.* Bethesda, Md: National Cancer Institute, US Department of Health and Human Services; 1991.

Epps RP, Manley MW. A physician's guide to preventing tobacco use during childhood and adolescence. *Pediatrics.* 1991;88:140-144.

Fiore MC, Bailey WC, Cohen SJ, et al. *Smoking Cessation. Clinical Practice Guideline No. 18.* Rockville, Md: US Department of Health and Human Services, Public Health Service, Agency for Health Care Policy and Research. AHCPR Publication No. 96-0692. April 1996.

Green M, ed. *Bright Futures: Guidelines for Health Supervision of Infants, Children, and Adolescents.* Arlington, Va: National Center for Education in Maternal and Child Health, 1994.

Mannino DM, Siegel M, Husten C, et al. Environmental tobacco smoke exposure and health effects in children: results from the 1991 National Health Interview Survey. *Tobacco Control.* 1996;5:13-18.

McGinnis JM, Shopland D, Brown C. Tobacco and health: trends in smoking and smokeless tobacco consumption in the United States. *Annu Rev Public Health.* 1987;8:441-467.

Schonberg KS, ed. *Substance Abuse: A Guide for Health Professionals.* Elk Grove Village, Ill: American Academy of Pediatrics; 1988.

University of Michigan. *Cigarette Smoking Continues to Rise Among American Teenagers in 1996.* Ann Arbor, Mich: The University of Michigan News and Information Services; December 19, 1996, news release, Monitoring the Future project.

US Department of Health and Human Services, Office of Inspector General. *Spit Tobacco and Youth.* Washington, DC: US Government Printing Office; 1992.

US Preventive Services Task Force. Counseling to prevent tobacco use. In: *Guide to Clinical Preventive Services.* 2nd ed. Washington, DC: US Department of Health and Human Services; 1996: chap 54.

25

UNINTENDED PREGNANCY

The rate of pregnancies among teenagers in the United States currently exceeds that of any other country in the western world. During the year 1990, one in 10 female adolescents in the United States aged 15 to 19 years became pregnant. Of teenage pregnancies, approximately 95% are unintended, and 40% are terminated by elective abortion. Among nonwhite teenagers, the rates of unintended pregnancies are nearly twice those of white teenagers. Young women with the least familial, educational, and financial resources are the most likely to become pregnant. As a result, teenage pregnancies are more likely than adult pregnancies to result in adverse health outcomes for both mother and baby, largely because of prenatal care delays, poor nutrition, and other lifestyle factors.

Recent data reveal a decrease in teenage sexual activity in the United States, with a concurrent increase in the rate of teenage contraceptive use. Previous surveys had demonstrated an increasing trend in teenage sexual activity since the 1970s. In 1995, 50% of females and 55% of males aged 15 to 19 years reported ever having sexual intercourse. These figures represent a decline from prior years (down from 55% of females in 1990 and 60% of males in 1988).

Approximately two-thirds of teenagers report using contraception (almost exclusively condoms) during their first sexual intercourse, and 78% report contraception usage during their most recent sexual intercourse. Younger adolescents are the least likely to use a contraceptive method when compared with either older teenagers or young adults.

See chapter 61 for information on counseling to prevent unintended pregnancy in adults. See chapters 23 and 59 for related information on counseling to prevent sexually transmitted diseases (STDs) and human immunodeficiency virus (HIV) infection among adolescents and adults, respectively. See chapters 14 and 48 for related information on hepatitis B in children and adults.

Recommendations of Major Authorities

All major authorities, including **American Academy of Pediatrics (AAP), American College of Obstetricians and Gynecologists (ACOG), American Medical Association (AMA), Canadian Task Force on the Periodic Health Examination,** and **US Preventive Services Task Force (USPSTF)**—Primary care providers should routinely counsel adolescents in the prevention of unintended pregnancies. **AAP** recommends that all pediatricians who choose to see teenagers should be able to provide counseling about sexual behavior, education on contraceptive methods and prevention of STDs, and assistance with access to contraception, preferably in the office or, if necessary, by referral. **ACOG** recommends that special attention be given to ensure that sexually active adolescents have access to suitable methods of contraception. **AMA** recommends that all adolescents should be asked annually about involvement in sexual behaviors that may result in unintended pregnancy and STDs, including HIV infection. **USPSTF** recommends that counseling be based on information from a careful history that includes direct questions about sexual history, current and past use of contraception, level of concern about pregnancy, and past history of unintended pregnancies. The **USPSTF** also recommends that clinicians inform adolescent patients that abstinence is the most effective way to prevent unintended pregnancy and sexually transmitted diseases; the effectiveness of abstinence counseling has not yet been established. Clinicians should involve young pubertal patients (and their parents, when appropriate) in early, open discussion of sexual development and effective methods to prevent unintended pregnancy and sexually transmitted diseases.

Basics of Counseling To Prevent Unintended Pregnancy

1. Ask all adolescents about their sexual experiences and use of contraceptives. Attempt to maintain a nonjudgmental, empathetic manner. This discussion can begin with questions about the patient's peer group before moving on to more explicit questions about the patient's own sexual behavior. State your willingness to answer any questions and to provide contraceptive advice and prescriptions. Provide adolescents with explicit information about the consequences of pregnancy and STDs and about effective methods to prevent them.

2. Counsel adolescents individually, assuring the patient that you will maintain confidentiality to the maximum extent possible. State laws vary regarding the minimum age at which an adolescent may consent to treatment, receive prescription contraceptives, or both. Become familiar with the laws in your state regarding these issues. Inform adolescents about their legal rights to confidentiality regarding pregnancy prevention and STD testing and treatment.

3. Counsel parents about the role of emerging sexuality in teenagers' lives, desire for privacy, and the options for contraception. Fostering effective communication between adolescents and their families regarding responsible sexual behavior is very important.

4. Support the decision of adolescents who choose to be sexually abstinent.

5. All patients should be encouraged and supported in their efforts to resist unwelcome or coercive sexual relationships.

6. Assist sexually active adolescents in choosing an effective, appropriate primary method of contraception. The choice should take into consideration the patients' personal preferences and motivation, religious beliefs, cultural norms, and relationship with their partner(s).

   See Table 61.1 for the pregnancy ("failure") rates of women during the first year of contraceptive use. The two most popular contraceptive methods among adolescents are oral contraceptives and condoms. Oral contraceptives can confer the benefits of less painful menstrual periods and regular, predictable cycles. Implants or injectable contraceptives may also be appropriate choices for teens. In general, diaphragms, cervical caps, withdrawal, and periodic abstinence are technically more difficult methods for teenagers to use effectively. Intrauterine devices (IUDs) are not recommended for adolescents because of the increased risk of pelvic inflammatory disease, which may lead to sterility. Permanent sterilization procedures are not appropriate for adolescents and are prohibited for individuals under age 21 years when Federal funds are involved. In situations of unprotected intercourse, suggesting use of emergency oral contraceptives (morning-after pills) may be appropriate if treatment can be initiated within 72 hours after sexual contact. See chapter 61 for a discussion on emergency contraception.

7. Encourage all sexually active adolescents to use condoms as a means of preventing STDs and HIV infection, even if they are using another form of contraception. Stress that latex condoms used consistently and correctly are an effective method for both pregnancy protection and disease prevention. Many teenagers, particularly those at younger ages, are hesitant to purchase condoms. Educating teenagers about their rights to purchase condoms and about access to other sources of condoms can be helpful. Some authorities recommend making condoms available to teenagers during office visits.

8. Encourage adolescents of both sexes to talk frankly with their partners about STDs, HIV, and hepatitis B infection, and the use of contraceptives. Encourage adolescents to be assertive with their partners about using contraception and protective measures against STDs. Also stress that saying "no," is every person's right each and every time.

9. Provide male adolescents with as much counseling as that provided to females about contraception and STD prevention. Instruct young adolescent males about responsible sexual behavior at an early age, particularly regarding the importance of condom use.

10. Provide adolescents with close follow-up after they begin using contraceptives. Adolescents often discontinue contraceptive use unnecessarily because of concerns about side effects and misconceptions about proper technique. Many such concerns and misconceptions can be easily dealt with in follow-up counseling. Table 25.1 provides sample responses to some common concerns of adolescents about oral contraceptives.

Table 25.1. Addressing Adolescents' Common Concerns About Oral Contraceptives

Concern	Response
Weight gain	Women are as likely to lose weight as gain weight while using oral contraceptives.
Irregular bleeding	This is a common side effect that tends to resolve after a few cycles of use if oral contraceptives are taken consistently and at the same time each day.
Nausea, acne, vaginal discharge	These are uncommon side effects. They can usually be eliminated by changing to a different type of pill.
Cancer risk	Oral contraceptive use decreases risk of endometrial and ovarian cancer. An increased risk of breast cancer is unproven.
Sexually transmitted diseases	Oral contraceptive use does not prevent STDs but does decrease the risk of developing pelvic inflammatory disease. Latex condoms are the only form of birth control that can help prevent STDs and HIV infection.
Ovarian cysts, benign breast disease	The incidence and severity of these are decreased by oral contraceptive use.
Blood clots	While the risk of thromboembolism in oral contraceptive users may be increased over that of the general population, the risk to teenagers, especially those who do not smoke, is minimal.

Adapted from: American College of Obstetricians and Gynecologists. Safety of Oral Contraceptives for Teenagers. Washington, DC: American College of Obstetricians and Gynecologists; 1991. ACOG Committee Opinion No 90. Reproduced by permission of the publisher; copyright © 1991.

Patient Resources

Being a Teenager: You and Your Sexuality; Teaching Your Children About Sexuality, Growing Up. American College of Obstetricians and Gynecologists, 409 12th St SW, Washington, DC 20024; (800)762-2264. Internet address: http://www.acog.com

Birth Control: Choosing the Method That's Right for You. American Academy of Family Physicians, 8880 Ward Pkwy, Kansas City, MO 64114-2797; (800)944-0000. Internet address: http://www.aafp.org

Emergency Contraception Website. The Office of Population Research at Princeton University. Internet address: http://opr.princeto.edu.ec/ec.html

Emergency Contraception Hotline. The Office of Population Research at Princeton University. (800)584-9911.

How to Talk With Your Child About Sexuality, Decisions About Sex; How to Talk to Your Teenagers About the Facts of Life. Planned Parenthood, 810 Seventh Ave, New York, NY 10019; (212)541-7800.

Making the Right Choice: Facts Young People Need to Know About Avoiding Pregnancy; Talking to Your Teen About Sex; The Correct Use of Condoms: A Message to Teens. American Academy of Pediatrics, 141 Northwest Point Blvd, PO Box 927, Elk Grove Village, IL 60009-0927; (800)433-9016. Internet address: http://www.aap.org

Provider Resources

The Adolescent and Young Adult Fact Book; Evaluating Your Adolescent Pregnancy Program: How to Get Started; Teenage Pregnancy Prevention Strategies; What About the Boys? Children's Defense Fund, 25 E St NW, Washington, DC 20001; (202)628-8787.

Selected References

Abma J, Chandra A, Mosher W, et al. *Fertility family planning, and women's health: new data from the 1995 National Survey of Family Growth.* National Center for Health Statistics. Vital Health Stat 23(19); 1997.

American Academy of Family Physicians. *Summary of Policy Recommendations for Periodic Health Examination.* Kansas City, Mo: American Academy of Family Physicians; 1997.

American Academy of Pediatrics. Counseling the Adolescent About Pregnancy Options. *Pediatrics.* 1989;83:135-137.

American Academy of Pediatrics. Committee on Adolescence: Contraception and Adolescents. *Pediatrics.* 1990;86:134-138.

American Academy of Pediatrics. Committee on Adolescence: condom availability and youth. *Pediatrics.* 1995;95:281-285.

American College of Obstetricians and Gynecologists. *Safety of Oral Contraceptives for Teenagers.* Washington, DC: American College of Obstetricians and Gynecologists; 1991. ACOG Committee Opinion No. 90.

American College of Obstetricians and Gynecologists. *The Adolescent Obstetric-Gynecologic Patient.* Washington, DC: American College of Obstetricians and Gynecologists; 1990. ACOG Technical Bulletin No. 145.

American Medical Association. Rationale and recommendations: psychosexual development and the negative health consequences of sexual behavior. In: *AMA Guidelines for Adolescent Preventive Services (GAPS): Recommendations and Rationale.* Chicago, Ill: American Medical Association; 1994: chap 7.

Canadian Task Force on the Periodic Health Examination. Prevention of unintended pregnancy and sexually transmitted diseases in adolescents. In: *The Canadian Guide to Clinical Preventive Health Care.* Ottawa, Canada: Minister of Supply and Services; 1994: chap 46.

Canadian Task Force on the Periodic Health Examination. The periodic health examination: 2. 1987 update. *Can Med Assoc J.* 1988;138:618-626.

Centers for Disease Control. Sexual behavior among high school students: United States, 1990. *MMWR.* 1991;40:85-88.

Center for Population Options. *Teenage Pregnancy and Too-Early Childbearing: Public Costs, Personal Consequences.* 5th ed. Washington, DC: Center for Population Options; 1990.

Hatcher RA, Stewart F, Trussell J, et al. *Contraceptive Technology 1994-1996 16th rev. ed.* New York, NY: Irvington Publishers, 1996.

Hatcher RA, Trussell J, Stewart F, et al. *Contraceptive Technology.* 17th rev ed. New York, NY: Irvington Publishers; 1998, in press.

Healthy People 2000: Midcourse Review and 1995 Revisions. Washington, DC: US Department of Health and Human Services. Public Health Service; 1995.

Spitz AM, Velbil P, Koonin LM, et al. Pregnancy, abortion, and birth rates among US adolescents-1908, 1985, and 1990. *JAMA.* 1996;275:989-994.

US Preventive Services Task Force. Counseling to prevent unintended pregnancy. In: *Guide to Clinical Preventive Services.* 2nd ed. Washington, DC: US Department of Health and Human Services; 1996: chap 63.

Ventura SJ, Taffel SM, Mosher WD, Henshaw S. Trends in pregnancies and pregnancy rates, United States, 1980-88. *Monthly Vital Statistics Report.* Hyattsville, Md: National Center for Health Statistics. 1993;41:6(suppl). US Department of Health and Human Services publication PHS 93-1120.

26

VIOLENT BEHAVIOR AND FIREARMS

Violence is a major health and social problem affecting children and adolescents in the United States. Homicide is the second leading cause of death among all 15- to 24-year-olds. For African-American males and females aged 15 to 24 years and Hispanic males aged 15 to 24 years, homicide is the leading cause of death. Firearms are involved in more than two thirds of homicides involving children and adolescents. A high percentage (41%) of school-aged boys report having easy access to a gun; handguns are in one of every four homes in the United States. According to Kellerman (1986), for every report of a gun being used in self-defense within the home, 40 shooting deaths of family members or acquaintances, by suicide, nonjustifiable homicide, and accidents, are reported.

For adolescent males, the risk of dying as a result of homicide is more than twice that of adolescent females, and their risk of victimization from other violent crimes is three times greater. However, adolescent females should not be overlooked as victims of violence, in particular dating violence, sexual assault, and rape. Urban adolescents, both males and females, of low socioeconomic status and low educational achievement are at greatest risk of being affected by violence. Other risk factors include a history of juvenile detention or incarceration, alcohol or other drug use, access to firearms, homelessness, mental illness, social isolation, and violence in the home. The risk factors for victims and perpetrators of violence are similar.

For information about depression and suicide, see chapter 5 (for children and adolescents) and chapter 33 (for adults). For information about alcohol and other drug abuse, see chapter 18 (for children and adolescents) and chapter 53 (for adults). For information about safety and injury prevention, see chapter 22 (for children and adolescents) and chapter 55 (for adults).

Recommendations of Major Authorities

American Academy of Pediatrics and **Bright Futures**—Children, adolescents, and their parents should be questioned about impulsiveness, antisocial behavior, and methods of dealing with anger. The clinician should be concerned about adolescents who display aggressive or acting-out behaviors, such as lying, stealing, temper outbursts, vandalism, excessive fighting, and destructiveness. Health-care providers should encourage families who own firearms to create a gun-safe home environment, with particular emphasis placed on high-risk homes—those with alcohol or drug-prone or drug-addicted individuals and those with adolescent boys. This should include asking about the presence of guns in the home; counseling patients, parents, and relatives (particularly male relatives) on the dangers of having a gun, especially a handgun, in the home; advising the removal or a reduction in the number of guns in the household; providing office literature on the risks of guns; and emphasizing gun safety rules when patients visit friends' homes. Asking about the presence of a gun in the home and, if one is present, counseling on its removal or secured storage may be the most effective action the primary care clinician can take.

American Medical Association—Parents or other adult care-givers of adolescents should be given health guidance during their children's early, middle, and late adolescence (more often if necessary) to avoid having weapons in the home and, if weapons are kept in the home, to make them inaccessible to adolescents. Adolescents should be counseled to avoid the use of weapons. Weapons should be removed from homes of adolescents with suicidal intent.

US Preventive Services Task Force—There is currently insufficient evidence to recommend for or against clinician counseling to prevent morbidity and mortality from youth violence. Adolescent patients should be screened for problem drinking. Clinicians may wish to inform patients (and the parents of child and adolescent patients) of the risk to household members associated with the presence of firearms in the home. Clinicians should also be alert for symptoms and signs of drug abuse and dependence, the various presentations of family violence, and suicidal ideation in persons with established risk factors. In settings where the prevalence of violence is high, clinicians should ask adolescents and young adults about previous violent behavior or victimization, current alcohol and drug use, and the availability of handguns and other firearms. Clinicians should inform those identified as being at high risk for violence about the risks of violent injury associated with easy access to firearms and with intoxication with alcohol or other drugs.

Basics of Counseling about Violent Behavior and Firearms

1. Make preventing violence-related injuries a priority. Assess every child and family for the potential for injury from violence. Factors to consider include:

   Is there a history of violent injury to the child or other family members?

Is there a history of alcohol or other drug abuse by the child or other family members?

Are guns or other weapons kept in the home?

Are violence-related injuries prevalent in the community?

2. Advise all parents about the dangers of keeping a gun in the home. This advice may be better accepted if it is given as part of general counseling on safety-related issues. The following model intervention has been suggested by the American Academy of Pediatrics and the Center To Prevent Handgun Violence (1994):

> You are doing all you can to make sure your children are not hurt—by using a car seat, buckling up safety belts in the car, locking away poisonous chemicals, and putting safety latches on kitchen cabinets. Along with these safety measures, I urge you to take another. Easy-to-reach, loaded guns at home are risky. The safest thing for your family is not to have a gun at home. If you keep a gun at home, be sure to empty it out and lock it up at all times. Lock and store the bullets in a separate location.

From: American Academy of Pediatrics, Center To Prevent Handgun Violence. STOP: Steps to Prevent Firearm Injury. Washington, DC: Center To Prevent Handgun Violence; 1996, 2nd edition. Reproduced by permission of the publisher; copyright 1996.

3. Urge parents who keep a gun in the home to follow basic rules of safety:

Never keep a loaded gun in the house or car.

Keep guns and ammunition locked in separate places.

Always treat a gun as if it were loaded and ready to fire.

Never allow children access to guns.

Have a gunsmith check antique and souvenir guns to be sure they are not loaded. Fix these guns so they cannot be fired.

From: American Academy of Pediatrics, Committee on Injury Control for Children and Youth. Firearms. In: Injury Control for Children and Youth. Elk Grove Village, Ill: American Academy of Pediatrics; 1987. Reproduced by permission of the American Academy of Pediatrics; copyright 1987.

4. Advise parents to inquire about the availability of guns in places their children spend time, such as at friends' houses, schools, and recreation facilities. Suggest to parents that limiting their children's access to these places may be wise until guns are no longer available. Encourage parents to take an active role in limiting the availability of guns in their children's environment.

5. Asking first about violence in an adolescent's environment (at school, at friends' houses) before asking specifically about their personal experiences may be less threatening.

6. When treating patients who have injuries that may have been caused by violence, ask specific questions about the cause of the injury. If the injury was caused by violence, attempt to determine if the conflict has been settled or has the potential to lead to further violence. The following sample questions have been suggested for use in this situation*:

   Have you settled it?

   Is there anyone who can settle this—someone who can talk for you and explain your side?

   Do you know where to go if this is not settled?

   Are you safe?

7. Despite the desirability of maintaining confidentiality, consulting parents, police, and other authorities may be necessary to protect the safety of children and adolescents involved in potentially violent situations.

8. Ask patients about ways in which they deal with anger*.

   Emphasize that anger is a normal emotion.

   Encourage young people to consider alternative ways of dealing with anger.

   Offer positive ways to deal with anger and arguments, the leading precipitators of homicide.

*From: Violence Prevention Project. Identification and Prevention of Youth Violence: A Protocol for Health Care Providers. Boston, Mass: Violence Prevention Project, Department of Health & Hospitals; 1992. Reproduced by permission of the publisher; copyright 1992.

9. Provide facts about violence with a variety of media in the office or clinic, such as posters, videotapes, and brochures.

10. Encourage participation in activities aimed at ensuring safe communities.

Patient Resources

Raising Children to Resist Violence: What You Can Do; Child Sexual Abuse: What It Is and How to Avert It. American Academy of Pediatrics, 141 Northwest Point Blvd, PO Box 927, Elk Grove Village, IL 60009-0927; (800)433-9016; Internet address: http://www.aap.org

The Abused Woman. American College of Obstetricians and Gynecologists, 409 12th St SW, Washington, DC 20024-2188; (202)638-5577; Internet address: http://www.acog.com

What Can You Do About Family Violence? (#NC110992) American Medical Association, 515 N State St, Chicago, IL 60610; (800)621-8335; Internet address: http://www.ama-assn.org

STOP: Steps to Prevent Firearm Injury. American Academy of Pediatrics and the Center To Prevent Handgun Violence. To order, contact the Center To Prevent Handgun Violence, 1225 I St NW, Suite 1100, Washington, DC 20005; (202)289-7319.

Provider Resources

Bright Futures: Guidelines for Health Supervision of Infants, Children and Adolescents; Bright Futures Pocket Guide; Bright Futures Anticipatory Guidance. Available from the National Center for Education in Maternal and Child Health, 2000 15th Street North, Suite 701, Arlington VA, 22201-2617; (703)524-7802. Internet address: http://www.brightfutures.org

Identification and Prevention of Youth Violence: A Protocol for Health Care Providers; Assessment and Treatment of Hospitalized Adolescent Victims of Interpersonal Violence. These materials, audiotapes, slides, a script on the process of interviewing youth on violence-related issues, and office posters on violence prevention are available from the Adolescent Wellness Program (formerly the Violence Prevention Project), Department of Health & Hospitals, 1010 Massachusetts Ave, 2nd Floor, Boston, MA 02118; (617)534-5196.

Diagnostic and Treatment Guidelines on Domestic Violence. American Medical Association, Department of Mental Health, 515 N State St, Chicago, IL 60610; (312)464-5066. Internet address: http://www.ama-assn.org

Selected References

American Academy of Family Physicians. *Summary of Policy Recommendations for Periodic Health Examination.* Kansas City, Mo: American Academy of Family Physicians; 1997.

American Academy of Pediatrics, Center To Prevent Handgun Violence. *Rx for Safety: Preventing Firearms Injuries Among Children and Adolescents.* Washington, DC: Center To Prevent Handgun Violence; 1992.

American Academy of Pediatrics, Committee on Adolescence. Firearms and adolescents. *Pediatrics.* 1992;89:784-787.

American Academy of Pediatrics, Committee on Injury and Poison Prevention. Firearm injuries affecting the pediatric population. *Pediatrics.* 1992;89:788-790.

American Academy of Pediatrics, Committee on Injury Control for Children and Youth. Firearms. In: *Injury Control for Children and Youth.* Elk Grove Village, Ill: American Academy of Pediatrics; 1987.

American Academy of Pediatrics, Committee on Psychosocial Aspects of Child and Family Health. *Guidelines for Health Supervision.* 2nd ed. Elk Grove Village, Ill: American Academy of Pediatrics; 1988.

American Medical Association. Rationale and recommendations: intentional and unintentional injuries. In: *AMA Guidelines for Adolescent Preventive Services (GAPS): Recommendations and Rationale.* Chicago, Ill: American Medical Association; 1994: chap 4.

American Psychiatric Association Task Force. *Clinical Aspects of the Violent Individual.* Washington, DC: American Psychiatric Association; 1974.

Centers for Disease Control. Weapon-carrying among high school students. *MMWR.* 1991;40:681.

Children's Safety Network. *A Data Book of Child and Adolescent Injury.* Washington, DC: National Center for Education in Maternal and Child Health; 1991.

Christoffel KK. Violent death and injury in US children and adolescents. *Am J Dis Child.* 1990;144:697-706.

Cohall AT, Mayer R, Cohall K, et al. Teen violence: the reasons why. *Contemporary Pediatrics.* October 1991:54-77.

Cohall AT, Mayer R, Cohall K, et al. Teen violence: the new mortality. *Contemporary Pediatrics.* September 1991:76-86.

Gardner P, Rosenberg HM, Wilson RW. *Leading Causes of Death by Age, Sex and Hispanic Origin: United States 1992.* National Center for Health Statistics. Vital Health Statistics 1996; 20 (29).

Green M, ed. *Bright Futures: Guidelines for Health Supervision of Infants, Children, and Adolescents.* Arlington, Va: National Center for Education in Maternal and Child Health; 1994.

Kellerman AL, Reay DT Protection or Peril? An Analysis of Firearm-Related Deaths in the Home. *N Engl J Med.* 1986; 31 14(24):1557-1560.

Rosenberg ML, Gelles RJ, Holinger PC, et al. Violence: homicide, assault, and suicide. In: Amber RW, Dull HB, eds. *Closing the Gap: The Burden of Unnecessary Illness.* New York, NY: Oxford University Press; 1987.

Singh GK, Kochanek KD, MacDorman MF. Advance Report of Final Mortality Statistics, 1994. *Monthly Vital Statistics Report.* 1996;45(3,S) pp 23, 31, 32.

US Department of Health and Human Services, US Department of Justice. *Report of the Surgeon General's Workshop on Violence and Public Health.* Leesburg, Va: Health Resources and Services Administration, US Department of Health and Human Services; 1986.

US Preventive Services Task Force. Counseling to prevent youth violence. In: *Guide to Clinical Preventive Services.* 2nd ed. Washington, DC: US Department of Health and Human Services; 1996: chap 59.

Adults and Older Adults

27

ANEMIA AND HEMOGLOBINOPATHIES

Anemia in adults, defined as a hemoglobin level below the 5th percentile of the reference distribution range for age and gender, is most prevalent in young women (4.5%) and elderly men (4.8%). Anemia is also more common in individuals of low socioeconomic status and in African Americans. Common causes of anemia include iron and vitamin deficiencies (folate and vitamin B-12), occult blood loss, chronic illness, and hemoglobinopathies. Although most forms of anemia are treatable, the benefits of treating asymptomatic individuals are unclear. For this reason, most authorities either recommend against routine screening of adults for anemia or recommend screening only high-risk adults (eg, elderly men, pregnant women, adults with chronic disease).

The hemoglobinopathies are genetic disorders that affect the production and function of hemoglobin molecules. These disorders include sickle cell disease and trait, the thalassemias, and other rarer conditions. Hemoglobinopathies tend to occur in defined ethnic and racial groups, predominantly African Americans in this country. However, they are also found in individuals of Caribbean, Latin American, Asian, and Mediterranean descent. Approximately 50,000 African Americans are affected by sickle cell disease, and another 2 million carry the trait. Fewer than 1000 Americans have beta-thalassemia major, but sizable numbers of Italian Americans, Greek Americans, and immigrants from Southeast Asia carry the genetic trait. In adult populations, screening is useful primarily for providing preconception and prenatal genetic counseling to carriers.

See chapters 1 and 8 for discussions about screening for anemia and hemoglobinopathies in children and adolescents.

Recommendations of Major Authorities

Screening for Anemia

American College of Physicians—Routine screening for anemia is not recommended in adults without clinical indications.

American College of Obstetricians and Gynecologists—
Hemoglobin levels should be measured as part of routine preventive care
for women with a history of excessive menstrual flow and for women 65
years of age or older at high risk.

US Preventive Services Task Force—There is insufficient evidence to
recommend for or against routine screening of asymptomatic, nonpregnant adults, although recommendations against can be made on the
grounds of low prevalence, cost, and potential adverse effects of iron
therapy.

Screening for Hemoglobinopathies

American College of Obstetricians and Gynecologists—Screening
should be provided to women of reproductive age who are of Caribbean,
Latin American, Asian, Mediterranean, or African descent.

Canadian Task Force on the Periodic Health Examination—A
family and genetic history should be obtained from all patients of
Mediterranean, African, Middle Eastern, East Indian, Hispanic, or Asian
ancestry who may become parents. Screening with hemoglobin electrophoresis or thin layer isoelectric focusing is recommended for pregnant, at-risk women but not for other adults.

US Preventive Services Task Force—There is insufficient evidence to
recommend for or against screening for hemoglobinopathies by
hemoglobin electrophoresis in young adults from ethnic and racial
groups known to be at increased risk for sickle cell disease, thalassemias,
and other hemoglobinopathies in order for them to be able to make informed reproductive choices. Recommendations to offer such testing may
be made on other grounds, including burden of suffering and patient
preference. If provided, testing should be accompanied by counseling,
which should include a description of the significance of the disease,
how it is inherited, the availability of a screening test, and the implications to the individual and their offspring of a positive result.

Basics of Screening for Anemia and Hemoglobinopathies

Anemia

1. The primary screening tests for anemia are measurements of hemoglobin
   (Hb) concentration and hematocrit (Hct), preferably measured from a venous blood specimen. Measuring venous samples yields more accurate and
   reliable results compared with analysis of a capillary sample by centrifuge
   or hemoglobinometer.

Table 27.1. Adjustments for Hemoglobin and Hematocrit Cut Points for Anemia in Smokers

Smoking Status	Hb (g/dL)	Hct (%)
Nonsmoker	0.0	0.0
Smoker (all)	+0.3	+1.0
0.5-<1.0 pack per day	+0.3	+1.0
1.0-2.0 packs per day	+0.5	+1.5
>2.0 packs per day	+0.7	+2.0

From: Centers for Disease Control. Reference criteria for anemia screening. MMWR. 1989;38:400-404.

2. In men, anemia is defined as a hemoglobin level of less than 13 g/dL or a hematocrit of less than 41%. In nonpregnant women, the cut-off values are 12 g/dL for hemoglobin and 36% for hematocrit. Cigarette smokers and persons living at altitudes above 3000 feet (1000 meters) tend to have higher levels of hemoglobin and higher hematocrits. Adjust cut-off points for anemia in smokers and persons living at high altitudes by using the correction factors given in Tables 27.1 and 27.2.

Table 27.2. Altitude Adjustments for Hemoglobin and Hematocrit Cut Points for Anemia

Altitude (Ft)	Hb (g/dL)	Hct (%)
<3000	0.0	0.0
3000-3999	+0.2	+0.5
4000-4999	+0.3	+1.0
5000-5999	+0.5	+1.5
6000-6999	+0.7	+2.0
7000-7999	+1.0	+3.0
8000-8999	+1.3	+4.0
9000-9999	+1.6	+5.0
≥10,000	+2.0	+6.0

From: Centers for Disease Control. Reference criteria for anemia screening. MMWR. 1989;38:400-404.

Hemoglobinopathies

1. Hemoglobin electrophoresis is the screening test of choice for hemoglobinopathies. This test is very accurate in identifying the types of hemoglobin in a blood sample. It can distinguish among affected homozygotes, heterozygous carriers, and persons who are unaffected by sickle cell disease, beta-thalassemia, and other hemoglobin disorders. Alpha-thalassemia trait may not be detectable. Sickle cell disease and trait can also be detected by using a sickle preparation that demonstrates red blood cell sickling under reduced oxygen concentration. After sickling is demonstrated, however, hemoglobin electrophoresis is still necessary to distinguish between the carrier and affected state and to determine if other hemoglobins are present. Measurement of mean corpuscular volume (MCV) can also be used to screen for thalassemia, but this method is much less sensitive than is hemoglobin electrophoresis.

2. Offer appropriate genetic counseling to adults who are screened for hemoglobinopathies, both before and after laboratory testing. At a minimum, this counseling should address: (1) a description of the disease process and its pattern of inheritance; (2) the availability and accuracy of screening and prenatal detection techniques; (3) the implications of possible results for the individual, partner, and potential offspring.

Patient Resource

Sickle Cell Anemia (New Hope for People With). This and other publications are available from the FDA Office of Consumer Affairs, HFE 88 Room 1675, 5600 Fishers Ln, Rockville, MD 20857; (800)532-4440.

Selected References

American College of Obstetricians and Gynecologists. *Hemoglobinopathies in Pregnancy: ACOG Technical Bulletin #220.* Washington, DC: American College of Obstetricians and Gynecologists; 1996.

American College of Obstetricians and Gynecologists. *Guidelines for Women's Health Care.* Washington, DC: American College of Obstetricians and Gynecologists; 1996.

Canadian Task Force on the Periodic Health Examination. Screening for hemoglobinopathies in Canada. In: *The Canadian Guide to Clinical Preventive Health Care.* Ottawa, Canada: Minister of Supply and Services; 1994: chap 20.

Centers for Disease Control. Reference criteria for anemia screening. *MMWR.* 1989;38:400-404.

Dallman P, Ray Y, Johnson C. Prevalence and causes of anemia in the United States, 1976 to 1980. *Am J Clin Nutr.* 1984;39:437-445.

Lipkin M, Fisher L, Rowley PT, Loader S, Iker HP. Genetic counseling of asymptomatic carriers in a primary care setting. *Ann Intern Med.* 1985;105:115-123.

Shapiro MF, Greenfield S. The complete blood count and leukocyte differential count: an approach to their rational application. *Ann Intern Med.* 1987;106:65-74.

US Preventive Services Task Force. Screening for hemoglobinopathies. In: *Guide to Clinical Preventive Services.* 2nd ed. Baltimore, Md: Williams & Wilkins; 1996: chap 22.

28

BLOOD PRESSURE

Approximately 50 million Americans have blood pressure elevations that warrant monitoring or drug therapy. These persons are at increased risk for coronary artery disease, peripheral vascular disease, stroke, renal disease, and retinopathy. Treatment of hypertension is very effective. Use of antihypertensive therapy has contributed to a 59% reduction in age-adjusted stroke mortality and a 50% reduction in mortality from coronary artery disease since 1972. The benefits of antihypertensive therapy are greatest for persons with the most markedly elevated blood pressure; however, even patients with stage 1, or mild hypertension, benefit from treatment. Recent research has demonstrated the importance of treating "isolated" systolic hypertension, especially in older adults.

Recommendations of Major Authorities

American Academy of Family Physicians—Blood pressure should be measured periodically in all patients over 21 years of age.

American College of Obstetrics and Gynecology—Blood pressure should be measured as part of periodic evaluation visits, which should occur yearly or as appropriate.

American College of Physicians—Blood pressure should be measured in adults every 1 to 2 years. Normotensive patients should have blood pressure measurements at least yearly if any of the following pertains: (1) diastolic blood pressure between 85 and 89 mm Hg; (2) African-American heritage; (3) moderate or extreme obesity; (4) a first-degree relative with hypertension; (5) a personal history of hypertension.

Canadian Task Force on the Periodic Health Examination—Case-finding (screening patients seen for any reason) should be considered in all persons aged 21 to 84 years; individual clinical judgement should be exercised in all other cases except pregnant women (for whom blood pressure should be measured as part of prenatal care).

National High Blood Pressure Education Program (NHBPEP) of the National Heart, Lung, and Blood Institute—Blood pressure measurements should be performed on adults at least every 2 years and at each patient visit if possible. Patients with diastolic blood pressures of 85 to 89 mm Hg should have their blood pressure rechecked within 1 year. See Tables 28.1 and 28.2 for classification of blood pressure and recommendations for follow-up.

US Preventive Services Task Force—Adults should have blood pressure measured periodically, with the optimal interval left to clinical discretion.

Table 28.1. Classification of Blood Pressure for Adults Aged 18 Years and Older*

Category	Systolic (mm Hg)	Diastolic (mm Hg)
Normal†	<130	<85
High normal	130-139	85-89
Hypertension‡		
Stage 1 (Mild)	140-159	90-99
Stage 2 (Moderate)	160-179	100-109
Stage 3 (Severe)	180-209	110-119
Stage 4 (Very Severe)	≥210	≥120

*Not taking antihypertensive drugs and not acutely ill. When systolic and diastolic pressures fall into different categories, the higher category should be selected to classify the individual's blood pressure status. For instance, 160/92 mm Hg should be classified as Stage 2, and 180/120 mm Hg should be classified as Stage 4. Isolated systolic hypertension (ISH) is defined as SBP≥140 mm Hg and DBP <90 mm Hg and staged appropriately (eg, 170/85 mm Hg is defined as stage 2 ISH).

†Optimal blood pressure with respect to cardiovascular risk is SBP <120 mm Hg and DBP <80 mm Hg. However, unusually low readings should be evaluated for clinical significance.

‡Based on the average of two or more readings taken at each of two or more visits following an initial screening.

Note: In addition to classifying stages of hypertension based on average blood pressure levels, the clinician should specify presence or absence of target-organ disease and additional risk factors. For example, a patient with diabetes and a blood pressure of 142/94 mm Hg plus left ventricular hypertrophy should be classified as "stage 1 hypertension with target-organ disease (left ventricular hypertrophy) and with another major risk factor (diabetes)." This specificity is important for risk classification and management.

From: Joint National Committee on Detection, Evaluation, and Treatment of High Blood Pressure. The Fifth Report of the Joint National Committee on Detection, Evaluation, and Treatment of High Blood Pressure. National High Blood Pressure Education Program, National Institutes of Health, National Heart, Lung, and Blood Institute. Bethesda, Md: The Institute; 1995.

Basics of Blood Pressure Screening

1. Instruct patients not to use tobacco or caffeine for 30 minutes before the measurement is performed.

2. Seat the patient in a quiet environment, free from temperature extremes, for at least 5 minutes before the measurement is performed.

3. Perform the measurement with a mercury sphygmomanometer, if available. An aneroid manometer may be used if it is periodically calibrated according to manufacturer's recommendations. A validated electronic device meeting the requirements of the American National Standard for Electronic or Automated Sphygmomanometers set forth by the Association for the Advancement of Medical Instruments may also be used.

4. Position the manometer at eye level, if possible, to assure accuracy in reading the measurement.

5. Use an appropriately sized cuff. The bladder of the cuff should encircle 80% to 100% of the arm. The cuff width should be 40% of the circumference of the upper arm. Use of narrow cuffs leads to falsely elevated readings. Use of wide cuffs may falsely lower the reading.

6. The patient's arm should be bare; avoid constricting the upper arm with a rolled shirt sleeve. Support the arm horizontally so the cuff is positioned at heart level (the fourth intercostal space).

7. Apply the stethoscope lightly to the antecubital fossa. Excess pressure results in falsely low diastolic blood pressure readings.

8. Rapidly increase cuff pressure to about 30 mm Hg beyond the point at which the radial pulse is no longer palpable. Decrease pressure at a rate of no more than 2 to 3 mm Hg per second.

9. In adults, the measured systolic blood pressure (SBP) and the diastolic blood pressure (DBP) readings are the pressures corresponding to the first of two consecutive sounds and the disappearance of sound (not muffling), respectively. Confirm the disappearance of sound by continuing to listen while decreasing pressure 10 to 20 mm Hg below the last sound heard.

10. Use the average of at least two readings unless the first two differ by more than 5 mm Hg, in which case obtain additional readings. To permit blood to be released from arm veins, allow an interval of 1 to 2 minutes before repeating pressure measurements in the same arm.

11. Measure blood pressure in both arms initially; at subsequent visits, remeasure using the arm with the higher initial pressures.

Table 28.2. Recommendations for Follow-Up Based on Initial Set of Blood Pressure Measurements for Adults Aged 18 and Over

Initial Screening Blood Pressure (mm Hg)*		Follow-up Recommended†
Systolic	Diastolic	
<130	<85	Recheck in 2 years
130-139	85-89	Recheck in 1 year‡
140-159	90-99	Confirm within 2 months
160-179	100-109	Evaluate or refer to source of care within 1 month
180-209	110-119	Evaluate or refer to source of care within 1 week
≥210	≥120	Evaluate or refer to source of care immediately

*If the systolic and diastolic recommendations are different, follow the recommendation for the shorter-time follow-up (eg, blood pressure of 160/85 mm Hg should be evaluated or referred to source of care within 1 month).

†Modify the scheduling of follow-ups according to reliable information about past blood pressure measurements, other cardiovascular risk factors, or the presence of target-organ disease.

‡Consider providing advice about lifestyle modifications.

From: Joint National Committee on Detection, Evaluation, and Treatment of High Blood Pressure. The Fifth Report of the Joint National Committee on Detection, Evaluation, and Treatment of High Blood Pressure. Arch Intern Med. 1993;153:154-188.

12. Confirming the diagnosis of hypertension requires high blood pressure readings during at least two subsequent visits (unless SBP is 210 mm Hg or higher, DBP is 120 mm Hg or higher, or both). See Table 28.2 for recommendations for follow-up from the Joint National Committee on Detection, Evaluation, and Treatment of High Blood Pressure.

13. Because blood pressure readings obtained in a medical setting may not be typical of a patient's usual blood pressure, monitoring at home or work by the patient, family, or friends may be valuable. Measurement devices must be calibrated initially and rechecked at least yearly. Instruct the person taking the blood pressure in proper technique, and recheck the technique periodically.

14. Lifestyle modifications can help prevent development of hypertension and should be the initial treatment modality for the first 3 to 4 months for patients with stage 1 (mild) hypertension. See Table 28.3 for a list of basic lifestyle modifications for controlling blood pressure.

Table 28.3. Life-style Modifications for Hypertension Control

Lose weight if overweight

Limit alcohol intake to no more than two drinks daily for men and one drink daily for women

Exercise (aerobic) regularly (3-5 times a week)

Reduce sodium intake to less than 100 mmol per day (<2.3 g sodium or <6 g sodium chloride; 1 tsp salt = 2 g sodium)

Maintain adequate dietary potassium, calcium, and magnesium intake

Adapted from: Joint National Committee on Detection, Evaluation, and Treatment of High Blood Pressure. The Fifth Report of the Joint National Committee on Detection, Evaluation, and Treatment of High Blood Pressure. Arch Intern Med. 1993;153:154-188.

Patient Resources

High Blood Pressure: Treat it for Life; Check Your Healthy Heart IQ; High Blood Pressure and What You Can Do About It; Six Good Reasons to Control Your High Blood Pressure; Eat Right to Lower Your Blood Pressure. To order these and other materials, in both English and Spanish, contact the National Heart, Lung, and Blood Institute Information Center, PO Box 30105, Bethesda, MD 20824-0105; (301) 251-1222. Internet address: http://www.nhlbi.nih.gov/nhlbi/nhlbi.htm.

Provider Resources

The Fifth Report of the Joint National Committee on Detection, Evaluation, and Treatment of High Blood Pressure. To order this report in either English or Spanish, contact the National Heart, Lung, and Blood Institute Information Center, PO Box 30105, Bethesda, MD 20824-0105; (301) 251-1222. Internet address: http://www.nhlbi.nih.gov/nhlbi/nhlbi.htm.

Selected References

American Academy of Family Physicians. *Summary of Policy Recommendations for Periodic Health Examination.* Kansas City, Mo: American Academy of Family Physicians; 1997.

American College of Obstetricians and Gynecologists. *Guidelines for Women's Care.* Washington, DC: American College of Obstetricians and Gynecologists; 1996.

American College of Physicians. Guidelines. In: Eddy DM, ed. *Common Screening Tests.* Philadelphia, Pa: American College of Physicians; 1991:396-397.

American College of Physicians. Automated ambulatory blood pressure and self-measured blood pressure monitoring devices: their role in the diagnosis and management of hypertension (position paper). *Ann Intern Med.* 1993;118:889-892.

Appel LJ, Stason WB. Ambulatory blood pressure monitoring and blood pressure self-measurement in the diagnosis and management of hypertension. *Ann Intern Med.* 1993;118:867-882.

Canadian Task Force on the Periodic Health Examination. Hypertension in the elderly: case-finding and treatment to prevent vascular disease. In: *The Canadian Guide to Clinical Preventive Health Care.* Ottawa, Canada: Minister of Supply and Services; 1994: chap 79.

Canadian Task Force on the Periodic Health Examination. Screening for hypertension in young and middle-aged adults. In: *The Canadian Guide to Clinical Preventive Health Care.* Ottawa, Canada: Minister of Supply and Services; 1994: chap 53.

Frohlich ED, Grim C, Labarthe DR, et al. Recommendations for human blood pressure determination by sphygmomanometers: report of a special task force appointed by the Steering Committee, American Heart Association. *Hypertension.* 1988;11:209A-222A.

Joint National Committee on Detection, Evaluation, and Treatment of High Blood Pressure. The fifth report of the Joint National Committee on Detection, Evaluation, and Treatment of High Blood Pressure. *Arch Intern Med.* 1993;153:154-188.

Littenberg B. A practice guideline revisited: screening for hypertension. *Ann Intern Med* 1995;122:937-939.

National High Blood Pressure Education Program (NHBPEP) Working Group. Report on ambulatory blood pressure monitoring. *Arch Intern Med.* 1990;150:2270-2280.

Systolic Hypertension in the Elderly Program (SHEP) Cooperative Research Group. Prevention of stroke by antihypertensive drug treatment in older persons with isolated systolic hypertension. *JAMA.* 1991;265:3255-3264.

US Preventive Services Task Force. Screening for hypertension. In: *Guide to Clinical Preventive Services.* 2nd ed. Washington, DC: US Department of Health and Human Services; 1996: chap 3.

Webster J, Newnham D, Petrie JC, Lovell HG. Influence of arm position on measurement of blood pressure. *Br Med J.* 1984;288:1574-157.

29

BODY MEASUREMENT

Obesity is a major public health concern in the United States. More than one-third of all American adults are overweight, and this proportion continues to increase. (**NOTE:** Obesity is an excess of body fat. Overweight refers to an excess of body weight relative to height. Because it is more readily quantified than obesity, overweight is often used as a proxy for obesity.) Overweight is associated with significantly increased mortality and multiple health risks, such as noninsulin-dependent diabetes mellitus (type 2), hypertension, hypercholesterolemia, stroke, and coronary heart disease, as well as several types of cancer. Abdominal adiposity, as measured by waist-to-hip circumference ratio (WHR) or absolute waist circumference, is associated with an increased risk of diabetes, hypertension, coronary heart disease, stroke, and death from all causes.

Even modest weight loss by overweight individuals, accomplished by changing the diet, increasing physical activity, and other interventions, can decrease the risk of most forms of morbidity associated with being overweight. The goal of any intervention should be making lifestyle changes that are permanent.

See chapter 3 for information on body measurement of children and adolescents. See chapters 56 and 57 for information on counseling adults about nutrition and physical activity.

Recommendations of Major Authorities

American Academy of Family Physicians—All patients should be measured for height and weight periodically.

American College of Obstetricians and Gynecologists—Height and weight should be measured as part of periodic evaluation visits, which should occur yearly or as appropriate.

Canadian Task Force on the Periodic Health Examination—There is insufficient evidence to recommend the inclusion or exclusion of height and weight measurement and BMI calculation in the periodic health examination, given the lack of long-term effectiveness of weight reduction therapy in the large majority of obese individuals. Weight reduction can be cautiously recommended in persons with obesity and coexistent diabetes, hypertension, or hyperlipidemia.

US Department of Agriculture, US Department of Health and Human Services—Calculation of the ratio of waist circumference to hip circumference can be used, in addition to height and weight measurements, to help evaluate body weight.

US Preventive Services Task Force—All adults should receive periodic measurement of height and weight. The optimal frequency for measuring height and weight in adults is a matter of clinical discretion. There is insufficient evidence to recommend for or against determination of the waist/hip ratio (WHR) as a routine screening test for obesity.

Basics of Body Measurement Screening

1. To ensure accuracy, measure height while the patient is barefoot or in socks or stockings only. Make sure that the patient is standing as erect as possible, with feet flat on the floor. Height-measuring rods attached to scales should be regularly checked for accuracy, because they become inaccurate with use.

2. Use a balance beam or electronic scale (not a spring-type scale) to measure weight. The measurement will be most accurate if the patient is wearing minimal or no clothing. Calibrate scales on a regular basis.

3. Historically, the definition of "healthy" weight has been a subject of debate. Typically, two different methods have been used for evaluating weight: (1) comparison with the Metropolitan Life Insurance Tables, and (2) calculation of body mass index (BMI).

   Clinicians have been most accustomed to using height-weight tables. Early tables were adapted from those developed in 1959 by the Metropolitan Life Insurance Company and were based on weights associated with minimal mortality. Although these tables were widely circulated and used, they had significant limitations: they included subjective estimates of body frame size and were based on an insured population, which may not be representative of the overall US population.

   Today, most authorities endorse using BMI to evaluate healthy weight for adults. The formula for calculating BMI is:

$$\frac{\text{Weight (kg)}}{\text{Height (m)}^2}$$

Table 29.1. Body Weights in Pounds According to Height and Body Mass Index*

Directions: To use the table, find the appropriate height in the left-hand column. Move across the row to a given weight. The number at the bottom of the column is the body mass index for the height and weight

Body Weight (lb.)

Height (in.)

Height														
58	91	96	100	105	110	115	119	124	129	134	138	143	167	191
59	94	99	104	109	114	119	124	128	133	138	143	148	173	198
60	97	102	107	112	118	123	128	133	138	143	148	153	179	204
61	100	106	111	116	122	127	132	137	143	148	153	158	185	211
62	104	109	115	120	126	131	136	142	147	153	158	164	191	218
63	107	113	118	124	130	135	141	146	152	158	163	169	197	225
64	110	116	122	128	134	140	145	151	157	163	169	174	204	232
65	114	120	126	132	138	144	150	156	162	168	174	180	210	240
66	118	124	130	136	142	148	155	161	167	173	179	186	216	247
67	121	127	134	140	146	153	159	166	172	178	185	191	223	255
68	125	131	138	144	151	158	164	171	177	184	190	197	230	262
69	128	135	142	149	155	162	169	176	182	189	196	203	236	270
70	132	139	146	153	160	167	174	181	188	195	202	207	243	278
71	136	143	150	157	165	172	179	186	193	200	208	215	250	286
72	140	147	154	162	169	177	184	191	199	206	213	221	258	294
73	144	151	159	166	174	182	189	197	204	212	219	227	265	302
74	148	155	163	171	179	186	194	202	210	218	225	233	272	311
75	152	160	168	176	184	192	200	208	216	224	232	240	279	319
76	156	164	172	180	189	197	205	213	221	230	238	246	287	328
	19	**20**	**21**	**22**	**23**	**24**	**25**	**26**	**27**	**28**	**29**	**30**	**35**	**40**

Body Mass Index (kg/m^2)

---

* Each entry gives the body weight in pounds(lb.) for a person of a given height and body mass index. Pounds have been rounded off.

Reprinted with permission of the Western Journal of Medicine (Bray GA and Gray DS, Obesity. Part I. Pathogenesis, 1988;149:429-441).

Although authorities previously suggested that the ranges of "healthy" BMI and weight should increase with age, most authorities now do not believe that such age adjustments are valid. Table 29.1 presents an easy way to calculate an individual's BMI based on the person's height and weight.

In 1995, the US Departments of Agriculture and Health and Human Services published new healthy weight ranges for adult men and women in *Dietary Guidelines for Americans* (see Selected References). These ranges, proposed by an expert committee and adopted by the Departments, are based on an exten-

Table 29.2. Healthy Weight Ranges for Adult Men and Women

Height*	Weight in Pounds†
4' 10"	91-119
4' 11"	94-124
5' 0"	97-128
5' 1"	101-132
5' 2"	104-137
5' 3"	107-141
5' 4"	111-146
5' 5"	114-150
5' 6"	118-155
5' 7"	121-160
5' 8"	125-164
5' 9"	129-169
5' 10"	132-174
5' 11"	136-179
6' 0"	140-184
6' 1"	144-189
6' 2"	148-195
6' 3"	152-200
6' 4"	156-205
6' 5"	160-211
6' 6"	164-216

*Without shoes

†Without clothing. The higher weights apply to people with more muscle and bone, such as many men.

Source: US Department of Agriculture. Report of the Dietary Guidelines Advisory Committee on the Dietary Guidelines for Americans. Washington, DC: US Department of Agriculture; 1995.

sive review of the literature pertaining to weight-related risk of morbidity and mortality over a range of BMI values. The weight ranges are presented in Table 29.2 and Figure 29.1. Note that the higher weights apply to people with more muscle and bone.

The upper boundary of healthy weight corresponds to a BMI of about 25, based on the significant increase in risk of mortality that occurs among persons with BMI values above this cutoff point. The lower boundary of healthy weight represents a BMI of 19, although whether a weight below this level is unhealthy remains unclear. BMI values above 28 to 29, the boundary between moderate and severe overweight, are associated with an increasingly higher risk of disease and death.

Figure 29.1. Weight Chart for Adult Men and Women*

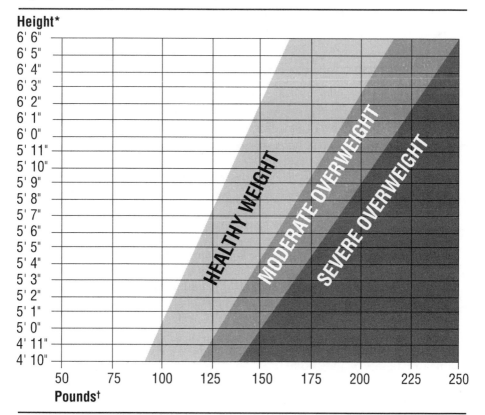

Height*

* The use of shading on the figure reflects the lack of consensus about exact cutoff points and emphasizes that disease risk varies with degree of overweight.

Note: To use this chart, find your height in feet and inches (without shoes) along the left side of the graph. Trace the line corresponding to your height across the figure until it intersects with the vertical line corresponding to your weight in pounds (without clothes). The point of intersection lies within a band that indicates whether your weight is healthy or is moderately or severely overweight. The higher weights apply mainly to men, who have more muscle and bone.

From: US Department of Agriculture, US Department of Health and Human Services. *Nutrition and Your Health: Dietary Guidelines for Americans.* Washington, DC: US Government Printing Office, 1995. Home and Garden Bulletin 232.

4. Research indicates that WHR or absolute weight circumference may be stronger predictors of mortality than are measures of general body adiposity. Determination of WHR is also useful for assessing patients, particularly those who have weight that is borderline-high and a personal or family medical history placing them at increased health risk. Determine the WHR by measuring the abdominal (waist) circumference and the hip circumference. Measure the abdominal circumference at the level of the umbilicus (or the level of greatest anterior extension of the abdomen) while the pa-

tient is standing. Determine the hip circumference by measuring the greatest circumference at the level of the buttocks. Obtain both measurements after a normal expiration by the patient and without indenting the skin. The formula for calculating WHR is:

$$\frac{\text{Abdominal Circumference}}{\text{Hip Circumference}}$$

WHR values above 1.0 for men and above 0.8 for women are associated with an increased risk of diabetes, hypertension, heart disease, and stroke. An absolute waist circumference measurement greater than 100 cm is also associated with an increased disease risk. However, evidence suggests that WHR or waist circumference and disease risk may not have as strong an association in some minority populations.

5. Bioelectric impedance analysis (BIA), a new technique for quickly estimating body composition, is currently used in many different practice settings. In theory, this technique measures the electrical impedance, or resistance, to the flow of electricity, in the body. From this measurement, an estimate of total body water (TBW) is calculated. An estimate of fat-free mass and body fat (adiposity) can then be determined. However, no industry standards for BIA currently exist, and a person's body fat measurement may vary by as much as 10% of body weight depending on the technique, machinery, conditions, and equations used. Variables that can affect the measurements include body position, hydration status, consumption of foods and beverages, ambient air and skin temperature, recent physical activity, and conductance of the examining table. Only when these variables become controlled and standardized may BIA prove to be a quick, accurate, and noninvasive way to determine body fat.

Patient Resources

Nutrition and Health: Dietary Guidelines for Americans. 4th ed. US Dept of Agriculture and US Dept of Health and Human Services, 1995. This material is available from the Consumer Information Center—3C, Dept 514-X, Pueblo, CO 81009.

Check Your Weight and Heart Disease I.Q. This information is available in both English and Spanish. National Heart, Lung, and Blood Institute Information Center, PO Box 30105, Bethesda, MD 20824-0105; (301)251-1222. Internet address: http://www.nhlbi.nih.gov/nhlbi/nhlbi.html

Weight Control: Losing Weight and Keeping It Off. American Academy of Family Physicians, 8880 Ward Parkway, Kansas City, MO 64114-2797; (800)944-0000. Internet address: http://www.aafp.org

Bioelectric Impedance Analysis in Body Composition Measurement; Understanding Adult Obesity; Weight Cycling. The National Institute of Diabetes and Digestive and Kidney Disease, 1 WIN Way, Bethesda, MD 20892-3665; (800)946-8098. Internet address: http://www.niddk.nih.gov/NutritionDocs.htm

Selected References

American Academy of Family Physicians. *Summary of Policy Recommendations for Periodic Health Examination.* Kansas City, Mo: American Academy of Family Physicians; 1997.

American College of Obstetricians and Gynecologists. *Guidelines for Women's Health Care.* Washington, DC: American College of Obstetricians and Gynecologists; 1996.

Bjorntorp P. Regional patterns of fat distribution. *Ann Intern Med.* 1985;103:994-995.

Bray GA, Gray DS. Obesity: part 1—pathogenesis. *West J Med.* 1988;149:429-441.

Canadian Task Force on the Periodic Health Examination. Prevention of obesity in adults. In: *The Canadian Guide to Clinical Preventive Health Care.* Ottawa, Canada: Minister of Supply and Services; 1994: chap 48.

Federation of American Societies for Experimental Biology, Life Sciences Research Office. *Third Report on Nutrition Monitoring in the United States.* Washington, DC: US Government Printing Office; 1995.

Folsom AR, Kaye SA, Sellers TA, et al. Body fat distribution and 5-year risk of death in older women. *JAMA.* 1993;269:483-487.

Hubert HB, Feinlieb M, McNamara PM, Castelli WP. Obesity as an independent risk factor for cardiovascular disease: a 26-year follow-up of participants in the Framingham Heart Study. *Circulation.* 1983;67:968-977.

Lissner L, Odell PM, D'Agostino RB, et al. Variability of body weight and health outcomes in the Framingham population. *N Engl J Med.* 1991;324:1839-1844.

Lohman TG, Roche AF, Martorell R. *Anthropometric Standardization Reference Manual.* Champaign, Ill: Human Kinetics Books; 1988.

Manson JE, Stampler MJ, Hennekens CH, Willet WC. Body weight and longevity: a reassessment. *JAMA.* 1987;257:353-358.

National Academy of Sciences, Committee on Diet and Health, Food and Nutrition Board, Commission on Life Sciences, National Research Council. *Diet and Health: Implications for Reducing Chronic Disease Risk.* Washington, DC: National Academy Press; 1989:564-565.

National Institutes of Health. National Institutes of Health Consensus Development Conference Statement: health implications of obesity. *Ann Intern Med.* 1985;103:1073-1077.

National Institutes of Health. *Bioelectric Impedance Analysis in Body Composition Measurement: Technology Assessment Conference Statement.* Bethesda, Md.: National Institutes of Health; 1994.

Rowland ML. A nomogram for computing body mass index. *Dietetic Currents.* 1989;16:5-12.

Simpoulos AP, Van Itallie TB. Body weight, health and longevity. *Ann Intern Med.* 1984;100:285-295.

US Department of Agriculture, Agricultural Research Service; Dietary Guidelines Advisory Committee, 1995. *Report of the Dietary Guidelines Advisory Committee on the Dietary Guidelines for Americans, 1995.* Washington, DC: US Department of Agriculture; 1995.

US Department of Agriculture, US Department of Health and Human Services. *Nutrition and Your Health: Dietary Guidelines for Americans*. Washington DC: US Government Printing Office; 1995. Home and Garden Bulletin 232.

US Preventive Services Task Force. Screening for obesity. In: *Guide to Clinical Preventive Services*. 2nd ed. Washington, DC: US Department of Health and Human Services; 1996: chap 21.

Van Itallie TB. Health implications of overweight and obesity in the United States. *Ann Intern Med*. 1985;103:983-988.

30

CANCER DETECTION BY PHYSICAL EXAMINATION

Cancer will eventually develop in approximately 30% of Americans; three of every four families will be affected. Many cancers can be cured if they are detected early and treated in the early stages. See Table 30.1 for data on the incidence and mortality of major types of cancer.

This chapter presents information regarding detection of several cancers through physical examination. Screening tests for early detection of specific cancers are addressed in separate chapters.

BREAST EXAMINATION

Cancer of the breast can manifest as visual and physical changes of the breast and axilla. Most clinical trials have evaluated the effectiveness of screening for breast cancer in women with either mammography alone or mammography combined with clinical breast examination (CBE). No direct evidence suggests superior effectiveness of CBE alone compared with no screening. When CBE is performed by a clinician, its sensitivity for detection of cancer is approximately 45%. The overall sensitivity of breast self-examination (BSE) is about 26%. The sensitivity of BSE decreases with advancing age: from 41% in women aged 35 to 39 years to only 21% for women aged 60 to 74 years. See chapter 36 for information on the epidemiology of breast cancer and screening mammography.

Recommendations of Major Authorities

Women Under 40 Years of Age

American Cancer Society—Women should have clinical breast examinations every 3 years from age 20 to 39 years.

American College of Obstetricians and Gynecologists—Women over age 18 years should have clinical breast examination during the periodic evaluation, yearly, or as appropriate.

Canadian Task Force on the Periodic Health Examination—
Clinical breast examination is not recommended for screening women less than 50 years of age.

Women 40 Years of Age and Over

American Academy of Family Physicians—Mammography and clinical breast examination should be offered to women aged 50 to 69 every 1 to 2 years.

American Cancer Society, American College of Obstetricians and Gynecologists, and **American College of Physicians—**Annual clinical breast examination should be performed on women 40 years of age and older.

Canadian Task Force on the Periodic Health Examination—
Clinical breast examination screening should be performed annually on women 50 to 69 years of age. Clinical breast examination should be used in conjunction with mammography for screening.

US Preventive Services Task Force—Breast cancer screening should be performed in women 50 to 69 years of age through mammography every one to two years with or without annual clinical breast examination. There is insufficient evidence to recommend for or against clinical breast examination alone in this age group or in any other age group. Although there is insufficient evidence, recommendations to screen high risk women beginning at age 40 and women over 70 may be made on other grounds.

There is no evidence specifically evaluating clinical breast examination in screening high-risk women under 50 years of age; recommendations for screening such women may be made on the basis of their high burden of suffering and the higher positive predictive value of screening. There is limited and conflicting evidence of the value of clinical breast examination screening in women 70 to 74 years of age and no evidence for women over 75; however, recommendations for screening women 70 years of age and older who have a reasonable life expectancy can be made on the basis of the high burden of suffering of this age group. There is insufficient evidence to recommend the use of clinical breast exam alone, without mammography, for screening.

Table 30.1. Leading Sites of Cancer Incidence and Death—1997 Estimates*

Rank	Cancer Incidence*		Cancer Deaths	
	Male	Female	Male	Female
1	Prostate 209,900	Breast 180,200	Lung 94,400	Lung 66,000
2	Lung 98,300	Lung 79,800	Prostate 41,800	Breast 43,900
3	Colon/Rectum 66,400	Colon/Rectum 64,800	Colon/Rectum 27,000	Colon/Rectum 27,900
4	Bladder 39,500	Corpus Uteri 34,900	Pancreas 13,500	Ovary 14,200
5	Non-Hodgkin's Lymphoma 30,300	Ovary 26,800	Non-Hodgkin's Lymphoma 12,400	Pancreas 14,600
6	Melanoma 22,900	Non-Hodgkin's Lymphoma 23,300	Leukemia 11,770	Non-Hodgkin's Lymphoma 11,400
7	Oral 20,900	Melanoma 17,400	Esophagus 8,700	Leukemia 9,540
8	Kidney 17,100	Cervix 14,500	Liver 7,500	Liver 4,900
9	Leukemia 15,900	Bladder 15,000	Stomach 8,300	Brain 6,000
10	Stomach 14,000	Pancreas 14,200	Bladder 7,800	Corpus Uteri 6,000
11	Pancreas 13,400	Leukemia 12,400	Kidney 7,500	Stomach 5,700
12	Liver 9,100	Kidney 11,700	Brain 7,200	Multiple Myeloma 5,400
All Sites†	661,200	596,600	292,300	262,440

*Excluding basal and squamous cell skin cancer and in situ carcinomas except bladder

†Including sites not listed in the table

Adapted from: American Cancer Society. Cancer Facts and Figures-1997. Atlanta, Ga: American Cancer Society; 1997, and from Parker SL, Tong T, Bolden S, Wingo PA. Cancer statistics 1997. CA. 47 (1), 5-27, Jan/Feb 1997. Reprinted by permission of the American Cancer Society, Inc. Copyright 1997.

Basics of Breast Examination

1. General Considerations: Breast examination involves bilateral inspection and palpation of the breasts (and areolae) and the axillary and supraclavicular areas. Perform examination while the patient is in the upright position and again in the supine position.

2. Inspection: Visually examine the breasts under good lighting with the patient sitting or standing with her hands on her hips. Focus on the symmetry and contour of the breasts; position of the nipples; skin changes such as puckering, dimpling, or scaling of the skin; scars; nipple discharge; nipple retraction; and appearance of a mass. Note any bulging, discoloration, or edema of the lymphatic drainage areas (ie, the supraclavicular and axillary regions).

3. Screening for Retraction: Observe the breast tissue for signs of retraction while the patient lifts her arms slowly over her head. Both breasts should move symmetrically. With the patient's arms lowered and palms pressed together at waist level, observe the breast tissue again for signs of retraction. Ask patients with large breasts to lean forward, and note the symmetric forward movement of the breasts. No evidence of fixation to the chest wall should be evident.

4. Breast Palpation: Palpation must be systematic. Two commonly used patterns of palpation are to start with the nipple and move out radially to the periphery—much like spokes on a wheel—or to move outward from the nipple and around the breast in a spiral, or corkscrew, pattern. Regardless of the pattern used, be thorough, and do not miss any areas. A careful, thorough examination requires 5 to 10 minutes. Take care to palpate the tail of Spence, which extends from the upper outer quadrant to the axilla. Use the first three fingers to press firmly in a small circular motion. The amount of pressure should vary from firm, to detect deep masses, to light, to detect superficial ones. Palpate all of the breast tissue when the patient is upright and again while she is supine. First, with the woman in an upright position, palpate the breast using a bimanual technique. Support the inferior aspect of the breast with one hand while the other hand palpates the breast. Next, palpate each breast with the patient in a supine position; the arm on the side to be examined should be raised over her head.

5. Axillary and Supraclavicular Node Palpation: Palpate the axillary and supraclavicular areas for adenopathy while the patient is sitting. While lifting and supporting the woman's arm, place the fingers high into the axilla and move them down firmly to palpate in four directions: along the chest wall, along the anterior border of the axilla, along the posterior border of the axilla, and along the inner aspect of the upper arm. It may be helpful to move the patient's arm through the full range of motion to increase the

surface area that can be reached. Palpate the supraclavicular nodes while the patient is sitting and relaxed, with neck flexed slightly forward. It may help to have the patient's head turned slightly toward the side being examined. The supraclavicular nodes may be felt in the angle formed by the clavicle and the sternocleidomastoid muscle.

6. Areolae: Check the nipple for discharge by gently squeezing the nipple. Discharge is easier to elicit when the patient is in an upright position. Nipple inversion may be normal. However, changes in nipple inversion should not occur after puberty, and inverted nipples should not be fixed (ie, it should be possible to pull the nipple out).

7. Breast Self-Examination: The American Cancer Society and the American College of Obstetricians and Gynecologists recommend encouraging women to examine their breasts every month. Instructing female patients in breast self-examination may be desirable. See "Patient Resources" for information about ordering pamphlets on breast self-examination.

ORAL CAVITY EXAMINATION

An estimated 30,750 new cases of oral cavity and pharyngeal cancer will be diagnosed in 1997, and approximately 8440 deaths are expected to occur during that period. Most deaths occur within 3 or 4 years of diagnosis. The incidence of oral cancer among men is more than twice that among women; the highest rates are seen among men over age 40 years. In the United States, 90% of oral cancer cases are attributable to the use of tobacco and to a lesser extent, alcohol.

Recommendations of Major Authorities

American Cancer Society—Individuals 20 to 39 years of age should have a cancer checkup, including examination of the oral region, every 3 years; those 40 years of age and older should have one yearly.

American College of Obstetricians and Gynecologists—Examinations of the oral cavity in women 40 years of age and older should be part of periodic health examinations performed annually, as appropriate.

Canadian Task Force on the Periodic Health Examination—There is insufficient evidence for inclusion or exclusion of oral cancer screening in the periodic health examination. Annual examination by physicians and/or dentists should be considered for men and women over 60 years of age who have a known risk factor for oral premalignancy and invasive oral cancers, such as tobacco use in any form and regular alcohol consumption.

US Preventive Services Task Force—There is insufficient evidence to recommend for or against routine screening of asymptomatic persons for oral cancer by primary care clinicians. Although direct evidence of a benefit is lacking, clinicians may wish to include an examination for cancerous and precancerous lesions of the oral cavity in the periodic health examination of persons who chew or smoke tobacco (or did so previously), older persons who drink regularly, and anyone with suspicious symptoms or lesions detected through self-examination. All patients, especially those over 65 years of age, should be advised to receive a complete dental examination on a regular basis.

Basics of Oral Cavity Examination

1. General Considerations: Examination of the oral cavity is intended to identify the presence of lesions that are precancerous or may predispose to cancer. Lesions that have the potential for malignant transformation tend to be flat and white (leukoplakia), white-red (erythroleukoplakia), or red (erythroplakia). The examination should include inspection and palpation of the lips, gingivae, buccal mucosa, palate, floor of the mouth, tongue, and pharynx. If the patient is wearing dentures, these should be removed before examination. Work systematically from anterior to posterior, omitting no areas. Use a bright light for optimal visualization.

2. Lips: Inspect the lips closely, noting symmetry, color, moisture, and the presence of cracking and lesions.

3. Gingivae: Inspect the gums for bleeding, sponginess, and discoloration. Normal gums appear pink or coral with a stippled surface.

4. Buccal Mucosa: Ask the patient to hold his or her mouth open widely. Holding the cheek open with a wooden tongue blade, inspect the buccal mucosa, noting color and the presence of nodules and lesions. The normal buccal surface appears pink, smooth, and moist. Leukoplakia appears as white plaque on the mucous membranes of the cheeks, gums, and tongue. Squamous cell carcinoma in its earliest stages may present as an erythematous, indurated lesion.

5. Palate: Inspect the palate for plaques, ulceration, and masses. A normal variation is a torus palatinus, a nodular bony ridge down the middle of the hard palate.

6. Floor of the Mouth: Closely examine the entire U-shaped area under the patient's tongue; this is the most common location for oral malignancies. Inspect the mouth for white patches, nodules, and ulcerations. Palpate the floor of the mouth bimanually with one finger under the tongue and the other hand under the jaw to stabilize the tissue, feeling for induration, thickening, and masses.

7. Tongue: Note color, surface characteristics, and moisture. Ask the patient to touch the tongue to the roof of the mouth to permit examination of its undersurface. While the patient's tongue is protruded, gently grasp it with a piece of gauze, using the other hand to palpate the tongue. More than 85% of all lingual cancers arise in the lateral margins of the tongue. Neoplasms may limit a patient's ability to protrude the tongue. Induration and ulceration are suggestive of carcinoma.

8. Pharynx: Depress the middle third of the patient's tongue with a tongue blade to increase visualization of the posterior pharynx. Note any asymmetry, discharge, mass, or ulceration of the pharynx.

PELVIC EXAMINATION AND OVARIAN CANCER

Pelvic examination is used to detect and identify cancers of the female genital tract. Use of the Pap smear testing during pelvic examination to identify cervical neoplasms and premalignant lesions (chapter 37) has been an unqualified success. Some authors have advocated performing bimanual examination during the pelvic examination to detect some pelvic neoplasms, including ovarian cancer, which has the highest mortality of all the gynecologic cancers. Approximately 26,800 new cases of ovarian cancer will occur in the United States in 1997, with an estimated 14,600 deaths occurring in that period. Ovarian cancer will develop in one of every 70 women. A woman's risk of ovarian cancer is increased by nulliparity; older age at the time of first pregnancy or live birth; fewer pregnancies; and a personal history of breast, endometrial, or colorectal cancer. Often, no signs or symptoms of ovarian cancer occur until late in the course of disease, and the cancer is often of considerable size by the time it is detectable by pelvic examination.

Recommendations of Major Authorities

American Cancer Society—Pelvic examination should be performed every 1 to 3 years for women aged 18 to 39 and annually for women over age 40.

American College of Obstetricians and Gynecologists—Women who have become sexually active or are 18 years of age and older should have annual pelvic examinations as part of a periodic health examination.

Canadian Task Force on the Periodic Health Examination (CTF-PHE) and **US Preventive Services Task Force**—Routine pelvic examination is not recommended for the detection of ovarian cancer. There is insufficient evidence to recommend for or against screening of asymptomatic women at increased risk for ovarian cancer. The **CTFPHE** states that it would be reasonable to examine the adnexa if a pelvic examination were being done for another reason, such as cervical inspection or Pap smear.

Basics of Pelvic Examination

1. General Considerations: Use good lighting and proper examination procedure. Instruct the patient to empty her bladder and rectum before examination.

2. Inspection: Perform a general inspection of the external genitalia with the patient in the lithotomy position. Inspect the skin of the vulva for redness, excoriation, masses, leukoplakia, and pigmentation.

3. Femoral Nodes: Palpate the horizontal chain of nodes inferior to the inguinal ligament and the vertical chain along the upper inner thigh. Nodes in this area that are smaller than 1 cm in diameter may be normal if they are soft, discrete, and movable.

4. Vagina and Cervix: Use a speculum to inspect the vagina and cervix. Warm the speculum, and lubricate it with water, not a lubricating jelly, because the jelly may interfere with interpretation of cervical cytology. Separate the labia with two fingers, and apply pressure posteriorly in the introitus. Introduce the speculum at an oblique angle, avoiding pain-sensitive anterior structures, then rotate the speculum to the transverse position. Open the blades slowly, and lock the speculum open. Use a cotton-tipped applicator or swab to remove any discharge that obscures the vaginal walls or cervix. Visually inspect the vagina and cervix for erosion, ulceration, leukoplakia, and masses. At this point, obtain a specimen for Pap smear testing (chapter 37). As the speculum is removed, examine the vaginal sidewalls again for leukoplakia, masses, and other abnormalities.

5. Bimanual Palpation: Place the lubricated index and middle fingers of one hand into the vaginal vault; place the other hand on top of the abdomen. Use the fingers within the vaginal vault to palpate the cervix and sidewalls of the vagina for induration, masses, and tenderness. Next, use the fingers within the vagina to lift the reproductive organs out of the pelvis so they can be palpated with the hand on the abdomen. Note the size, location, contour, and mobility of the uterus, ovaries, and adnexa.

6. Rectovaginal Septum: Partially withdraw the hand from the vagina, moving the middle finger to insert it into the rectum. This maneuver allows for palpation of the rectovaginal septum to detect tumors, inflammatory or granulomatous masses, and for better evaluation of the uterus in obese individuals or in those in whom the uterus is retroverted.

DIGITAL RECTAL EXAMINATION FOR COLORECTAL AND PROSTATE CANCER

Digital rectal examination (DRE) can be used to identify colorectal and prostate cancers. The DRE is of limited value as a screening test for colorectal cancer, because fewer than 10% of colorectal cancers can be palpated. See chapter 34 for information on the epidemiology of colorectal cancer and screening with fecal occult blood testing.

Rectal examination does afford an opportunity for limited palpation of the prostate gland in men. See chapter 39 for information on the epidemiology of prostate cancer and screening with prostate-specific antigen (PSA). The sensitivity and specificity of digital rectal examination for detecting prostate cancer are 33% to 69% and 49% to 97%, respectively. Scant evidence exists suggesting that screening by digital rectal examination decreases mortality from prostate cancer. Some authorities believe that the limited effectiveness of DRE may be attributable to either its inability to detect tumors at an early, treatable stage or the fact that some tumors grow so rapidly that yearly screening cannot detect most of them at an early, treatable stage, or both.

Recommendations of Major Authorities

American Academy of Family Physicians—Clinicians should counsel men age 50 to 65 about the known risks and uncertain benefits of screening for prostate cancer.

American Cancer Society—Annual digital rectal examination should be performed for men aged 50 and over as part of prostate cancer screening (chapter 39). In men and women age 50 and over, a rectal examination should be done as part of colorectal cancer screening every 5 to 10 years, depending on the type of screening test used.

American College of Obstetricians and Gynecologists—Digital rectal examination should be included in the periodic health examination of women 50 years of age and older as part of the pelvic exam.

American Society of Colon and Rectal Surgeons—Annual digital rectal examination should be performed for asymptomatic, low-risk individuals 40 years of age and older and for asymptomatic individuals over 35 years of age with either a family history of colorectal adenomatous polyps or cancer in one or more first-degree relatives.

American Urological Association—Annual digital rectal examination is recommended as part of prostate cancer screening for all men age 50 and over and for those at high risk starting at age 40 (chapter 39).

Canadian Task Force on the Periodic Health Examination (CTFPHE)—There is insufficient evidence to recommend for or against the use of digital rectal examination to screen for prostate cancer. The **CTFPHE** has stated that evidence is insufficient to advise physicians who currently include digital rectal exam in examination on men 50 to 70 years of age to discontinue the practice.

US Preventive Services Task Force—There is insufficient evidence to recommend for or against routine digital rectal examination as an effective screening test for prostate cancer in asymptomatic men. No recommendation has been made regarding the use of the examination for colorectal cancer screening.

Basics of Rectum and Prostate Examination

1. General Considerations: Examine male and female patients while they are in the left lateral decubitus position or are standing, bent over the examination table. Female patients may also be examined while they are in the lithotomy position during a pelvic examination.

2. Inspection: Inspect the anal opening visually, noting any skin breakdown, fissures, and protrusions from the anal opening.

3. Palpation: To perform the examination, insert the lubricated, gloved index finger into the anal opening. Insert the gloved finger just past the rectal sphincter; do not advance it until the sphincter relaxes. The procedure can be uncomfortable for the patient but usually is not painful. Be sure to palpate all sides of the rectum for polyps, which may be sessile (attached by a base) or pedunculated (attached by a stalk). Intraperitoneal metastases may be felt anterior to the rectum as hard, shelf-like projections into the rectum. In men, thoroughly palpate the posterior and lateral lobes of the prostate gland. The normal prostate gland is approximately 2.5 cm by 4 cm and does not protrude into the rectum by more than 1 cm. It should feel smooth and rubbery throughout and have a palpable central groove. Asymmetry of the prostate gland or the presence of a hard, irregular nodule, or both, is typical of prostate cancer.

SKIN EXAMINATION

Skin cancer is the most common type of cancer in the United States. Approximately 900,000 new cases of basal and squamous cell carcinoma, as well as 40,300 cases of malignant melanoma, will be diagnosed in 1997. An estimated 7300 deaths from malignant melanoma and approximately 2190 deaths from other types of skin cancer will occur in 1997. The incidence of malignant melanoma is increasing at the rate of 4% per year. Virtually 100% of skin cancers are curable if they are diagnosed and excised early. Skin cancers occur more commonly in fair-skinned individuals who have been exposed to the sun, radiation, or ultraviolet light for prolonged periods of time. Chronic overexposure to sunlight is the cause of 95% of all basal cell carcinomas. Other risk factors for basal cell and squamous cell carcinomas include exposure to radiation, complications of burning or scarring, and contact with arsenic. Basal cell cancer is more common in older adults and affects men more frequently than women. Both basal cell and squamous cell cancers can occur in anyone with a history of prolonged sun exposure, and both are most likely to occur in sun-exposed areas. Factors placing individuals at increased risk for malignant melanoma include the presence of atypical moles and a personal or family history of skin cancer, especially malignant melanoma.

Recommendations of Major Authorities

American Academy of Dermatology and Skin Cancer Foundation—Annual skin examinations are recommended for all patients.

Canadian Task Force on the Periodic Health Examination (CTF-PHE), and **US Preventive Services Task Force (USPSTF)**—There is insufficient evidence to recommend for or against routine screening for skin cancer by primary care clinicians with total skin examination. Clinicians should remain alert for skin lesions with malignant features when examining patients for other reasons, particularly in those with established risk factors. Risk factors include: melanocytic precursor or marker lesions (eg, atypical moles), large numbers of common moles, immunosuppression, a family or personal history of skin cancer, substantial cumulative lifetime sun exposure, intermittent intense sun exposure or severe sunburns in childhood, freckles, poor tanning ability, and light skin, hair, and eye color. The **USPSTF** states that clinicians should consider referring patients with melanocytic precursor or marker lesions to skin care specialists. The **CTFPHE** states that patients with family melanoma syndrome should receive total body skin examinations and be considered for referral to a specialist. Both the **CTFPHE** and the **USPSTF** state that there is insufficient evidence to recommend for or against routine counseling of patients to perform skin self-examination or to use sunscreens to prevent skin cancer. The **CTFPHE** states that use of sunscreen is recommended for patients with prior history of solar keratosis. The **USPSTF** states that use of sunscreen may be appropriate for such patients.

American Cancer Society—Patients should undergo a cancer checkup that includes examination of the skin every 3 years for those 20 to 39 years of age, and yearly after age 40.

American College of Obstetricians and Gynecologists—Skin examination should be performed for individuals with a family or personal history of skin cancer, increased occupational or recreational exposure to sunlight, or clinical evidence of precursor lesions (eg, dysplastic nevi and certain congenital nevi).

Basics of Skin Examination

1. General Considerations: Perform the examination in a room that is comfortably warm; adjust lighting to produce optimal illumination. Basal cell or squamous cell carcinomas are likely to present in one of the following ways: as an open sore that bleeds, oozes, or crusts and is present for more than 3 weeks; as an irritated red patch that may itch or hurt; as a growth with a rolled border and central indentation; as a shiny bump or nodule; or as a scar-like area. Characteristics that may make a lesion suspicious for malignant melanoma may be remembered by following the ABCDs: **A**—**A**symmetry; **B**—irregular **B**orders; **C**—variation in **C**olor from one area to another within the same lesion; and **D**—a **D**iameter greater than 6 mm, about the size of a pencil eraser. Additional warning signs for malignant melanoma include sudden or continuous enlargement of a lesion; elevation of a previously macular pigmented lesion; surface changes, such as bleeding, crusting, erosion, oozing, scaliness, or ulceration; changes in the surrounding skin, such as redness, swelling, or satellite pigmentation; changes in sensation, such as itching, tenderness, or pain; changes in consistency, such as softening or friability; and the development of a new pigmented lesion, particularly in patients older than 40 years of age. Carefully evaluate all pigmented lesions.

2. With the Patient Seated: Examine the skin of the head, upper torso, and upper extremities while the patient is seated. Part the hair and inspect the scalp thoroughly and carefully. While examining the skin of the face and neck, take special note of the eyelids, forehead, ears, nose, and lips. Examine the upper extremities, shoulders, and back completely.

3. With the Patient Supine: Inspect the skin of the chest and abdomen with particular attention to the inguinal and genital areas. Elevate the scrotum to allow inspection of the perineal area. Carefully examine the feet, including the soles and the area between the toes.

4. With the Patient Lying on the Left Side: Examine the remaining skin of the back, legs, gluteal and perianal areas.

TESTICULAR EXAMINATION

Testicular cancer accounts for only about 1% of all cancers in men. However, it is the most common cancer in white men aged 20 to 34 years; 7200 new cases and 350 deaths are expected to occur in 1997. The prognosis for testicular cancer is very good, especially if it is treated early. The major risk factor is a history of cryptorchidism. Other risk factors include a previous history of testicular cancer, gonadal dysgenesis, Klinefelter's syndrome, and in utero exposure to diethylstilbestrol (DES). Testicular cancer is more common in white men than in African Americans; incidence rates are intermediate in Hispanics, American Indians, and Asians.

The two screening tests proposed for testicular cancer are health provider palpation of the testes and patient self-examination of the testes. No information is available on the sensitivity, specificity, or positive predictive value of testicular examination in asymptomatic men by either modality. Published evidence that self-examination can detect testicular cancer in asymptomatic men is limited to a small number of case reports.

Recommendations of Major Authorities

> **American Cancer Society**—Testicular examination should be a part of the cancer checkup received by men every 3 years from 20 to 39 years of age and annually beginning at age 40.

> **American Urological Association**—Yearly clinical examinations should begin at age 15.

> **Canadian Task Force on the Periodic Health Examination** and **US Preventive Services Task Force (USPSTF)**—There is insufficient evidence to recommend for or against routine screening of asymptomatic men for testicular cancer by physician examination or patient self-examination. The **USPSTF** has stated that recommendations against such screening can be made on other grounds, such as the current excellent prognosis of testicular cancer patients and the likelihood that a large number of false-positive results would result from screening. Patients with an increased risk of testicular cancer (those with a history of cryptorchidism or testicular atrophy) should be informed of their increased risk of testicular cancer and counseled about the options for screening (physician or self-examination). Adolescent and young adult males should be advised to seek prompt medical attention if they notice a testicular or intrascrotal abnormality.

Basics of Testicular Examination

1. Inspection: With the patient standing, inspect the genital area for swelling, edema, and other visible abnormalities. Elevate the scrotum to permit inspection of the perineum.

2. Femoral Nodes: Palpate the horizontal chain of nodes inferior to the inguinal ligament and the vertical chain along the upper inner thigh. Nodes smaller than 1 cm in diameter may be normal if they are soft, discrete, and movable.

3. Palpation: With the patient standing, use both hands to examine each testicle individually. One hand holds the superior and inferior poles of the testicle while the other hand palpates the anterior, posterior, medial, and lateral surfaces. If any masses are noted, attempt to place a finger between

the mass and the testicle. This will help differentiate between masses that originate from the testicle and those that arise from other structures within the scrotum. Next, attempt to transilluminate the mass. A tumor should not transilluminate. When a neoplasm is present, the testicle is usually enlarged, firm, and heavier than normal. If any abnormalities are noted, examine the patient while he is in the supine position to try to distinguish between solid masses (which will remain) and varicoceles (which may resolve).

4. Testicular Self-Examination: Authorities disagree about whether to encourage patients to examine their testes regularly. Clinicians wishing to do so may refer to pamphlets on self-examination listed in "Patient Resources" below.

THYROID EXAMINATION

Approximately 16,100 cases of thyroid cancer will be diagnosed in 1997 in the United States; approximately 1239 deaths will be attributable to the disease. Persons at increased risk include those who have undergone irradiation of the head and neck as children and persons with a family history of multiple endocrine neoplasia, type II. Thyroid malignancy occurs twice as frequently in women as in men.

Recommendations of Major Authorities

American Academy of Family Physicians—Use of ultrasound screening in asymptomatic persons for detection of thyroid cancer is not recommended.

American Cancer Society—A cancer checkup, including palpation of the thyroid, should be performed every 3 years on individuals 20 to 39 years of age and yearly for individuals aged 40 years and over.

American College of Obstetricians and Gynecologists—Thyroid palpation should be part of the periodic health examination for all women over the age of 18 years.

Canadian Task Force on the Periodic Health Examination and **US Preventive Services Task Force (USPSTF)**—There is insufficient evidence for or against the performance of thyroid palpation for screening for thyroid cancer. The **USPSTF** has stated that a recommendation for screening patients with a history of external upper-body (primarily head and neck) irradiation in infancy and childhood can be made on other grounds, such as patient preference or anxiety.

Basics of Thyroid Examination

1. Inspection: The patient should be seated with the neck flexed slightly in order to relax the sternocleidomastoid muscles. To highlight any swelling, position a standing lamp so that it shines tangentially across the neck. Observe the neck as the patient takes a sip of water. Thyroid masses will move up and down with swallowing because of the thyroid's location within the fascial sheath of the trachea. A midline mass may also be a thyroglossal duct cyst.

2. Palpation: The patient should be sitting straight, with the neck flexed slightly forward and to the right. While standing behind the patient, use the fingertips of the left hand to push the trachea slightly to the right and the fingers of the right hand to retract the sternocleidomastoid muscle. While the patient takes a sip of water, palpate the medial and lateral margins of the thyroid with the fingertips of the right hand. Reverse the procedure on the left side. A malignancy may present as a discrete area of firmness or hardness. Thyroid gland tenderness may also be suggestive of malignancy.

3. Lymph Nodes: Examine the thyroid for the presence of lymphadenopathy. The uppermost pretracheal node that lies above or over the thyroid isthmus is called the Delphian node. An enlarged Delphian node may be the earliest sign of metastatic papillary cancer. Also examine the pre- and postauricular nodes, as well as the anterior and posterior cervical nodes. The anterior cervical nodes are clustered in a 7-shaped configuration, with the horizontal axis just below the body of the mandible and the vertical axis along the anterior border of the sternocleidomastoid muscle. The posterior cervical nodes are clustered in an L-shaped configuration, with horizontal axis along the clavicle and the vertical axis along the anterior margin of the trapezius. Palpate the lymph nodes using a gentle circular motion of the finger pads. It is usually most efficient to palpate with both hands to permit comparison of the two. Normal nodes should feel movable, discrete, soft, and nontender.

Patient Resources - Breast Cancer

Breast Cancer: Steps to Finding Breast Lumps Early. American Academy of Family Physicians, 8880 Ward Pkwy, Kansas City, MO 64114-2797; (800)944-0000. Internet address: http://www.aafp.org

How To Do Breast Self Examination; Breast Cancer - Questions and Answers; Cancer Facts for Women. American Cancer Society, 1599 Clifton Rd, NE, Atlanta, GA 30329-4251; 1-800-ACS-2345. Internet address: http://www.cancer.org

Mammography. American College of Obstetricians and Gynecologists, 409 12th St, SW, Washington, DC 20024; (800)762-2264. Internet address: http://acog.com

Questions and Answers About Evaluating Breast Changes; Benign Breast Lumps and other Benign Breast Changes; What You Need To Know About Ovarian Cancer; The Pap Test: It Could Save Your Life (Spanish). Office of Cancer Communications, National Cancer Institute, Bldg 31, Room 10A16, Bethesda, MD 20892; 1-800-4-CANCER.

Chances are You Need a Mammogram; Are You Age 50 or Older? A Mammogram Could Save Your Life (English and Spanish). Office of Cancer Communications, National Cancer Institute, Bldg 31, Room 10A16, Bethesda, MD 20892; (800)4-CANCER. Internet address: http://wwwicic.nci.nih.gov

Provider Resources - Breast Cancer

Detecting and Treating Breast Problems. American College of Obstetricians and Gynecologists, 409 12th St, SW, Washington, DC 20024-2188; (202) 638-5577. Internet address: http://www.acog.com

Nonmalignant Conditions of the Breast (ACOG Technical Bulletin 156; 1991). American College of Obstetricians and Gynecologists, 409 12th St, SW, Washington, DC 20024; 1-800-762-2264. Internet address: http://www.acog.com

Mammography Awareness Kit. Office of Cancer Communications, National Cancer Institute, Bldg 31, Room 10A16, Bethesda, MD 20892; (800)4-CANCER. Internet address: http://wwwicic.nci.nih.gov

Patient Resources - Cancers of the Oral Cavity

Head & Neck Cancer: Know What the Warning Signs Are. American Academy of Otolaryngology-Head and Neck Surgery, Order Department, 1 Prince St, Alexandria, VA 22314; (703) 836-4444.

Facts on Oral Cancer; Self Oral Screen in Six Orderly Steps. American Cancer Society, 1599 Clifton Rd, NE, Atlanta, GA 30329-4251; (800)ACS-2345. Internet address: http://www.cancer.org

What You Need to Know about Oral Cancer. Office of Cancer Communications, National Cancer Institute, Bldg 31, Room 10A16, Bethesda, MD 20892; (800)4-CANCER. Internet address: http://wwwicic.nci.nih.gov

Patient Resources - Cancer of Pelvic Organs

Preventing Cancer; Cancer of the Ovary. American College of Obstetricians and Gynecologists, 409 12th St SW, Washington, DC 20024; (800)762-2264. Internet address: http://www.acog.com

What You Need To Know About Ovarian Cancer; The Pap Test: It Could Save Your Life (Spanish). Office of Cancer Communications, National Cancer Institute, Bldg 31, Room 10A16, Bethesda, MD 20892; 1-800-4-CANCER.

Preventing Cancer; Cancer of the Ovary. American College of Obstetricians and Gynecologists, 409 12th St, SW, Washington, DC 20024; (800)762-2264. Internet address: http://www.acog.com

Provider Resources - Cancer of Pelvic Organs

Cervical Cytology: Evaluation and Management of Abnormalities. Technical Bulletin 183. American College of Obstetricians and Gynecologists, 409 12th St, SW, Washington, DC 20024; 1-800-762-2264. Internet address: http://www.acog.com

The Pap Test. American College of Obstetricians and Gynecologists, 409 12th St, SW, Washington DC 20024; (800)762-2264. Internet address: http://www.acog.com

Patient Resources - Prostate Cancer

For Men Only: Prostate Cancer; Cancer Facts for Men. American Cancer Society, 1599 Clifton Rd, NE, Atlanta, GA 30329-4251; 1-800-ACS-2345. Internet address: http://www.cancer.org

Prostate Disease: What Every Man Over 40 Should Know. Prostate Health Council, c/o American Foundation for Urologic Disease, Inc, 1128 N Charles St, Baltimore, MD 21201. Written requests only.

The prostate puzzle. *Consumer Reports.* 1993;58(7):459-465.

Patient Resources - Colorectal Cancer

Colorectal Cancer, Questions & Answers. American Society of Colon and Rectal Surgeons, 800 E Northwest Hwy, Suite 1080, Palatine, IL 60067; (708) 359-9184.

Colonoscopy: Questions and Answers; Polyps of the Colon and Rectum: Questions and Answers. American Society of Colon and Rectal Surgeons, 800 E Northwest Hwy, Suite 1080, Palatine, IL 60067; (708) 359-9184.

What You Need to Know about Cancer of the Colon and Rectum. Office of Cancer Communications, National Cancer Institute, Bethesda, MD 20892; (800)4-CANCER. Internet address: http://wwwicic.nci.nih.gov

Patient Resources - Skin Cancer

Skin Cancer: Saving Your Skin From Sun Damage. American Academy of Family Physicians, 8880 Ward Pkwy, Kansas City, MO 64114-2797; (800)944-0000. Internet address: http://www.aafp.org

The ABCDs of Moles & Melanomas; Dysplastic Nevi and Malignant Melanoma: A Patient's Guide; Skin Cancer: If You Can Spot It, You Can Stop It. The Skin Cancer Foundation, PO Box 561, New York, NY 10156; (212) 725-5176.

Facts on Skin Cancer. American Cancer Society, 1599 Clifton Rd, NE, Atlanta, GA 30329-4251. (800)ACS-2345. Internet address: http://www.cancer.org

Provider Resource - Skin Cancer

Prevention and Early Detection of Malignant Melanoma. American Cancer Society, 1599 Clifton Rd, NE, Atlanta, GA 30329-4251. (800)ACS-2345. Internet address: http://www.cancer.org

Patient Resource - Testicular Cancer

Testicular Cancer & Testicular Self-Examination. American Urological Association, Inc, 1120 N Charles St, Baltimore, MD 21201-5559; (410) 727-1100.

Provider Resource - General

PDQ: The Physician Data Query System for Cancer Information. PDQ is the National Cancer Institute's computerized database providing the most up-to-date cancer information available. Access to the system can be gained 24 hours a day, 7 days a week, using a personal computer and standard telephone line or through medical libraries. Ask a medical librarian for assistance or call (800)4-CANCER (line 3). In Hawaii, on Oahu, call 524-1234.

OncoLink - The University of Pennsylvania Cancer Center Resource. Internet address: http://cancer.med.upenn.edu

Selected References

American Academy of Family Physicians. *Summary of Policy Recommendations for Periodic Health Examination.* Kansas City, Mo: American Academy of Family Physicians; 1997.

American Cancer Society. *Cancer Facts & Figures-1997.* Atlanta, Ga: American Cancer Society; 1997.

American Cancer Society. *Summary of American Cancer Society recommendations for the early detection of cancer in asymptomatic people*. CA. 1993;43:45.

American Cancer Society. *Cancer Information Database*. Atlanta, Ga: American Cancer Society; June 1997.

American College of Obstetricians and Gynecologists. *Routine Cancer Screening*. ACOG Committee Opinion #128. Washington, DC: American College of Obstetricians and Gynecologists; 1993.

American College of Obstetricians and Gynecologists. *Guidelines for Women's Health Care*. Washington, DC: American College of Obstetricians and Gynecologists; 1996.

American College of Physicians. Guidelines. In Eddy DM, ed. *Common Screening Tests*. Philadelphia, Pa: American College of Physicians; 1991:411-416.

American Society of Colon and Rectal Surgeons. *Practice Parameters for the Detection of Colorectal Neoplasms*. Palatine, Ill: American Society of Colon and Rectal Surgeons; 1992.

American Urological Association. *Early Detection of Prostate Cancer*. Baltimore, Md: American Urological Association; 1995.

Canadian Task Force on the Periodic Health Examination. Prevention of skin cancer. In: *The Canadian Guide to Clinical Preventive Health Care*. Ottawa, Canada: Minister of Supply and Services; 1994: chap 70.

Canadian Task Force on the Periodic Health Examination. Screening for breast cancer. In: *The Canadian Guide to Clinical Preventive Health Care*. Ottawa, Canada: Minister of Supply and Services; 1994: chap 65.

Canadian Task Force on the Periodic Health Examination. Screening for colorectal cancer. In: *The Canadian Guide to Clinical Preventive Health Care*. Ottawa, Canada: Minister of Supply and Services; 1994: chap 66.

Canadian Task Force on the Periodic Health Examination. Screening for oral cancer. In: *The Canadian Guide to Clinical Preventive Health Care*. Ottawa, Canada: Minister of Supply and Services; 1994: chap 69.

Canadian Task Force on the Periodic Health Examination. Screening for ovarian cancer. In: *The Canadian Guide to Clinical Preventive Health Care*. Ottawa, Canada: Minister of Supply and Services; 1994: chap 72.

Canadian Task Force on the Periodic Health Examination. Screening for prostate cancer. In: *The Canadian Guide to Clinical Preventive Health Care*. Ottawa, Canada: Minister of Supply and Services; 1994: chap 67.

Canadian Task Force on the Periodic Health Examination. Screening for testicular cancer. In: *The Canadian Guide to Clinical Preventive Health Care*. Ottawa, Canada: Minister of Supply and Services; 1994: chap 74.

Canadian Task Force on the Periodic Health Examination. Screening for thyroid disorders and thyroid cancer in asymptomatic adults. In: *The Canadian Guide to Clinical Preventive Health Care*. Ottawa, Canada: Minister of Supply and Services; 1994: chap 51.

Canadian Task Force on the Periodic Health Examination. The periodic health examination: 2. 1987 update: endometrial cancer. *Can Med Assoc J*. 1988;138:620–621.

DeGowin EL, DeGowin RL. *Bedside Diagnostic Examination*. 5th ed. New York, NY: Macmillan Publishing Co; 1987.

Eddy DM, Gordon MA, Bredt A. Screening for breast cancer. *Ann Intern Med*. In press.

Fink DJ, Mettlin CJ. Cancer detection: the cancer-related checkup guidelines. In: Murphy GP, Lawrence W, Jr., Lenhard RE, Jr., eds. *American Cancer Society Textbook of Clinical Oncology*. 2nd ed. Atlanta, Ga: American Cancer Society; 1995: chap 10.

Friedman RJ, Rigel DS, Silverman MK, Kopf AW, Vossaert KA. Malignant melanoma in the 1990s: the continued importance of early detection and the role of physician examination and self-examination of the skin. *CA*. 1991;41:201–227.

Gerber GS, Thompson IM, Thisted R, Chodak GW. Disease-specific survival following routine prostate cancer screening by digital rectal examination. *JAMA*. 1993;269:61–64.

Jarvis C. *Physical Examination and Health Assessment*. Philadelphia, Pa: WB Saunders Co; 1992.

MacLeod J, Munro J, eds. *Clinical Examination*. 7th ed. New York, NY: Churchill Livingstone; 1986.

Mettlin C, Jones G, Averette H, et al. Defining and updating the American Cancer Society guidelines for the cancer-related checkup: prostate and endometrial cancers. *CA*. 1993;43:42-46.

Moloy PJ. How to (and how not to) manage the patient with a lump in the neck. In: *Common Problems of the Head and Neck Region*. Philadelphia, Pa: WB Saunders Co; 1992:129–150.

Parker SL, Tong T, Bolden S, Wingo PA. Cancer statistics, 1997. *CA*. 1997;47:5-27.

Rhodes AR, Weinstock MA, Fitzpatrick TB, Mihm MC, Sober AJ. Risk factors for cutaneous melanoma: a practical method of recognizing predisposed individuals. *JAMA*. 1987;258:3146–3153.

Garnick MB, Mayer RJ, Richie JP. Testicular self-examination. *N Engl J Med*. 1980;302:297.

Smart CR, Chu K, Conley V, Henson DE, Pommerenke F, Srivastova S. Cancer screening and early detection. In: Holland JF, Frei EF III, Bast RC Sr. , Kufe DW, Morton DL, Weichselbaum RR, eds. *Cancer Med*. 3rd ed. Vol 1. Philadelphia, Pa: Lea and Febiger, 1993;408-431.

Swartz MH. *Textbook of Physical Diagnosis*. Philadelphia, Pa: WB Saunders Co; 1989.

US Preventive Services Task Force. Screening for breast cancer. In: *Guide to Clinical Preventive Services*. 2nd ed. Washington, DC: US Department of Health and Human Services; 1996: chap 7.

US Preventive Services Task Force. Screening for colorectal cancer. In: *Guide to Clinical Preventive Services*. 2nd ed. Washington, DC: US Department of Health and Human Services; 1996: chap 8.

US Preventive Services Task Force. Screening for oral cancer. In: *Guide to Clinical Preventive Services*. 2nd ed. Washington, DC: US Department of Health and Human Services; 1996: chap 17.

US Preventive Services Task Force. Screening for ovarian cancer. In: *Guide to Clinical Preventive Services*. 2nd ed. Washington, DC: US Department of Health and Human Services; 1996: chap 14.

US Preventive Services Task Force. Screening for prostate cancer. In: *Guide to Clinical Preventive Services*. 2nd ed. Washington, DC: US Department of Health and Human Services; 1996: chap 10.

US Preventive Services Task Force. Screening for skin cancer. In: *Guide to Clinical Preventive Services*. 2nd ed. Washington, DC: US Department of Health and Human Services; 1996: chap 12.

US Preventive Services Task Force. Screening for testicular cancer. In: *Guide to Clinical Preventive Services*. 2nd ed. Washington, DC: US Department of Health and Human Services; 1996: chap 13.

US Preventive Services Task Force. Screening for thyroid cancer. In: *Guide to Clinical Preventive Services*. 2nd ed. Washington, DC: US Department of Health and Human Services; 1996: chap 18.

Wartofsky L. Examination of the thyroid. In: Becker KL, ed. *Principles and Practice of Endocrinology & Metabolism*. New York, NY: JB Lippincott; 1990.

Wingo PA, Landis S, Ries LAG. An adjustment to the 1997 estimate for new prostate cancer cases. *CA*. 1997;47(4):239-242.

31

CHOLESTEROL

High blood cholesterol is an important modifiable risk factor for coronary heart disease (CHD)—the leading cause of death for both men and women in the United States. This year, as many as 1.5 million Americans will have a new or recurrent myocardial infarction, and about one third of these individuals will die. Large, population-based studies have demonstrated that total cholesterol levels are directly related to the incidence of CHD. The Multiple Risk Factor Intervention Trial (MRFIT) found that the 6-year risk of death from CHD in normotensive, nonsmoking, middle-aged men with blood cholesterol levels less than 182 mg/dL was one fourth that of men with blood cholesterol levels of 245 mg/dL or higher. An analysis of 22 epidemiologic studies has shown that elevated cholesterol is also a risk factor for CHD in women and in individuals ≥ 65 years of age. Epidemiologic studies have also shown that cholesterol lipoprotein subfractions play an important role in CHD. LDL-cholesterol is directly, and HDL-cholesterol is inversely, associated with the incidence of CHD.

No long-term study has compared interventions to reduce cholesterol levels and CHD incidence based on routine cholesterol screening with interventions based on selective case-finding or with universal dietary advice. Because the recent increase in cholesterol screening had been accompanied by an improved knowledge and public awareness of dietary risk factors, isolating the contribution of screening from other factors that may account for improved outcomes may be difficult. The major evidence to support cholesterol screening is the ability of cholesterol-lowering interventions to reduce the risk of CHD in patients with high cholesterol.

A meta-analysis of cholesterol-lowering trials performed mainly in middle-aged men found that lowering blood cholesterol levels through dietary management or drug therapy significantly reduces the risk of CHD death and nonfatal myocardial infarction. The West of Scotland Coronary Prevention Study Group, a primary prevention trial, showed a reduction in cardiovascular mortality associated with drug treatment with no difference between treatment groups in the rate of death due to noncardiovascular causes. Similarly, the Scandinavian Simvastatin Survival Study, a secondary prevention trial, showed that in patients with a history of myocardial infarction, the reduction in CHD mortality associated with drug treatment was accompanied by a reduction in total mortality.

See chapter 4 for information on cholesterol screening for children and adolescents.

Recommendations of Major Authorities

American Academy of Family Physicians—Males aged 35 to 65 years and females aged 45 to 65 years should be screened periodically for high cholesterol levels.

American College of Obstetricians and Gynecologists—Adults (19 years of age and older) should have cholesterol measured every 5 years until 64 years of age, then every 3 to 5 years thereafter. (These are currently under review for a possible change to recommendations consistent with the US Preventive Services Task Force.)

American College of Physicians—Screening for total cholesterol in the primary prevention of CHD is appropriate but not mandatory in men between 35 and 65 years of age and for women between 45 and 65 years of age. Screening for total cholesterol is not recommended for men younger than 35 years of age or women younger than 45 years of age unless the history or physical examination suggests a familial lipoprotein disorder, or at least two other characteristics place them at increased risk for developing CHD. There is insufficient evidence to recommend for or against screening in men and women between the ages of 65 and 75. Screening of individuals over 75 years of age is not recommended. In those individuals who are screened for the primary prevention of CHD, the total cholesterol level should be measured once. It should be repeated periodically if the measured value is near a treatment threshold. All patients with known CHD or whose history of other kinds of vascular disease places them at very high risk of CHD should have measurements of total cholesterol.

Canadian Task Force on the Periodic Health Examination—There is insufficient evidence for the inclusion or exclusion of universal screening for hypercholesterolemia in a periodic health examination. Nonetheless, case-finding through repeated measurements of the non-fasting total blood cholesterol level should be considered in men 30 to 59 years of age.

National Cholesterol Education Program (NCEP) of the National Heart, Lung, and Blood Institute—Adults (20 years of age and older) should have a measurement of total blood cholesterol at least once every 5 years; HDL-cholesterol should be measured at the same time if accurate results are available. Lipoprotein analysis should be performed for all patients with CHD. In patients without CHD, lipoprotein analysis should be performed in any of the following circumstances: (1) if the total cholesterol is 240 mg/dL or above; (2) if the total cholesterol is 200 to

239 mg/dL and the patient also has two or more CHD risk factors; (3) if the patient has an HDL-cholesterol less than 35 mg/dL. See Tables 31.1 and 31.2 and Figures 31.1, 31.2, and 31.3 for **NCEP** recommendations on CHD risk factors and patient classification and identification.

US Preventive Services Task Force—Periodic screening for high serum cholesterol is recommended for all men 35-65 years of age and women 45-65 years of age. There is insufficient evidence to recommend for or against screening asymptomatic persons after 65 year of age, but screening may be considered on a case-by-case basis. Older persons with major CHD risk factors (smoking, hypertension, diabetes) who are otherwise healthy may be more likely to benefit from screening, based on their high risk of CHD and the proven benefits of lowering cholesterol in older persons with symptomatic CHD. Cholesterol levels are not a reliable predictor of risk after age 75, however. There is also insufficient evidence to recommend for or against screening of young adults, although this may be recommended on other grounds to young adults at high risk, such as the greater absolute risk attributable to high cholesterol and potential long-term benefits of early lifestyle interventions. Risk factors include: family history of very high cholesterol, premature CHD in a first-degree relative (before age 50 in men or age 60 in women), diabetes, smoking, or hypertension. The appropriate interval for periodic screening is not known. Periodic screening is most important when cholesterol levels are increasing (eg, middle-aged men, perimenopausal women, and persons who have gained weight). An interval of five years has been recommended by experts, but longer intervals may be reasonable for low-risk subjects (including those with previously desirable cholesterol levels). There is insufficient evidence to recommend for or against routine measurement of HDL-cholesterol or triglycerides at initial screening.

Basics of Cholesterol Screening

1. Do not screen patients who are acutely ill, losing weight, pregnant, or breast-feeding, because their cholesterol levels may not be representative of their usual levels. Cholesterol levels in patients who have had a myocardial infarction within the past 3 months are likely to be lower than usual. Therefore, recheck any results obtained during this period.

2. Inform patients that they need not vary their usual eating habits before undergoing screening for total blood cholesterol or HDL-cholesterol levels. Instruct patients undergoing lipoprotein analysis to fast for 12 hours before testing. Water and black coffee are acceptable, however.

3. If possible, perform cholesterol tests on venous blood samples, because cholesterol concentrations measured from finger-stick blood samples may be unreliable. The NCEP cut-off values for diagnostic and therapeutic actions refer to venous serum samples.

4. To prevent an effect of posture or stasis on the cholesterol value, perform venipuncture only after the patient has been in the sitting position for at least 5 minutes; apply the tourniquet for as brief a period as possible.

5. When interpreting results, be aware of the effects of medications on blood cholesterol levels. Anabolic steroids, progestins, bile salts, and chlorpromazine increase blood cholesterol levels. Be knowledgeable about conditions that may cause increased cholesterol levels, such as hypothyroidism, nephrotic syndrome, diabetes mellitus, and obstructive liver disease.

6. Cholesterol tests should be analyzed by an accredited laboratory that meets current standards for precision and accuracy. The Laboratory Standardization Panel of the National Cholesterol Education Program has set a goal that laboratories have systematic and precision errors of less than 3% each in processing total cholesterol samples. Inquire about a laboratory's performance history and its quality-control methods before using it for screening.

7. Cholesterol values in plasma samples tend to be lower than serum samples because of the effects of EDTA in plasma samples. NCEP has determined cholesterol level cut-off values based on serum samples and has designated that cholesterol levels obtained from plasma samples be multiplied by 1.03 to arrive at a serum equivalent.

8. Convert cholesterol values in mg/dL to mmol/L by multiplying by 0.02584. Convert triglyceride levels similarly by multiplying by 0.01129.

9. See Table 56.3 for information about NCEP's Step I and Step II Diet for treatment of patients with elevated cholesterol levels.

10. Provide dietary and weight-reduction counseling to all patients who are obese, regardless of their cholesterol levels (chapters 29 and 56). Provide advice about increasing physical activity to all patients who are physically inactive, regardless of their cholesterol levels (chapter 57).

Table 31.1. NCEP Coronary Heart Disease Risk Factors Other Than LDL-Cholesterol*

Positive Risk Factors

Age   Male ≥45 years
        Female ≥55 years or premature menopause without estrogen replacement therapy

Family history of premature CHD (definite myocardial infarction or sudden death)
    father/first-degree male relative <55 years
    mother/first-degree female relative <65 years

Cigarette smoking

Hypertension
    ≥140/90 mmHg† or on antihypertensive medication

Low HDL-cholesterol (<35 mg/dL)

Diabetes mellitus

Negative Risk Factor‡

HDL Cholesterol ≥60 mg/dL

---

* High risk, defined as two or more CHD risk factors (after positive and negative factors have been summed), leads to more vigorous intervention (see Figs 31-1 and 31-2). Age, defined differently for men and for women, is treated as a risk factor, because rates of CHD are higher in the elderly than in the young and are higher in men than in women of the same age. Obesity is not listed as a risk factor, because it operates through other risk factors (eg hypertension, hyperlipidemia, decreased HDL-cholesterol, and diabetes mellitus). Obesity should, however, be considered a target for intervention. Physical inactivity is similarly not listed as a risk factor, but it too should be considered a target for intervention, and physical activity is recommended as desirable for everyone. High risk attributable to coronary or peripheral atherosclerosis is addressed directly in Fig 31-3.

† Confirmed by measurements on several occasions

‡ If the HDL-cholesterol level is ≥60 mg/dL, subtract one risk factor (because HDL-cholesterol levels decrease CHD risk)

Adapted from: National Cholesterol Education Program. *Second Report of the National Cholesterol Education Program Expert Panel on Detection, Evaluation, and Treatment of High Blood Cholesterol in Adults (Adult Treatment Panel II).* Bethesda, Md: National Institutes of Health, National Heart, Lung, and Blood Institute; 1993. USDHHS Publication NIH 93-3095.

Table 31.2. Treatment Decisions Based on LDL-Cholesterol

Dietary Therapy

	Initiation Level	LDL Goal
Without CHD and with fewer than 2 risk factors	≥160mg/dL	<160 mg/dL
Without CHD and with 2 or more risk factors	≥130 mg/dL	<130 mg/dL
With CHD	>100 mg/dL	≤100 mg/dL

Drug Treatment

	Consideration Level	LDL Goal
Without CHD and with fewer than 2 risk factors	≥190mg/dL*	<160 mg/dL
Without CHD and with 2 or more risk factors	≥160 mg/dL	<130 mg/dL
With CHD	≥130 mg/dL†	≤100 mg/dL

* In men under 35 years of age and premenopausal women with LDL-cholestrol levels 190-219 mg/dL, drug therapy should be delayed except in high-risk patients such as those with diabetes.

† In CHD patients with LDL-cholestrol levels 100-129 mg/dL, the physician should exercise clinical judgment in deciding whether to initiate drug treatment.

Figure 31.1.   Primary Prevention in Adults Without Evidence of CHD: Initial Classification Based on Total Cholesterol and HDL-Cholesterol

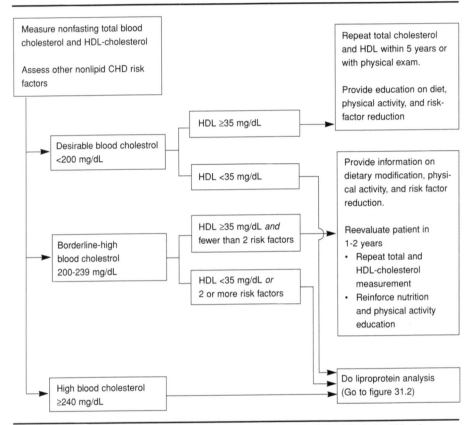

Adapted from: National Cholesterol Education Program. *Second Report of the National Cholesterol Education Program Expert Panel on Detection, Evaluation, and Treatment of High Blood Cholesterol in Adults (Adult Treatment Panel II)*. Bethesda, Md: National Institutes of Health, National Heart, Lung, and Blood Institute; 1993. USDHHS Publication NIH 93-3095.

Figure 31.2. Primary Prevention in Adults Without Evidence of CHD: Subsequent Classification Based on LDL-Cholesterol

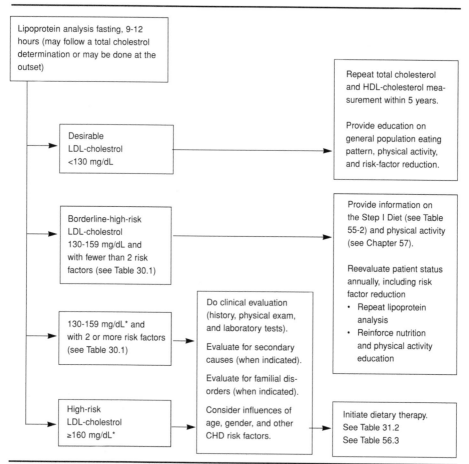

*On the basis of the average of two determinations. If the first two LDL-cholesterol levels differ by more than 30 mg/dL, perform a third test within 1 to 8 weeks, and use the average value of the three tests.

Adapted from: National Cholesterol Education Program. *Second Report of the National Cholesterol Education Program Expert Panel on Detection, Evaluation, and Treatment of High Blood Cholesterol in Adults (Adult Treatment Panel II)*. Bethesda, Md: National Institutes of Health, National Heart, Lung, and Blood Institute; 1993. USDHHS Publication NIH 93-3095.

Figure 31.3. Secondary Prevention in Adults With Evidence of CHD: Classification Based on LDL-Cholesterol

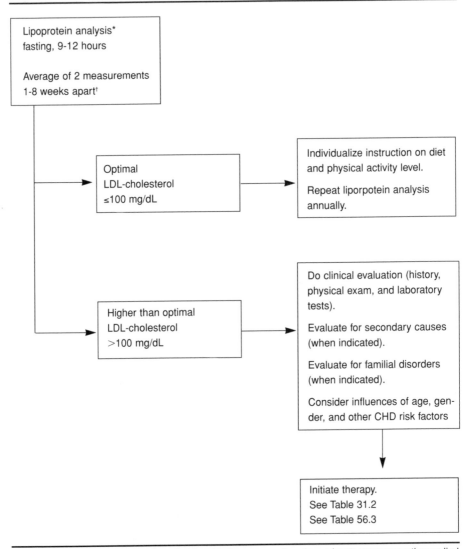

*Perform lipoprotein analysis when the patient is not in the recovery phase from an acute coronary or other medical event that would lower the patient's usual LDL-cholesterol level.

†If the first two LDL-cholesterol levels differ by more than 30 mg/dL, perform a third test within 1 to 8 weeks, and use the average value of the three tests.

Adapted from: National Cholesterol Education Program. *Second Report of the National Cholesterol Education Program Expert Panel on Detection, Evaluation, and Treatment of High Blood Cholesterol in Adults (Adult Treatment Panel II).* Bethesda, Md: National Institutes of Health, National Heart, Lung, and Blood Institute; 1993. USDHHS Publication NIH 93-3095.

Patient Resources

Cholesterol: What You Can Do to Lower Your Level. American Academy of Family Physicians, 8880 Ward Parkway, Kansas City, MO 64114-2797; (800)944-0000; http://www.aafp.org

Cholesterol and Your Health. American College of Obstetricians and Gynecologists, 409 12th St, SW, Washington, DC 20024-2188; (800)762-2264. Internet address: http://www.acog.com

Cholesterol and Your Heart; Dietary Treatment of Hypercholesterolemia: A Manual for Patients; Eat Less Fat and High Cholesterol Foods; Heart Rx (a kit of materials for patients, providers, and staff). To order these and many other materials, contact the American Heart Association, 7320 Greenville Ave, Dallas, TX 75231. To receive the telephone number of your state office, call the main office at: (800)242-8721; materials vary by state. Internet address: http://www.amhrt.org

American Heart Association Low-Fat, Low-Cholesterol Cookbook. This publication is available at retail bookstores. Internet address: http://www.amhrt.org

Eat Right to Lower Your High Blood Cholesterol and *Step by Step: Eating to Lower Your High Blood Cholesterol; So You Have High Blood Cholesterol.* National Heart, Lung, and Blood Institute Information Center, PO Box 30105, Bethesda, MD 20824-0105; (301) 251-1222. Internet address: http://www.nhlbi.nih.gov/nhlbi/nhlbi.html. Information is available in both English and Spanish. The following materials are available in Spanish: *Learn Your Cholesterol Number (Conozca su nivel de colesterol); Protect Your Health-Lower Your Blood Cholesterol (Proteja su corazon-baje su colesterol);* and *Heart-Healthy Latino Recipes (Platillos Latinos).*

Provider Resource

Summary of the Second Report of the National Cholesterol Education Program Expert Panel on Detection, Evaluation, and Treatment of High Blood Cholesterol in Adults (Adult Treatment Panel II). Full report: *National Cholesterol Education Program: Second Report of the Expert Panel on Detection, Evaluation, and Treatment of High Blood Cholesterol in Adults (Adult Treatment Panel II).* National Heart, Lung, and Blood Institute Information Center, PO Box 30105, Bethesda, MD 20824-0105; (301) 251-1222. Information is available in both English and Spanish. Internet address: http://www.nhlbi.nih.gov/nhlbi/nhlbi.html

Selected References

American Academy of Family Physicians. *Summary of Policy Recommendations for Periodic Health Examination.* Kansas City, Mo: American Academy of Family Physicians; 1997.

American College of Obstetricians and Gynecologists. *Guidelines for Women's Health Care.* Washington, DC: American College of Obstetricians and Gynecologists; 1996.

American College of Physicians, Clinical Efficacy Assessment Project. Using serum cholesterol, high-density lipoprotein cholesterol, and triglycerides as screening tests for the prevention of coronary heart disease in adults. *Ann Intern Med.* In press.

American College of Physicians. Guidelines. In: Eddy DM, ed. *Common Screening Tests.* Philadelphia, Pa: American College of Physicians; 1991:402-403.

American Heart Association. *Heart and Stroke Facts: 1996 Statistical Supplement.* Dallas, TX: American Heart Association; 1995.

Canadian Task Force on the Periodic Health Examination. Lowering the total blood cholesterol level to prevent coronary heart disease. In: *The Canadian Guide to Clinical Preventive Health Care.* Ottawa, Canada: Minister of Supply and Services; 1994: chap 54.

Expert Panel on Detection, Evaluation, and Treatment of High Blood Cholesterol in Adults. Summary of the second report of the National Cholesterol Education Program (NCEP) Expert Panel on Detection, Evaluation, and Treatment of High Blood Cholesterol in Adults (Adult Treatment Panel II). *JAMA.* 1993;269:3015-3023.

Greenland P, Bowley NL, Meiklejohn B, Doane KL, Sparks CE. Blood cholesterol concentration: fingerstick plasma vs venous serum sampling. *Clin Chem.* 1990;36:628-630.

National Cholesterol Education Program. *Second Report of the National Cholesterol Education Program Expert Panel on Detection, Evaluation, and Treatment of High Blood Cholesterol in Adults (Adult Treatment Panel II).* Bethesda, Md: National Heart, Lung, and Blood Institute. 1993. The full Adult Treatment Panel II report is also available in *Circulation.* 1994;89:1329-1445.

National Cholesterol Education Program. *Report of the Expert Panel on Population Strategies for Blood Cholesterol Reduction.* Bethesda, Md: National Institutes of Health, National Heart, Lung, and Blood Institute; 1990. US Dept of Health and Human Services, PHS publication NIH 90-3046.

NIH Consensus Development Panel on Triglyceride, High-Density Lipoprotein, and Coronary Heart Disease. Triglyceride, high-density lipoprotein, and coronary heart disease. *JAMA.* 1993;269:505-510.

Sempos CT, Cleeman JI, Carroll MD, et al. Prevalence of high blood cholesterol among US adults: an update based on guidelines from the second report of the National Cholesterol Education Program Adult Treatment Panel. *JAMA.* 1993;269:3009-3014.

Shepherd J, Cobbe SM, Ford I, et al. Prevention of coronary heart disease with pravastatin in men with hypercholesterolemia. *N Engl J Med.* 1995;333:1301-7.

US Preventive Services Task Force. Screening for blood cholesterol. In: *Guide to Clinical Preventive Services.* 2nd ed. Washington, DC: US Department of Health and Human Services; 1996: chap 2.

32

COGNITIVE AND FUNCTIONAL IMPAIRMENT

Cognitive impairment includes deficits in memory, abstract thinking, judgement, speech, coordination, planning, or organization. A functional impairment is a deficit in an individual's ability to perform either the basic activities of daily living (ADLs), such as as dressing, bathing, and eating, or instrumental activities of daily living (IADLs) — such as using transportation, shopping, or handling finances. A functional impairment can be the result of a cognitive, physical, social, or psychological disorder. Dementia is a syndrome of progressive decline in multiple cognitive abilities that eventually leads to functional impairment. The most common form of dementia is Alzheimer's disease.

It is estimated that between 5% and 10% of persons older than 65 years of age suffer from some form of cognitive impairment, and this increases dramatically with age. The most common causes of cognitive impairment, Alzheimer's disease and vascular infarctions, are largely untreatable. However, approximately 10% to 15% of cases of cognitive impairment in older adults are attributable to treatable causes, such as hypothyroidism and drug intoxications. In some instances, early intervention can result in the arrest or reversal of cognitive defects. Approximately 2% to 8% of community-dwelling elderly persons suffer from impairments of ADLs. As many as 25% of community-dwelling older adults may suffer from functional impairment in carrying out IADLs.

Cognitive and functional impairment are growing health concerns in the United States because of the aging population. In some instances, early identification of these impairments can lead to the reversal or slowing of the progression of the impairment. In other instances, early identification alerts affected persons and their families to potentially hazardous situations and is of value in terms of planning support services.

See chapter 58 on polypharmacy.

Recommendations of Major Authorities

The Alzheimer's Disease and Related Dementias Panel of the Agency of Health Care Policy and Research—Health care providers should perform an initial assessment of dementia on clients with symptoms of increasing difficulties in the following areas: learning and retaining new information; handling complex tasks; reasoning ability; spatial ability and orientation; language or behavior.

American College of Obstetricians and Gynecologists—Women over 65 years of age should be screened for changes in cognitive function as part of their routine preventive visits.

American College of Physicians—Functional assessment screening by the clinician is useful for evaluating the health status of elderly patients and determining their needs for in-home assistance, home health services, or institutional placement. In the acute-care setting, functional assessment in selected patients facilitates discharge planning and is essential in patients over 75 years of age. Primary care providers should incorporate into the routine medical management of older adults procedures for measuring functional deficits and identifying dependency needs. Employing a comprehensive screening instrument followed by targeted screening instruments can be useful in systematically assessing functional deficits that otherwise might be overlooked by conventional examination methods.

Canadian Task Force on the Periodic Health Examination—There is insufficient evidence to recommend for or against active screening for cognitive impairment in people over 65 years of age. However, prudent clinicians should be alert for symptoms suggestive of cognitive impairment and conduct appropriate assessments.

US Preventive Services Task Force—There is insufficient evidence to recommend for or against routine screening for dementia in asymptomatic elderly persons. Clinicians should periodically ask patients about their functional status at home and at work, and they should remain alert to changes in performance with age. When possible, information about daily activities should be solicited from family members and other persons. Brief tests, such as the Mini-Mental State Exam, should be used to assess cognitive function in patients in whom the suspicion of dementia is raised by restrictions in daily activities, concerns of family members, or other evidence of worsening function (eg, trouble with finances, medications, transportation). Possible effects of education and cultural differences should be considered when interpreting abnormal results.

Basics of Cognitive and Functional Impairment Screening

Cognitive Impairment

1. Effective screening for cognitive impairment requires assessment of multiple aspects of mental functioning, including orientation, short-term mem-

ory, receptive and expressive language ability, attention, and visual-spatial ability.

2. Orientation can be rapidly assessed by asking the patient to give the day of the week, the month, the year, and current location. Short-term memory can be rapidly assessed by asking the patient to repeat a seven-digit number or recall three objects. Language ability can be rapidly assessed by asking the patient to name simple objects, repeat a phrase, or write a sentence. Attention can be rapidly assessed by asking the patient to count backward from 100 to 65 by subtracting 7, or to name the months of the year in reverse order. Visual-spatial ability can be rapidly assessed by asking the patient to draw a complex figure, such as the face of a clock or a three-dimensional cube.

3. Use of a short, standardized screening instrument can accomplish this basic assessment and provide a baseline for assessing changes in cognitive function in the future. No single screening instrument best addresses all areas of cognition or is appropriate for all patients. The most widely used and studied brief screening instrument is the Mini-Mental State Examination (Table 32.1).

4. Any assessment of cognitive functioning must take into consideration the patient's level and clarity of consciousness (is the patient delirious?), affective state (is the patient depressed?), effects of medications and drugs (is the patient intoxicated?), level of education and baseline intelligence (would the patient have understood as a young person?), and native language (is the patient fluent in English?).

5. Patients with indications of cognitive impairment should be considered for referral to a specialist for more definitive evaluation before the diagnosis of dementia is made and treatment begun.

Functional Impairment

1. Assessment of functional impairment can be performed by a variety of methods, including observation of the patient in the home; observation of the patient in the office; questioning of the patient, family, or both; and use of brief, structured questionnaires. Within the limits of time and resources, use a variety of methods of assessment.

2. Use structured questions to supplement, not replace, clinical observation and more extensive forms of assessment.

3. IADLs can be briefly evaluated by using the following five structured questions in Table 32.2.

Table 32.1. Mini-Mental State Examination*

Maximum Score	Patient's Score	Questions
5		"What is the (year) (season) (date) (day) (month)?"
5		"Where are we?" Name of (state) (county) (city or town) (place, such as hospital or clinic) (specific location, such as floor or room)
3		The examiner names three unrelated objects clearly and slowly, then asks the patient to name all three of them. The patient's response is used for scoring. The examiner repeats them until patient learns all of them, if possible.
5		"Begin with 100 and count backwards by subtracting 7." Stop at 65. (5 responses)
3		If the patient learned the three objects above, ask the patient to recall them now.
2		The examiner shows the patient two simple objects, such as a wrist watch and pencil, and asks the patient to name them.
1		"Repeat the phrase, 'No ifs, ands, or buts.'"
3		The examiner gives the patient a piece of blank paper and asks him or her to follow the three-step command: "Take the paper in your right hand, fold it in half, and put it on the floor."
1		On a blank piece of paper the examiner prints the command "Close your eyes," in letters large enough for the patient to see clearly, then asks the patient to read it and follow the command.
1		"Make up and write a sentence about anything." This sentence must contain a noun and verb.
1		The examiner gives the patient a blank piece of paper and asks him or her to draw this symbol. All 10 angles must be present and two must intersect.
Total Possible = 30	Patient's Total =	If total score is 23 or less, further evaluation may be indicated.

*Instructions: Score one point for each correct response within each question or activity.

Reprinted with permission from: *The Journal of Psychiatric Research*, 12:189–198, Folstein MF, Folstein SE, McHugh P. "Mini-mental state": a practical method for grading the cognitive state of patients for the clinician, 1975, Elsevier Science.

Table 32.2. Questions for Evaluating Instrumental Activities of Daily Living (IADLs)

---

1. Can you get to places outside of walking distance without help? (For example, travel alone on buses, taxis, or drive a car)
2. Can you go shopping for groceries or clothes without help? (Assumes that the patient has transportation.)
3. Can you prepare your own meals without help? (For example, plan and cook full meals without help)
4. Can you do your housework without help?
5. Can you handle your own money without help? (For example, write checks, pay bills)

Adapted from: Fillenbaum GG. Screening the elderly: a brief instrumental activities of daily living measure. *J Am Geriatr Soc.* 1985;33:698–706. Reproduced with permission of the American Geriatrics Society; copyright 1985.

4. ADLs can be briefly assessed using the six structured questions in Table 32.3

5. Investigate any identified impairments in function for etiology (physical, psychological, environmental) and possible means of treatment or amelioration (in-home support services, speech and language therapy, physical and occupational therapy).

Table 32.3. Questions for Evaluating Activities of Daily Living (ADLs)

---

1. Do you bathe yourself without help?
2. Do you dress yourself without help?
3. Do you use the toilet without help?
4. Do you move in and out of bed or a chair without help?
5. Do you have any trouble controlling your bladder or your bowels?
6. Do you feed yourself without help?

Adapted from: Katz S, Ford AB, Moskowitz RW, Jackson BA, Jaffe MW, Cleveland MA. The index of ADL: a standardized measure of biological and psychosocial function. *JAMA.* 1963;185:914–919. Reproduced by permission of the American Medical Association; copyright 1963.

Patient Resources

Memory and Aging: Alzheimer's Disease and Related Disorders. To order this and many other materials, contact the Alzheimer's Association, 919 N Michigan Ave, Suite 1000, Chicago, IL 60611;(800)272-3900.

Memory Loss: What's Normal, What's Not. American Academy of Family Physicians, 8880 Ward Pkwy, Kansas City, MO 64114; (800)944-0000. Internet address: http://www.aafp.org

Where Did I Put My Keys? American Association of Retired Persons, Fulfillment Services, 601 E St, NW, Washington, DC 20049; (202) 434-2534.

Age Page—Senility: Myth or Madness; Age Page—Confusion and Memory Loss in Old Age: It's Not What You Think. National Institute on Aging, Bldg 31, Room 5C27, Bethesda, MD 20892; (301) 496-1752. Internet address: http://www.nih.gov/nia/health/pubpub/pubpub.htm

Early Alzheimer's Disease. AHCPR Publication no. 96-0704. Agency for Health Care Policy and Research, Publications Clearinghouse, P.O. Box 8547, Silver Spring MD 20907; (800)358-9295. Internet address: http://www.ahcpr.gov

Administration on Aging. 330 Independence Ave., SW, Washington, DC 20201, (202)619-1006. The national office can provide phone numbers and addresses for state and local agencies on aging. Internet address: http://www.aoa.dhhs.gov

The Elder Care Locator (800)667-1116 provides toll-free access to state agency networks.

Provider Resources

Older Voices. To order this trainer's manual and resource materials for communication problems of older persons, contact the American Speech-Language-Hearing Association, 10801 Rockville Pike, Rockville, MD 20852; (301)897-5700.

Early Identification of Alzheimer's Disease and Related Dementias: Quick Reference Guide for Clinicians (Number 19). AHCPR Publication no. 97-0703. Agency for Health Care Policy and Research, Publications Clearinghouse, P.O. Box 8547, Silver Spring Md 20907; (800)358-9295. The full text of guideline documents for online retrieval is available on the AHCPR Home Page. Click on "Clinical Practice Guidelines Online." Internet address: http://www.ahcpr.gov/guide

Selected References

American College of Physicians, Health and Public Policy Committee. Comprehensive functional assessment for elderly patients. *Ann Intern Med.* 1988;109:70-72.

Calkins DR, Rubenstein LV, Cleary PD, Davies AR, Jette AM, Fink A, Kosecoff J, et al. Failure of physicians to recognize functional disability in ambulatory patients. *Ann Intern Med.* 1991;114:451-454.

Canadian Task Force on the Periodic Health Examination. The periodic health examination. *Can Med Assoc J.* 1979;121:1193-1254.

Canadian Task Force on the Periodic Health Examination. *Periodic Health Examination Monograph.* Hull, Quebec: Ministry of Supply and Services; 1980.

Canadian Task Force on the Periodic Health Examination. Screening for cognitive impairment in the elderly. In: *The Canadian Guide to Clinical Preventive Health Care.* Ottawa, Canada: Minister of Supply and Services; 1994: chap 75.

Costa PT Jr, Williams TF, Somerfield M, et al. *Recognition and Initial Assessment of Alzheimer's Disease and Related Dementias.* Clinical Practice Guideline No. 19. Rockville, Md: US Department of Health and Human Services, Public Health Service, Agency for Health Care Policy and Research, AHCPR Publication No. 97-0702. November 1996.

Fillenbaum GG. Screening the elderly: a brief instrumental activities of daily living measure. *J Amer Geriatr Soc.* 1985;33:698-706.

Folstein MF, Folstein SE, McHugh P. "Mini-mental state": a practical method for grading the cognitive state of patients for the clinician. *J Psychiatr Res.* 1975;12:189-198.

Katz S, Ford AB, Moskowitz RW, Jackson BA, Jaffe MW, Cleveland MA. The index of ADL: a standardized measure of biological and psychosocial function. *JAMA.* 1963;185:914-919.

National Institutes of Health, Consensus Development Panel. Differential diagnosis of dementing diseases. *JAMA.* 1987;258:3411-3416.

Patterson CJ. Detecting cognitive impairment in the elderly. In: Goldbloom RB, Lawrence RS. *Preventing Disease: Beyond the Rhetoric.* New York, NY: Springer-Verlag; 1990: chap 18.

Pfeiffer E. A short portable mental status questionnaire for the assessment of organic brain deficit in elderly patients. *J Amer Geriatr Soc.* 1975;23:433-441.

Siu AL. Screening for dementia and investigating its causes. *Ann Intern Med.* 1991;115:122-132.

Siu AL, Reubens DB, Hays RD. Hierarchical measures of physical function in ambulatory geriatrics. *J Amer Geriatr Soc.* 1990;38:1113-1119.

Rubenstein LV, Calkins DR, Greenfield S, et al. Health status assessment for elderly patients: report of the Task Force on Health Assessment, Society of General Internal Medicine. *J Amer Geriatr Soc.* 1988;37:562-569.

US Preventive Services Task Force. Screening for dementia. In: *Guide to Clinical Preventive Services.* 2nd ed. Washington, DC: US Department of Health and Human Services; 1996: chap 48.

Weiner JM, Hanley RJ, Clark R, Van Nostrand JF. Measuring the activities of daily living: comparisons across national surveys. *Journal of Gerontology.* 1990;45(6):S229-237.

33

DEPRESSION

Major depressive episodes are common in adults, affecting more than 9 million Americans and costing between $33 million and $40 billion yearly. Depression affects persons of all ages, genders, and races. See Table 33.1 for a list of risk factors for major depression.

Between 5% and 10% of patients in primary care practices and 10% to 14% of medical inpatients meet the criteria for major depression, and many patients with depressive disorders are seen only by nonpsychiatric health-care providers. Research has shown that up to 50% of depressed persons seen in primary care settings are not recognized as having this disorder. Patients with major depressive disorders have a great deal of functional impairment, resulting in lost time on the job, decreased job performance, and decreased family and social functioning. Effective medical treatments are available for major depression.

Recommendations of Major Authorities

American College of Obstetricians and Gynecology—All women should receive age-specific psychosocial evaluations to detect depression and other problems.

American College of Physicians—Elderly patients should undergo functional assessment screening, including measures of emotional status.

Canadian Task Force on the Periodic Health Examination—There is fair evidence to exclude the use of depression detection tests from the periodic health examination of asymptomatic people. However, physicians should be sensitive to the possibility of depression in their patients, particularly those at high risk.

US Preventive Services Task Force—There is insufficient evidence to recommend for or against performance of routine screening tests for depression in asymptomatic primary care patients. Clinicians should, however, maintain an especially high index of suspicion for depressive symptoms in adolescents and young adults, persons with a family or personal history of depression, those with chronic illnesses, those who have or

Table 33.1. Risk Factors for Depression

Prior episode(s) of depression

Family history of depressive disorder

Prior suicide attempt(s)

Female gender

Postpartum period

Medical co-morbidity

Lack of social support

Stressful life events

Personal history of sexual abuse

Current substance abuse

From: Agency for Health Care Policy and Research, Depression Guideline Panel. *Depression in Primary Care: Detection, Diagnosis, and Treatment.* Rockville, Md: US Department of Health and Human Services, Public Health Service. Technical Report 5.

perceive they have experienced a recent loss, and those with sleep disorders, chronic pain, or multiple unexplained somatic complaints.

Basics of Depression Screening

1. The diagnostic criteria for a major depressive episode, as defined in the *Diagnostic and Statistical Manual of Mental Disorders* (DSM-IV), are given in Table 33.2. Because the essential feature is either depressed mood or loss of pleasure in usual activities for at least 2 weeks, these symptoms should be discussed first when taking a history.

2. Some features of depression in elderly persons may be confused with symptoms of dementia, resulting in what has been called pseudodementia due to depression. Keep in mind that disorientation, memory loss, and distractibility in the elderly may be signs of depression rather than dementia.

3. Basic steps for detecting depression in primary care patients include:

   ■ Maintaining a high index of suspicion, especially with patients who have risk factors

   ■ Using the clinical interview or a written questionnaire (see item 4 below)

Table 33.2. Criteria for Major Depressive Disorder

At least five of the following symptoms are present during the same period and represent a change from previous functioning; depressed mood or loss of interest or pleasure must be present. Symptoms are present most of the day, nearly daily for at least 2 weeks.

Depressed mood (can be irritable in children and adolescents) most of the day, nearly every day

Markedly diminished interest or pleasure in almost all activities most of the day, nearly every day (as indicated either by subjective account or observation by others of apathy most of the time)

Significant weight loss or gain

Insomnia or hypersomnia

Psychomotor agitation or retardation

Fatigue (loss of energy)

Feelings of worthlessness (guilt)

Impaired concentration (indecisiveness)

Recurrent thoughts of death or suicide

Reprinted with permission from: *The Diagnostic and Statistical Manual of Mental Disorders*, Fourth Edition. Copyright 1994, American Psychiatric Association.

- Eliciting additional information by questioning family or caretakers (with patient consent)
- Identifying (and treating, if present) other possible causes for mood disorders, such as medical illness, medication use, or substance abuse
- Making the diagnosis of major depressive disorder and proceeding to treatment or referral if no other causes for the mood changes are found (or if the depression continues after treatment of other causes of mood changes)

4. Several short self-report questionnaires for depression have been evaluated and found to be useful in primary care settings (Coulehan et al, 1989). These include the Short Beck Depression Inventory (BDI), the Zung Self-Rating Depression Scale (SDS), and the Center for Epidemiologic Studies Depression Scale (CES-D). The CES-D is given in Table 33.3. Self-report questionnaires are helpful in finding patients with depressive symptoms, but they are not diagnostic instruments. Many patients with mild depression who do not meet diagnostic criteria for a major depressive episode

Table 33.3. Center for Epidemiologic Studies Depression Scale*

DURING THE PAST WEEK	RARELY or NONE of the time (< day)	SOME or a LITTLE of the time (1–2 days)	OCCASIONALLY or a MODERATE amount of the time (3–4 days)	MOST or ALL of the time (5–7 days)
1. I was bothered by things that don't usually bother me.	0	1	2	3
2. I did not feel like eating; my appetite was poor.	0	1	2	3
3. I felt that I could not shake off the blues even with the help of my family and friends.	0	1	2	3
4. I felt that I was just as good as other people.	3	2	1	0
5. I had trouble keeping my mind on what I was doing.	0	1	2	3
6. I felt depressed.	0	1	2	3
7. I felt everything I did was an effort.	0	1	2	3
8. I felt hopeful about the future.	3	2	1	0
9. I thought my life had been a failure.	0	1	2	3
10. I felt fearful.	0	1	2	3
11. My sleep was restless.	0	1	2	3
12. I was happy.	3	2	1	0
13. I talked less than usual.	0	1	2	3
14. I felt lonely.	0	1	2	3
15. People were unfriendly.	0	1	2	3
16. I enjoyed life.	3	2	1	0
17. I had crying spells.	0	1	2	3
18. I felt sad.	0	1	2	3
19. I felt that people disliked me.	0	1	2	3
20. I could not get "going."	0	1	2	3

* Interpretation: A total score of 22 or higher is indicative of depression when this scale is used in primary care.

From: Radloff LS. The CES-D Scale: a self-report depression scale for research in the general population. *Appl Psychol Meas*. 1977;1:385–401. Copyright 1977, West Publishing Company/Applied Psychological Measurement, Inc. Reproduced by permission.

will be identified with these questionnaires. If a patient scores above the cut-off point on a questionnaire, use the clinical interview to elicit the criterion symptoms of a major depressive episode. Because self-report questionnaires are very sensitive to depressive symptoms, they can also be used appropriately to exclude major depression in patients who score below the cut-off points.

Patient Resources

Depression Is a Treatable Illness: A Patient's Guide. Agency for Health Care Policy and Research Publications Clearinghouse, PO Box 8547, Silver Spring, MD 20907; 1-800-358-9295.

Depression. ACOG Patient Education Pamphlet AP106. Washington, DC: American College of Obstetricians and Gynecologists, 1994. Internet address: http://www.acog.com

To obtain free brochures about clinical depression, including information on depression in women, depression in the workplace, and depression co-morbid with medical, psychiatric, and substance abuse disorders, contact the National Institute of Mental Health, 5600 Fishers Ln, Room 10-85, Rockville, MD 20857; (800)421-4211. Internet address: http://www.nimh.nih.gov

Many types of materials are available from the National Mental Health Association, 1021 Prince St, Alexandria, VA 22314; (800)969-6642.

The National Depressive and Manic Depressive Association, 730 North Franklin Street, Suite 501, Chicago, IL 60610. (800)826-3632.

The National Mental Health Services Knowledge Exchange Network (KEN), P.O. Box 42490, Washington, DC 20015. KEN is a national, one-stop resource for mental health information and referrals that is accessible through a toll-free telephone number, (800)789-CMHS (2647); a toll-free electronic bulletin board system (BBS), (800)790-CMHS (2647). Internet address: http://www.mentalhealth.org/

Provider Resources

Depression in Primary Care: Detection and Diagnosis (vol 1; AHCPR publication 93-0550); *Treatment of Major Depression* (vol 2; AHCPR publication 93-0551). These publications are available through the US Government Printing Office; call (202) 510-1800.

Diagnosis and Treatment (Quick Reference Guide for Clinicians; AHCPR publication 93-0552). Agency for Health Care Policy and Research Publications Clearinghouse, PO Box 8547, Silver Spring, MD 20907; (800)358-9295.

Depression in Women. American College of Obstetricians and Gynecologists Technical Bulletin #182, 1992. ACOG Resource Center, 409 12th St., SW, Washington, DC 20024-2188; 1-800-762-2264. Internet address: http://www.acog.com

Diagnosis and Treatment of Depression in Late Life (NIH Consensus Development Conference, November 4-6, 1991; NIH Consensus Statements vol 9, no 3). NIH Consensus Clearing House, PO Box 2577, Kensington, MD 20891, 1-888-644-2667.

Selected References

Agency for Health Care Policy and Research, Depression Guideline Panel. *Depression in primary care: detection, diagnosis, and treatment quick reference guide for clinicians 5.* Rockville, Md: US Department of Health and Human Services, Public Health Service, Agency for Health Care Policy and Research, AHCPR Publication 93-0552; April 1993.

American College of Obstetricians and Gynecologists. *Depression in Women.* Washington, DC: American College of Obstetricians and Gynecologists; 1993.

American College of Obstetricians and Gynecologists. *Guidelines for Women's Health Care.* Washington, DC: American College of Obstetricians and Gynecologists; 1996.

American College of Physicians, Health and Public Policy Committee. Comprehensive functional assessment for elderly patients. *Ann Intern Med.* 1988;109:70-72.

American Psychiatric Association. *Diagnostic and Statistical Manual of Mental Disorders.* 3rd ed, rev. Washington, DC: American Psychiatric Association; 1987.

Beck AT, Rial WY, Rickels K. Short form of depression inventory: cross validation. *Psychological Reports.* 1974;34:1184-1186.

Canadian Task Force on the Periodic Health Examination. Early detection of depression. In: *The Canadian Guide to Clinical Preventive Health Care.* Ottawa, Canada: Minister of Supply and Services; 1994: chap 39.

Coulehan JL, Schulberg HC, Block MR. The efficiency of depression questionnaires for case-finding in primary medical care. *J Gen Intern Med.* 1989;4:542-547.

Kamerow DB, Pincus HA, Macdonald DI. Alcohol abuse, other drug abuse, and mental disorders in medical practice: prevalence, costs, recognition, and treatment. *JAMA.* 1986;255: 2054-2057.

Radloff LS. The CES-D Scale: a self-report depression scale for research in the general population. *Appl Psychol Meas.* 1977;1:385-401.

US Preventive Services Task Force. Screening for depression. In: *Guide to Clinical Preventive Services.* 2nd ed. Washington, DC: US Department of Health and Human Services; 1996: chap 49.

Wells KB, Stewart A, Hays RD, et al. The functioning and well-being of depressed patients: results from the Medical Outcomes Study. *JAMA.* 1989;4:7-13.

Zung WWK. A self-rating depression scale. *Arch Gen Psychiatry.* 1965;12:63-70.

34

FECAL OCCULT BLOOD

In 1997, approximately 131,200 new cases of colorectal cancer will occur, resulting in 54,900 deaths. Principal risk factors for colorectal cancer include a history of one of the familial polyposis syndromes, familial cancer syndromes, colorectal cancer in first-degree relatives, or a personal history of ulcerative colitis, adenomatous polyps, or endometrial, ovarian, or breast cancer. Colorectal cancer detected at an early stage can be successfully treated with surgery.

Malignancies and, to a lesser extent, polyps, bleed intermittently. Fecal occult blood tests (FOBT) can detect this bleeding by identifying occult blood or breakdown products of blood in fecal material. The reported sensitivity of FOBT for detecting colorectal cancer in asymptomatic individuals ranges from 26% to 92% but with most data suggesting a sensitivity of less than 40%. The specificity ranges form 90% to 99%. Measures of sensitivity and specificity are usually based on two samples from three consecutive and easily passed stools.

Until recently, no studies had shown that fecal occult blood testing resulted in decreased mortality. In 1993, however, Mandel et al found that yearly fecal occult blood testing using rehydrated stool specimens decreased mortality from colorectal cancer by about one third. In that study, guaiac-impregnated paper slides were used to test for fecal blood.

Rehydration of dried samples before testing can increase sensitivity but also produces more false-positive results. The predictive value of a positive fecal occult blood test for colorectal cancer in general populations is only 5% to 10%. Thus, up to 75% of cancers will be missed, and for every case of colorectal cancer that is detected by fecal occult blood testing, up to 20 patients will undergo workups that will be negative.

See chapters 30 and 41 for information about other methods of screening for colorectal cancer.

Recommendations of Major Authorities

American Academy of Family Physicians—Adults aged 40 years and older with a family history of early colorectal cancer and all adults aged 50 years and older should be screened for colorectal cancer with fecal occult blood testing (annually), sigmoidoscopy, colonoscopy, or barium enema.

American Cancer Society—Annual fecal occult blood testing is recommended in combination with flexible sigmoidoscopy every 5 years in normal risk individuals beginning at 50 years of age. The American Cancer Society further recommends that digital rectal examination be performed along with sigmoidoscopy. (See chapter 41 for details.)

American College of Obstetrics and Gynecology—Fecal occult blood testing should be done for all women 50 years of age and older as part of their periodic health examination.

American College of Physicians—Persons who decline screening colonoscopies and barium enemas, and especially people who decline screening flexible sigmoidoscopies, should be offered annual fecal occult blood testing from 50 to 70 or 80 years of age. No recommendation is made about the optimal frequency for screening with FOBT. In general, persons who have positive results on a fecal occult blood test should have a full colonic examination. More research is needed to understand and improve the sensitivity and specificity of the fecal occult blood test.

Canadian Task Force on the Periodic Health Examination (CTFPHE)—There is insufficient evidence to recommend including or excluding fecal occult blood testing in the periodic health examination of individuals over 40 years of age. There is also insufficient evidence to provide fecal occult blood testing to adults at risk because of family history. Patients with true cancer family syndrome should be screened with colonoscopy, not fecal occult blood testing.

US Preventive Services Task Force—Screening for colorectal cancer is recommended for all persons 50 years of age or older. This can be accomplished with annual fecal occult blood testing or sigmoidoscopy (frequency unspecified). There is insufficient evidence to determine which method is preferable or whether combining both methods produces results superior to either method alone.

Basics of Fecal Occult Blood Screening

1. Three types of tests are available for detecting fecal occult blood: guaiac-impregnated cards and other carriers that detect the peroxidase-like activity of hemoglobin (Hemoccult®); quantitative tests based on the conver-

sion of heme to fluorescent porphyrins (HemoQuant®); and immunoassay tests for human hemoglobin. Currently only the first two types are routinely used in practice. Guaiac-based tests have the disadvantage of giving false-negative and false-positive results because of dietary factors, and thus are more accurate if patients restrict their diets (see Table 34.1). Guaiac-based tests have the advantages of being relatively easy for patients and clinicians to use and relatively specific for lower gastrointestinal tract bleeding. The quantitative porphyrin tests are not affected by dietary factors and are potentially more sensitive than the other tests, depending on the cut point designated for a positive result. Recent evidence indicates, however, that at matched levels of specificity, the quantitative porphyrin tests are not significantly more sensitive than guaiac-based tests. Quantitative porphyrin tests have the potential disadvantages of not being specific for lower gastrointestinal tract bleeding and of requiring interpretation by a laboratory.

2. Do not collect a stool sample from patients with hematuria or obvious rectal bleeding (eg, from hemorrhoids). Instruct women to avoid collecting stool samples during or just after a menstrual period.

3. If possible, patients should avoid using medications that cause gastric irritation and bleeding for at least 48 hours before and during the testing period. Such medications include aspirin, nonsteroidal antiinflammatory drugs (NSAIDs), corticosteroids, anticoagulants, reserpine, antimetabolites, and chemotherapeutic agents. Consumption of excess amounts of alcohol should be avoided. The manufacturer of Hemoccult® recommends avoidance of aspirin and NSAIDs for 7 days before the test. When guaiac-based tests are used, patient adherence to the dietary guidelines in Table 34.1 for

---

Table 34.1. Additional Instructions for Patients Using Guaiac-Based Tests

Seven days prior to and during the test period, avoid aspirin and other non-steroidal anti-inflammatory drugs.

Three days prior to and during the test period, avoid Vitamin C in excess of 250 mg per day* (from all sources, dietary and supplemental).

Three days prior to and during the test period, do not consume red meat (beef, lamb) including processed meats and liver.

Three days prior to and during the test period, do not consume raw fruits and vegetables (especially broccoli, cauliflower, horseradish, parsnips, radishes, turnips and melons).

Remove toilet bowl cleaners from toilet tank and flush twice before proceeding.

---

*Caution: some iron supplements contain quantities of Vitamin C which exceed 250 mg per day.

Adapted from: SmithKline Diagnostic. *Product Instructions for Hemoccult®*. Palo Alto, Calif: SmithKline Diagnostics, Inc: 1994. Reproduced by permission of the publisher; copyright 1994.

at least 48 hours before and during the testing period can help avoid false-positive and false-negative results. Despite previous reports, dietary iron does not cause false-positive test results. To prevent false-positive test results, avoid applying antiseptic preparations containing iodine to the anal area immediately before and during the testing period.

4. When guaiac-impregnated cards are used, collect two separate samples from different sections of three consecutive bowel movements; use the supplied applicator and apply thin smears of the samples to the cards. Instruct patients to return samples as soon as possible for processing. Optimally, processing of the cards should occur within 6 days of collection but definitely not after 14 days. Rehydration of the samples with a drop of water before application of the developer increases sensitivity by approximately 30% to 40%, but it also decreases specificity by 2% to 3%, leading to significantly more false-positive results. For this reason, authorities disagree about the use of rehydration. A positive result on even one sample qualifies the entire test as positive. Store both cards and developer at room temperature, protected from heat and light.

5. Patients who return samples through the mail should use special US Postal Service-approved envelopes. These may be obtained by contacting the manufacturers of the fecal occult blood test system.

6. Because of the intermittent nature of bleeding in patients with colorectal cancer, malignancy cannot be conclusively ruled out by repeat fecal occult blood testing.

7. Follow-up of a positive fecal occult blood test requires diagnostic procedures such as sigmoidoscopy, colonoscopy, or barium enema.

Patient Resources

Colonoscopy: Questions and Answers; Colorectal Cancer: Questions & Answers; Polyps of the Colon and Rectum: Questions and Answers. American Society of Colon and Rectal Surgeons, 800 E Northwest Hwy, Suite 1080, Palatine, IL 60067; (708) 359-9184.

What You Need to Know about Cancer of the Colon and Rectum. Office of Cancer Communications, National Cancer Institute, Bethesda, MD 20892; (800)4-CANCER; Internet address: http://wwwicic.nci.nih.gov

Selected References

Ahlquist DA, Wieand HS, Moertal CG, et al. Accuracy of fecal occult blood screening for colorectal neoplasia. *JAMA.* 1993;269:1262-1267.

American Academy of Family Physicians. *Summary of Policy Recommendations for Periodic Health Examination.* Kansas City, Mo: American Academy of Family Physicians; 1997.

American Cancer Society. *Cancer Information Database.* Atlanta, Ga: American Cancer Society; June 1997.

American Cancer Society. *Cancer Facts & Figures-1997.* Atlanta, Ga: American Cancer Society; 1997.

American Cancer Society. Summary of American Cancer Society recommendations for the early detection of cancer in asymptomatic people. *CA.* 1993;43:45.

American College of Obstetricians and Gynecologists. *Guidelines for Women's Health Care.* Washington, DC: American College of Obstetricians and Gynecologists; 1996.

American College of Obstetricians and Gynecologists. *Routine Cancer Screening.* ACOG Committee Opinion. Washington, DC: American College of Obstetricians and Gynecologists; In press.

American College of Physicians. Guidelines. In: Eddy DM, ed. *Common Screening Tests.* Philadelphia, Pa: American College of Physicians; 1991:415-416.

American College of Physicians. Suggested technique for fecal occult blood testing and interpretation in colorectal cancer screening. *Ann Intern Med.* 1997;126:808-810.

American College of Physicians. Screening for colorectal cancer with the fecal occult blood test: a background paper. *Ann Intern Med.* 1997;126:811-822.

Canadian Task Force on the Periodic Health Examination. Screening for colorectal cancer. In: *The Canadian Guide to Clinical Preventive Health Care.* Ottawa, Canada: Minister of Supply and Services; 1994: chap 66.

Eddy DM. Screening for colorectal cancer. *Ann Intern Med.* 1990;113:373-384.

Eddy DM, Ferioli C, Anderson DS. Screening for colorectal cancer. *Ann Intern Med.* In press.

Fleischer DE, Goldberg SB, Browing TH, et al. Detection and surveillance of colorectal cancer. *JAMA.* 1989;261:580-585.

Gnauck R, Macrae FA, Fleisher M. How to perform the fecal occult blood test. *CA.* 1984;34: 134-137.

Kewenter J, Bjork S, Haglind E, Smith L, Svanvik J, Ahren C. Screening and rescreening for colorectal cancer: a controlled trial of fecal occult blood testing in 27,700 subjects. *Cancer.* 1988;62:645-651.

Knight KK, Fielding JE, Battista RN. Occult blood screening for colorectal cancer. *JAMA.* 1989;261:587-593.

Levin B, Murphy GP. Revision in American Cancer Society recommendations for the early detection of colorectal cancer. *CA.* 1992;42:296-299.

Mandel JS, Bond JH, Church TR, et al. Reducing mortality from colorectal cancer by screening for fecal occult blood. *N Engl J Med.* 1993;328:1365-1371.

McCrae FA, St John JB, Caligiore P, Taylor LS, Legge JW. Optimal dietary conditions for Hemoccult® testing. *Gastroenterology.* 1982;82:899-903.

Parker SL, Tong T, Bolden S, Wingo PA. Cancer statistics, 1997. *CA.* 1997;47:5-27.

Pye G, Thomas WM, Hardcastle JD. Comparison of coloscreen self-test and Haemoccult faecal occult blood tests in the detection of colorectal cancer in symptomatic patients. *Br J Surg.* 1990;77:630-631.

Ransohoff DF, Lang CA. Screening for Colorectal Cancer. *N Engl J Med.* 1991;325:37-41.

Selby JV, Friedman GD, Quesenberry CP, Weiss NS. Effect of fecal occult blood testing on mortality from colorectal cancer: a case-control study. *Ann Intern Med.* 1993;118:1-6.

Selby JV. How should we screen for colorectal cancer? *JAMA*. 1993;269:1294-1296.

SmithKline Diagnostics. *Product Instructions for Hemoccult®*. San Jose, Calif: SmithKline Diagnostics, Inc; 1994.

US Preventive Services Task Force. Screening for colorectal cancer. In: *Guide to Clinical Preventive Services*. 2nd ed. Washington, DC: US Department of Health and Human Services; 1996: chap 8.

Walter SD, Frommer DJ, Cook RJ. The estimation of sensitivity and specificity in colorectal cancer screening methods. *Cancer Detect Prev*. 1991;15:465-469.

Winawer SJ, Fletcher RH, Miller L, et al. Colorectal cancer screening: clinical guidelines and rationale. *Gastroenterology*. 1997;112:594-642.

Winawer SJ, Schottenfeld D, Flehinger BJ. Colorectal cancer screening. *J Natl Cancer Inst*. 1991;83:243-253.

35

HEARING

The prevalence of hearing loss increases with advancing age and is very common in older adults. Approximately one fourth of adults aged 65 to 74 years and half of adults aged 85 years and older report some degree of hearing loss. Hearing loss, particularly when it develops late in life and is progressive in nature, can compromise an individual's ability to perform many important activities, such as using the telephone, driving, and shopping. Hearing loss also may lead to social withdrawal, depression, and exacerbation of coexisting psychiatric problems. Some older people with hearing loss also have cognitive impairment, and evidence suggests that improvement of hearing may contribute to improvement in cognitive ability. Many types of hearing loss can be improved with the use of hearing aids; however, only 10% to 15% of patients who could benefit from a hearing aid actually use one.

See chapter 6 for information about hearing screening for children and adolescents.

Recommendations of Major Authorities

American Academy of Family Physicians—Clinicians should question elderly adults about hearing impairment and counsel about the availability of treatment when appropriate.

American College of Obstetricians and Gynecologists—Women 65 years and older should be evaluated for hearing loss.

American Speech-Language-Hearing Association—Considerable debate concerning the efficacy of selected screening protocols for older adults has taken place in recent years. Whether the choice of protocol actually influences compliance with the follow-up recommendations remains unclear. The clinician may choose to use a hearing handicap questionnaire, pure-tone audiometry, or both. The rationale for using a questionnaire and pure-tone audiometry in combination is that compliance with audiologic recommendations is often greater when individuals perceive their hearing loss to be a handicap. Selection of the protocol should take into consideration cost, compliance data for the particular population, and the specificity, sensitivity, and predictive values of screening. Equipment used should be appropriately calibrated, and self-assessment scales must be reliable. Compliance-improving strategies (eg, educational materials) should be an integral part of any screening program and appropriate follow-up services should be available.

Canadian Task Force on the Periodic Health Examination— There is fair justification for looking for hearing loss in adults seen for other reasons. Further study is warranted if adults report being hard of hearing or fail to respond to the normal spoken voice; have a medical or family history placing them at high risk for hearing loss (eg, family history of hearing loss, occupational history of exposure to noise, pursuit of noisy leisure activities, or history of recurring ear problems). Screening for hearing impairment using an audioscope, a single question about hearing difficulty, or whispered voice out of the patient's field of vision is recommended as part of the periodic health examination for persons 65 years of age and older.

US Preventive Services Task Force—Screen older patients for hearing impairment by periodically questioning them about their hearing. Counseling should be provided about the availability of hearing aid devices and referrals made for abnormalities as appropriate. The optimal frequency of such screening is left to clinical discretion. An otoscopic examination and audiometric testing should be performed on all persons with evidence of impaired hearing by patient inquiry. There is insufficient evidence to recommend routinely screening adults with audiometric testing. Screening of workers for noise-induced hearing loss should be performed in the context of existing worksite programs and occupational medicine guidelines.

Basics of Hearing Screening

1. Question all older adult patients about signs of hearing loss. Because patients may not be fully aware of impairment, also question their family members, if possible.

2. A screening questionnaire may be used to screen for communication problems and social and emotional handicaps stemming from hearing loss. Questionnaires may be filled out by the patient or administered by staff. One type of standardized questionnaire for this purpose is presented in Table 35.1. This instrument has been shown to have sensitivity and specificity values in the range of 60% to 80%; these values are almost as high as those attained by pure-tone audiometry screening. Some authorities recommend audiologic referral for patients who score 10 or higher on this questionnaire. Screening questionnaires have the advantage of identifying patients who perceive hearing loss to be a problem and who may be partic-

ularly motivated to use a hearing aid. Some authorities recommend using both a questionnaire and pure-tone testing for screening. This approach may modestly improve sensitivity and specificity.

3. Pure-tone screening can be administered using either a standard pure-tone audiometer or a hand-held audioscope (an otoscope that emits tones of calibrated frequencies and intensities). When using either method, keep the environment in which screening is administered as quiet as possible. Use frequencies that are within the speech range. Disagreement exists about the sound intensity that should be used for screening. Following are two examples of suggested screening protocols:

   ■ Present pure tones at 25 dB at 1000 Hz, 2000 Hz, and 4000 Hz. Failure to respond to any one frequency in either ear at 25 dB constitutes a "fail." For adults younger than age 65 years, this may be the preferred protocol, but the majority of persons aged 65 years and older who are screened with this protocol may fail. Because of this difference, some authorities recommend using a 40-dB tone at 4000 Hz.

   ■ Present pure tones at 25 dB at 1000 Hz, 2000 Hz and 4000 Hz (optional). Failure to respond to the 40-dB tone at any one frequency in either ear constitutes a "fail". Inability to hear any one frequency 25 dB places an individual "at risk" for hearing loss. A referral for audiologic assessment may be appropriate if the person reports being handicapped by hearing loss. Persons who fail the screening should be monitored annually to determine whether their hearing loss is progressive.

4. Simple physical examination procedures for hearing screening, such as the whispered voice and finger-rub tests, are not recommended by major authorities. Although these crude hearing tests are fairly accurate, they are insensitive to disorders of central auditory processing and the understanding of speech.

5. Patients with evidence of hearing loss should be considered for referral to a specialist for comprehensive audiologic evaluation, especially if they feel handicapped by hearing loss. Because approximately 10% of individuals with hearing loss are amenable to medical or surgical treatment, and some patients are incorrectly identified as having hearing loss by screening, do not refer patients directly to a hearing aid dealer.

6. Provide appropriate follow-up management for all patients who are referred for audiologic evaluation. Patients may need considerable support and training to use their hearing aids effectively.

Table 35.1. Hearing Handicap Inventory in the Elderly—Screening Questionnaire

Instructions: Check one answer for each question. Do not skip a question if you avoid a situation because of a hearing problem. If you use a hearing aid, please answer according to the way you hear without the aid.

Question	Yes	No	Sometimes
1. Does a hearing problem cause you to feel embarrassed when you meet new people?			
2. Does a hearing problem cause you to feel frustrated when talking to members of your family?			
3. Do you have difficulty hearing when someone speaks in a whisper?			
4. Do you feel handicapped by a hearing problem?			
5. Does a hearing problem cause you difficulty when visiting friends, relatives, or neighbors?			
6. Does a hearing problem cause you to attend religious services less often than you would like?			
7. Does a hearing problem cause you to have arguments with family members?			
8. Does a hearing problem cause you difficulty when listening to TV or radio?			
9. Do you feel that any difficulty with your hearing limits or hampers your personal or social life?			
10. Does a hearing problem cause you difficulty when in a restaurant with relatives or friends?			

Scoring: No = 0; Sometimes = 2; Yes = 4

Interpretation of Total Scores: 0–8 = no handicap; 10–24 = mild to moderate handicap; 26–40 = severe handicap.

Adapted from: Ventry I, Weinstein B. Identification of elderly people with hearing problems. *ASHA.* 1983; 25:37–42. Reproduced by permission of the author and the American Speech and Hearing Association; copyright © 1983.

Patient Resources

Answers to Questions About Noise and Hearing Loss; How to Buy a Hearing Aid. American Speech-Language-Hearing Association, 10801 Rockville Pike, Rockville, MD 20852; (800)638-TALK (voice or TTY); (301) 897-8682 (in Maryland). To order, call (301) 897-5700, ext. 218. Internet address: http://www2.asha.org

Age Page: Hearing and the Elderly. National Institute on Aging. Bldg 31, Room 5C27, 31 Center Drive, MSC 2922 Bethesda, MD 20892-2922; (301) 496-1752. Internet address: http://www.nih.gov/nia/health/pubpub/pubpub.htm

Provider Resources

Older Voices. To order this trainer's manual and resource materials for communication problems of older persons, contact the American Speech-Language-Hearing Association, 10801 Rockville Pike, Rockville, MD 20852; (301) 897-5700, ext 218. For general information, call (800)638-8255; http://www2.asha.org

Selected References

American Academy of Family Physicians. *Summary of Policy Recommendations for Periodic Health Examination*. Kansas City, Mo: American Academy of Family Physicians; 1997.

American College of Obstetricians and Gynecologists. *Guidelines for Women's Care.* Washington, DC: American College of Obstetricians and Gynecologists; 1996.

American Speech-Language-Hearing Association, Ad Hoc Committee on Hearing Screening in Adults. Considerations in screening adults/older persons for handicapping hearing impairments. *ASHA*. 1992;34:81-85.

Bess FH, Lichtenstein MJ, Logan SA, et al. Hearing impairment as a determinant of function in the elderly. *J Am Geriatr Soc*. 1989;37:123-128.

Canadian Task Force on the Periodic Health Examination. The periodic health examination: 2. 1984 update. *Can Med Assoc J*. 1984;130:1278-1285.

Canadian Task Force on the Periodic Health Examination. Prevention of hearing impairment and disability in the elderly. In: *The Canadian Guide to Clinical Preventive Health Care*. Ottawa, Canada: Minister of Supply and Services; 1994: chap 80.

Gennis V, Garry PJ, Haaland KY, Yeo RA, Goodwin JS. Hearing and cognition in the elderly; new findings and a review of the literature. *Arch Intern Med*. 1991; 151: 2259-2264.

Havlik RJ. Aging in the eighties: impaired senses for sound and light in persons aged 65 years and over: preliminary data from the Supplement on Aging to the National Health Interview Survey: United States; January-June 1984. *Vital and Health Statistics*. Hyattsville, Md: National Center for Health Statistics; 1986;125. US Department of Health and Human Services publication PHS 86-1250.

Lichtenstein ME, Bess FH, Logan SA. Screening for impaired hearing in the elderly. *JAMA*. 1988;260: 3589-3590.

Macphee GJ, Crowther JA, McAlpine CH. A simple screening test for hearing impairment in elderly patients. *Age Aging*. 1988:17:347-351.

Mulrow CD, Lichtenstien MJ. Screening for hearing impairment in the elderly: rationale and strategy. *J Gen Intern Med.* 1991;6:249-258.

Pappas JJ, Graham SS. *Hearing Aid Dispensing Within a Medical Setting.* Alexandria, Va: American Academy of Otolaryngology—Head and Neck Surgery Foundation; 1990.

Schow R, Nerbonne M. Communication screening profile uses with elderly clients. *Ear Hearing.* 1982;3:133-147.

Uhlman RF, Larson EB, Rees TS, Koepsel TD, Duckert LG. Relationship of hearing impairment to dementia and cognitive dysfunction in older adults. *JAMA.* 1989;262:1916-1919.

Uhlman RF, Rees TS, Psaty BM, Duckert LG. Validity and reliability of auditory screening tests in demented and non-demented older adults. *J Gen Intern Med.* 1980;4:90-96.

US Preventive Services Task Force. Screening for hearing impairment. In: *Guide to Clinical Preventive Services.* 2nd ed. Washington, DC: US Department of Health and Human Services; 1996: chap 35.

Ventry I, Weinstein B. Identification of elderly people with hearing problems. *ASHA.* 1983; 25:37-42.

36

MAMMOGRAPHY

Breast cancer is the most common type of cancer in women and the second leading cause of cancer death in American women after lung cancer. The American Cancer Society predicts that there will be an estimated 180,200 new cases of breast cancer in women and 43,900 related deaths in 1997. In the United States, a woman's average lifetime risk for developing breast cancer is approximately one in eight. Breast cancer mortality increases with age. Mortality from breast cancer does not plateau, even in extreme old age. After age, the next strongest risk factor is a family history of breast cancer in a first-degree relative (sister or mother). Very modest increases in risk are also associated with nulliparity, first pregnancy after 30 years of age, menarche before 12 years of age, menopause after 50 years of age, postmenopausal obesity, some types of benign breast disease, high socioeconomic status, and a personal history of ovarian or endometrial cancer.

Mortality from breast cancer is strongly influenced by stage at detection. The 5-year survival rate for women in whom local disease is found is 96%. In contrast, the 5-year survival rate for women with distant metastasis is only 20%. Survival rates at every stage of diagnosis are lower among African-American women compared with Caucasian women.

Mammography is the most effective approach to early detection of breast cancer and is associated with sensitivity of 70% to 90% and specificity of 90% to 95%. Although mammography can detect small tumors in younger women, controversy exists regarding whether mammography screening reduces mortality in women younger than age 50 years.

Well-maintained, modern mammography equipment is very safe, requiring very low levels of radiation. Screening does, however, carry the added risk of morbidity attributable to any unnecessary biopsies that are performed following false-positive mammography results.

See chapter 30 for information about clinical breast examination to detect breast cancer.

Recommendations of Major Authorities

Women Aged 50 Years and Older

American Academy of Family Physicians (AAFP), American Cancer Society (ACS), American College of Obstetricians and Gynecologists (ACOG), American College of Physicians (ACP), American College of Preventive Medicine (ACPM), American Medical Association, Canadian Task Force on the Periodic Health Examination (CTFPHE), National Cancer Institute (NCI) and the **US Preventive Services Task Force (USPSTF)**—Routine mammography screening is recommended. Yearly screening is recommended by **ACS, ACOG** and **CTFPHE**. **AAFP, ACP, ACPM, NCI,** and **USPSTE** recommend a frequency of 1 to 2 years. The **CTFPHE, AAFP** and **USPSTF** recommend screening until 70 years of age. The **AAFP** and **USPSTF** indicate that there is insufficient evidence to recommend for or against screening of women 70 years of age or older, although recommendations for this can be made on other grounds for women in this age category with a reasonable life expectancy. **ACPM** advises that women aged 70 or older should continue undergoing mammography screening provided their health status permits breast cancer treatment. **ACP** states that the use of mammography above 75 years of age should be discouraged. The **American Geriatrics Society** recommends that women over 65 years of age receive mammograms at least every 2 or 3 years until at least 85 years of age.

Women Under 50 Years of Age

American Academy of Family Physicians—Recommends counseling about potential risks and benefits of mammography and clinical breast exam for women ages 40 to 49 years.

American Cancer Society (ACS), American College of Obstetricians and Gynecologists (ACOG), American Medical Association (AMA), and National Cancer Institute (NCI)—The **ACS** recommends that women begin annual mammography at age 40. **ACOG, NCI,** and the **AMA** recommend screening mammograms every 1 to 2 years for women 40 to 49 years of age.

American College of Physicians and **Canadian Task Force on the Periodic Health Examination**—Women under 50 should not be screened.

American College of Preventive Medicine and **US Preventive Services Task Force**—There is insufficient evidence to recommend for or against routine screening in this age group, but screening high risk younger women may be appropriate despite the lack of direct evidence of benefit.

National Institutes of Health Consensus Development Panel on Breast Cancer Screening for Women Ages 40 to 49 (an independent panel)—Currently available data does not warrant a universal recommendation for mammography for all women in their forties. Each woman should decide whether to undergo mammography.

High-Risk Women

American College of Obstetricians and Gynecologists—Women with a family history of premenopausally diagnosed breast cancer in a first-degree relative should have mammography regularly beginning at 35 years of age.

American College of Physicians—High-risk women should receive the same recommendations as average-risk women, unless a woman expresses great anxiety about breast cancer and insists on more intensive screening.

American College of Preventive Medicine and US Preventive Services Task Force—Although there is no direct evidence evaluating mammography in high-risk women under 50 years of age, recommendations for screening such women can be made on other grounds. Women at high risk include those with a family history of premenopausal breast cancer in a first-degree relative or those with a history of breast and/or gynecologic cancer.

Canadian Task Force on the Periodic Health Examination—Physicians may elect to recommend mammography starting at age 35 for women at high risk, especially those whose first-degree relatives have had breast cancer diagnosed before menopause.

Basics of Mammography Screening

1. Emphasize the importance of mammography. A major reason reported by patients for not undergoing mammography is that they did not know they needed a mammogram. Counsel women on the need for regular mammography, not just one mammogram.

2. Use pamphlets, videotapes, and other media to educate and motivate patients to receive mammographic screening.

3. Because cost can be a significant barrier to patients obtaining mammography, the clinician should be knowledgeable about low-cost, high-quality mammography facilities available in the community and should make referrals to these facilities as needed. For information on the availability of low cost mammography at accredited facilities, contact your local office of

the American Cancer Society or call the national toll-free number: (800)ACS-2345.

4. Instruct the patient to wear pants or a skirt, because she will have to undress from the waist up. Instruct her to avoid use of deodorants, powders, or other topical agents on the breasts or in underarm areas, because these may cause artifacts on the mammogram.

5. Because of potential perimenstrual breast tenderness, scheduling mammography at other times in the patient's menstrual cycle is preferred.

6. Patients commonly experience mild discomfort during mammography. Instruct patients to tell the technician if the level of discomfort becomes unacceptable.

7. Verify that mammography facilities use only dedicated mammography equipment that meets minimum safety and image-quality standards. Facilities that receive Medicare reimbursement must use equipment that complies with minimum standards for patient safety. The American College of Radiology provides certification for compliance with minimum standards for image quality. As of October 1, 1994, all US mammography facilities must be certified by the Food and Drug Administration (FDA) as providing quality mammography. Certification requirements cover personnel, equipment, radiation exposure, quality assurance programs, and record-keeping and reporting. Further information on this program is available from the FDA Center for Devices and Radiological Health, Office of Training and Assistance, Division of Mammography Quality and Radiation Programs, HFZ-240, 5600 Fishers Ln, Rockville, MD 20857.

8. Establish a tracking system to ensure that mammograms that are ordered are actually performed, that results return in a timely fashion, and that patients who are not seen frequently can be called or contacted by letter about the importance of getting mammograms and other needed preventive care. Encourage patients to keep track of and prompt their own mammography through use of a patient-held record form or card.

9. Any palpable breast lump, even with a normal mammogram, requires careful evaluation, including possible biopsy.

Patient Resources

Breast Cancer: Steps to Finding Breast Lumps Early. American Academy of Family Physicians, 8880 Ward Pkwy, Kansas City, MO 64114-2797; (800)944-0000. Internet address: http://www.aafp.org

Mammography. American College of Obstetricians and Gynecologists, 409 12th St, SW, Washington, DC 20024; (800)762-2264. Internet address: http://www.acog.com

What You Need To Know About Breast Cancer; A Mammogram Once a Year for Life; Smart Advice for Women 40 and Over: Have a Mammogram. Office of Cancer Communications, National Cancer Institute, Bldg 31, Room 10A24, Bethesda, MD 20892; (800)4-CANCER.

Chances are You Need a Mammogram; Are you age 50 or Older? A Mammogram Could Save Your Life. Available in both English and Spanish. Office of Cancer Communications, National Cancer Institute, Bldg 31, Room 10A16, Bethesda, MD 20892; (800)4-CANCER. Internet address: http://wwwicic.nci.nih.gov

Provider Resources

Mammography. American College of Obstetricians and Gynecologists, 409 12th St, SW, Washington, DC 20024; (800)762-2264. Internet address: http://www.acog.com

Educating Older Women About Mammography: A Guide For Program Planners and Volunteer Leaders. American Association of Retired Persons, 1909 K Street, NW, Washington, DC 20049; (202) 434-2277.

Detecting and Treating Breast Problems. American College of Obstetricians and Gynecologists, 409 12th St, SW, Washington, DC 20024-2188; (202) 638-5577. Internet address: http://www.acog.com

Mammography Awareness Kit. Office of Cancer Communications, National Cancer Institute, Bldg 31, Room 10A16, Bethesda, MD 20892; (800)4-CANCER. Internet address: http://wwwicic.nci.nih.gov

OncoLink—The University of Pennsylvania Cancer Resource. Internet address: http://cancer.med.upenn.edu

PDQ: The Physician Data Query System for Cancer Information. PDQ is the National Cancer Institute's computerized database providing the most up-to-date cancer information available. Access to the system can be gained 24 hours a day, 7 days a week, using a personal computer and standard telephone line, or through medical libraries. Ask a medical librarian for assistance or call (800)4-CANCER (line 3). In Hawaii, on Oahu, call 524-1234.

Selected References

American Academy of Family Physicians. *Summary of Policy Recommendations for Periodic Health Examination.* Kansas City, Mo: American Academy of Family Physicians; 1997.

American Cancer Society. *Cancer Facts & Figures-1997.* Atlanta, Ga: American Cancer Society; 1997.

American Cancer Society. Summary of American Cancer Society recommendations for the early detection of cancer in asymptomatic people. *CA.* 1993;43;45.

American College of Obstetricians and Gynecologists. *Guidelines for Women's Health Care*. Washington, DC: American College of Obstetricians and Gynecologists; 1996.

American College of Physicians. Guidelines. In: Eddy DM, ed. *Common Screening Tests*. Philadelphia, Pa: American College of Physicians; 1991:411-412.

American Geriatrics Society, Clinical Practice Committee. Screening for breast cancer in elderly women. *J Amer Geriatr Soc*. 1989;37:883-884.

American Medical Association, Council on Scientific Affairs. Mammographic screening in asymptomatic women aged 40 years and older. *JAMA*. 1989;261:2535-2542.

Breast Cancer Screening for Women Ages 40-49. NIH Consensus Statement. 1997; Jan 21-23; 15(1):1-35.

Canadian Task Force on the Periodic Health Examination. Screening for breast cancer. In: *The Canadian Guide to Clinical Preventive Health Care*. Ottawa, Canada: Minister of Supply and Services; 1994: chap 65.

Eddy DM. Screening for breast cancer. In: Eddy DM, ed. *Common Screening Tests*. Philadelphia, Pa: American College of Physicians; 1991: chap 9.

Eddy DM, Gordon MA, Bredt A. Screening for breast cancer. *Ann Intern Med*. In press.

Ferrini R, Mannino E, Ramsdell E, et al. Screening mammography for breast cancer: American College of Preventive Medicine. *Am J Prev Med*. 1996;12(5):340-341.

National Cancer Institute. *Cancer Facts: Questions and Answers About Mammography Screening*. Bethesda, Md: National Institutes of Health; 1997.

US Preventive Services Task Force. Screening for breast cancer. In: *Guide to Clinical Preventive Services*. 2nd ed. Washington, DC: US Department of Health and Human Services; 1996: chap 7.

37

PAPANICOLAOU SMEAR

In 1997 approximately 14,500 cases of invasive cervical cancer are expected to be diagnosed in the United States and 4800 women are expected to die of the disease. The major risk factor for cervical cancer is sexually transmitted infection with human papillomavirus (HPV). Other risk factors include early age at first intercourse, having multiple sexual partners, long-term use ($\geq$5 years) of oral contraceptives, low socioeconomic status, and cigarette smoking. Rates for carcinoma in situ reach a peak in both African-American and white women between the ages of 20 and 30 years. After age 25 years, the incidence of invasive cancer in African-American women increases dramatically with advancing age. In Caucasian women, the incidence rises more slowly. Over 25% of invasive cervical cancers occur in women older than age 65 years, and 40% to 50% of all women who die of cervical cancer are older than age 65 years.

The effectiveness of early detection through Papanicolaou (Pap) smear testing and early treatment has been impressive, resulting in a marked decrease in mortality from cervical cancer. The incidence of invasive cervical cancer has decreased an estimated 70% because of screening. Nonetheless, a large proportion of women, particularly elderly African-American women and middle-aged women of lower socio-economic status, do not have regular Pap smears. In some geographic areas, as many as 75% of women over age 65 years report not having a Pap smear within the previous 5 years.

Depending on the technique used, Pap testing has a sensitivity of 50% to 90% and a specificity of 90% to 99%. A large proportion of false-negative Pap smear results are thought to be attributable to inadequate collection technique (up to 50% of all false-negative results) and inadequate laboratory interpretation. Because of the long lead time from development of precancerous changes until development of invasive carcinoma (8 to 9 years by some estimates), almost all precancerous or early-stage malignancies initially missed can be detected by repeat testing.

Recommendations of Major Authorities

American Academy of Family Physicians—All women who are or have been sexually active and who have a cervix should be offered a Pap smear at least every 3 years. Use of Pap smears is not recommended in women who have had hysterectomies for reasons other than cancer.

American Cancer Society and American College of Obstetricians and Gynecologists, and National Cancer Institute—All women should begin having annual Pap tests at the onset of sexual activity or at 18 years of age, whichever occurs first. After a woman has had three or more consecutive satisfactory normal annual examinations, the Pap test may be performed less frequently in low-risk women at the discretion of the patient and clinician.

American College of Physicians—Sexually active women between 20 and 65 years of age should be screened with a Pap smear every 3 years. Women 66 to 75 years of age who have not been screened within the 10 years prior to age 66 should be screened every 3 years. Women at increased risk for cervical cancer should be screened every 2 years. Initial screening tests may be done as frequently as annually for two or three examinations to ensure diagnostic accuracy.

American College of Preventive Medicine—Screening for cervical cancer by regular Pap tests should be performed in all women who are or have been sexually active, and should be instituted after a woman first engages in sexual intercourse. If the sexual history is unknown or considered unreliable, screening should begin at age 18. At least two initial screening tests should be performed one year apart. For women who have had at least two normal annual smears, the screening interval may be lengthened at the discretion of the patient and physician but should not exceed three years. Screening may be discontinued at age 65 if the following criteria are met: the women has been regularly screened, has had two satisfactory smears, and has had no abnormal smears within the previous nine years. For all women over age 65 who have not been previously screened, three normal annual smears should be documented prior to discontinuation of screening.

Canadian Task Force on the Periodic Health Examination—Pap smears to screen for cervical cancer are recommended for women who have been sexually active. The optimum frequency of screening is not known, but it is suggested that women in the general population be screened annually until two normal smears are reported and then every 3 years to age 69 years. More frequent screening should be considered for women with risk factors: age of first sexual intercourse less than 18 years, many sexual partners or a consort with many partners, smoking, or low socioeconomic status.

US Preventive Services Task Force—All women who are or have been sexually active should have regular Pap tests. Testing should begin at the age when the woman first engages in sexual intercourse. Adolescents whose sexual history is thought to be unreliable should be presumed to be sexually active at age 18. There is little evidence that annual screening achieves better outcomes than screening every 3 years. Pap tests should be performed at least every 3 years. The interval for each patient should be recommended by the physician based on risk factors (eg, early onset of sexual intercourse, history of multiple sexual partners, low socioeconomic status). Women infected with human immunodeficiency virus require more frequent screening according to established guidelines. There is insufficient evidence to recommend for or against an upper age limit for Pap testing, but recommendations can be made on other grounds to discontinue regular testing after 65 years of age in women who have had regular previous screening with consistently normal results. Women who have undergone a hysterectomy in which the cervix was removed do not require Pap testing, unless the hysterectomy was performed because of cervical cancer or its precursors.

Basics of Pap Smear Screening

1. Attempt to ensure that performance of a Pap smear is not an unpleasant or painful experience for the patient. Be sure to clearly explain the importance of the procedure and the steps used to carry it out.

2. Instruct patients not to douche on the day of the examination. Do not perform a Pap smear if the patient has significant menstrual flow or obvious inflammation.

3. Perform the Pap smear before performing the bimanual examination and before obtaining culture specimens. In general, do not lubricate the speculum with anything except water, because contamination of Pap smear specimens with lubrication jelly tends to obscure cellular detail. Use of a small amount of lubricating jelly may be necessary for speculum insertion in some older patients.

4. Visualize the cervix and vagina completely before collecting the specimen. Gently remove any excess cervical mucus with a swab.

5. The traditional gold standard for the adequacy of a Pap smear has been the presence of endocervical cells in the sample: 90% of cervical cancers develop at the junction of the squamous epithelium of the ectocervix and the columnar epithelium of the endocervix (located at the external os in young women and inside the endocervical canal in older women). Studies differ regarding whether the presence of endocervical cells actually improves detection rates of abnormalities, but the presence of endocervical

cells and/or squamous metaplastic cells remain widely accepted as a standard of adequacy for Pap smears.

6. A variety of implements have been used to obtain Pap smear samples, including simple cotton swabs, wooden and plastic spatulas, and endocervical and combined endocervical-exocervical brushes. The best sensitivity (defined as presence of endocervical cells) is achieved by using both a spatula (preferably Ayer's type) and an endocervical brush. Use the spatula first, because bleeding is commonly caused by the endocervical brush, and endocervical cells are susceptible to drying effects.

7. Gently yet firmly rotate the spatula around the os at least one complete turn to obtain a 360° sample. Promptly transfer the specimen to a glass slide (or to a preservative vial if your laboratory is using a thin layer technique). Patients who have been exposed to DES should also have smears taken circumferentially with a spatula from the upper two thirds of the vagina. To obtain the endocervical sample, insert the brush into the os no deeper than the length of the bristled section. Rotate the brush 360° (avoiding excessive rotation), then transfer the specimen by rolling the brush on a glass slide or by placing the material in a preservative vial as instructed by your laboratory for the thin layer technique.

8. Apply specimens to the slides uniformly and without clumping. Perform fixation promptly, and take care to minimize air drying of the specimens. If one slide is used for both specimens, collect, transfer, and fix the endocervical sample as quickly as possible. Use of two separate slides can help avoid prolonged air exposure of the spatula specimen while the endocervical specimen is being collected. Use of two slides does, however, double the amount of work for the cytotechnologist. Use of a combined endocervical-exocervical brush requires collection and fixation of only a single specimen (thus decreasing the risk of air drying), but such use has been shown to be somewhat less sensitive than use of a spatula and an endocervical brush.

9. Inquire about the quality control procedures of the laboratories to which specimens are sent. Laboratories should be certified by the American Society of Cytopathology, the College of American Pathologists, the Health Care Financing Administration, the Joint Commission on the Accreditation of Health Care Organizations, or the New York State Department of Health.

10. Many authorities recommend that laboratories use the new Bethesda System developed by a National Cancer Institute consensus conference for reporting results (Table 37.1). The Bethesda System attempts to standardize classification categories and provides for reporting on aspects of the sample not addressed in traditional Pap smear reports, such as adequacy of the sample submitted. In the Bethesda System, HPV infection is classi-

fied as a low-grade squamous intraepithelial lesion. Both moderate and severe dysplasia are classified as high-grade squamous intraepithelial lesions. Some concern exists, although unsubstantiated by research, that these classifications may lead to excessive use of colposcopic examination for patients with HPV infection or moderate dysplasia. The American College of Obstetricians and Gynecologists has issued guidelines for Pap smear reporting and follow-up in their publication *Cervical Cytology: Evaluation and Management of Abnormalities* (Selected References).

11. General recommendations for initial follow-up of abnormal PAP smears according to the American College of Obstetricians and Gynecologists include:

    ASCUS (Atypical Squamous Cells of Undetermined Significance): The prognosis of women with ASCUS varies depending on the cytopathologist or laboratory. Clinicians are encouraged to communicate with the cytopathologist or to monitor a number of patients with an ASCUS report to help determine the appropriate follow-up and the need for colposcopy.

    LSIL (Low-grade Squamous Intraepithelial Lesions): Repeat Pap test at intervals of 4 to 6 months and colposcopy if abnormalities persist.

    High-grade Squamous Intraepithelial Lesions: Colposcopy and directed biopsy.

12. Only about 60% of women with abnormal Pap smear results return for follow-up. Establish a tracking system to make sure that Pap smears are performed regularly, that results return in a timely fashion, that patients with abnormal results are contacted, and that women who are not seen frequently are called or contacted by letter about the importance of getting Pap smears and other needed preventive care. Encourage patients to keep track of the results and prompt their own Pap smears through use of a patient-held record form or card.

Table 37.1. The Revised Bethesda System for Reporting Cervical and/or Vaginal Cytologic Diagnoses

Adequacy of the specimen
    Satisfactory for evaluation
    Satisfactory for evaluation but limited by . . . (specify reason)
    Unsatisfactory for evaluation . . . (specify reason)

General categorization (optional)
    Within normal limits
    Benign cellular changes: See descriptive diagnosis
    Epithelial cell abnormality: See descriptive diagnosis

Descriptive diagnoses
    Benign cellular changes
        Infection
            Trichomonas vaginalis
            Fungal organisms morphologically consistent with *Candida* spp
            Predominance of coccobacilli consistent with shift in vaginal flora
            Bacteria morphologically consistent with *Actinomyces* spp
            Cellular changes associated with herpes simplex virus
            Other
        Reactive changes
            Reactive cellular changes associated with:
                Inflammation (includes typical repair)
                Atrophy with inflammation ("atrophic vaginalis")
                Radiation
                Intrauterine contraceptive device (IUD)
                Other
    Epithelial cell abnormalities
        Squamous cell
            Atypical squamous cells of undetermined significance: Qualify*
            Low-grade squamous intraepithelial lesion encompassing: HPV†, mild dysplasia/CIN 1
            High-grade squamous intraepithelial lesion encompassing: Moderate and severe
                dysplasia, CIS/CIN 2 and CIN 3
            Squamous cell carcinoma
        Grandular cell
            Endometrial cells, cytologically benign, in postmenopausal women
            Atypical glandular cells of undetermined significance: Qualify*
            Endocervical adenocarcinoma
            Endometrial adenocarcinoma
            Extrauterine adenocarcinoma
            Adenocarcinoma, NOS
    Other malignant neoplasms: Specify
    Hormonal evaluation (applies to vaginal smears only)
        Hormonal pattern compatible with age and history
        Hormonal pattern incompatible with age and history: Specify
        Hormonal evaluation not possible due to: Specify

*Atypical squamous or glandular cells of undetermined significance should be further qualified as to whether a reactive or premalignant/malignant process is favored.

†Cellular changes of human papillomavirus (HPV)—previously termed koilocytosis, koilocytotic atypia, or condylomatous atypia—are included in the category of low-grade squamous intraepithelial lesion.

From: National Cancer Institute Workshop. The revised Bethesda system for reporting cervical and/or vaginal cytologic diagnoses; report of the 1991 Bethesda workshop. *Acta Cytol.* 1992;36:273–275. Reproduced by permission of Science Printers and Publishers, Inc; copyright 1992.

Patient Resources

The Pap Test. American College of Obstetricians and Gynecologists, 409 12th St, SW, Washington DC 20024; (800)762-2264. Internet address: http://www.acog.com

The Pap Test: It Could Save Your Life. To order this information (in Spanish), contact the Office of Cancer Communications, National Cancer Institute, Bldg 31, Room 10A16, Bethesda, MD 20892; 1-800-4-CANCER.

Provider Resources

Cervical Cytology: Evaluation and Management of Abnormalities. Technical Bulletin 183. American College of Obstetricians and Gynecologists, 409 12th St, SW, Washington, DC 20024; 1-800-762-2264. Internet address: http://www.acog.com

Recommended Actions to Assure Quality Pap Tests (Pap Smears). The American Society of Clinical Pathologists. American Society of Clinical Pathologists, 1225 New York Ave, NW, Suite 250, Washington, DC 20005; 202-347-4450. Internet address: http://www.ascp.org

PDQ: The Physician Data Query System for Cancer Information. PDQ is the National Cancer Institute's computerized database providing the most up-to-date cancer information available. Access to the system can be gained 24 hours a day, 7 days a week, using a personal computer and a standard telephone line or through medical libraries. Ask a medical librarian for assistance or call (800)4-CANCER (line 3). In Hawaii, on Oahu, call 524-1234.

Selected References

American Academy of Family Physicians. *Summary of Policy Recommendations for Periodic Health Examination.* Kansas City, Mo: American Academy of Family Physicians; 1997.

American Cancer Society. *Cancer Facts and Figures—1997.* Atlanta, Ga: American Cancer Society; 1997.

American Cancer Society. Summary of American Cancer Society recommendations for the early detection of cancer in asymptomatic people. *CA.* 1993;43:45.

American College of Obstetricians and Gynecologists. *Guidelines for Women's Health Care.* Washington, DC: American College of Obstetricians and Gynecologists; 1996.

American College of Physicians. Guidelines. In: Eddy DM, ed. *Common Screening Tests.* Philadelphia, Pa: American College of Physicians; 1991:413-414.

Appleby J. Management of the abnormal Papanicolaou smear. *Med Clin North Am.* 1995;79: 345-360.

Boon ME, de Graaff Guilloud JC, Rietveld WJ. Analysis of five sampling methods for the preparation of cervical smears. *Acta Cytol.* 1989;33:843-848.

Canadian Task Force on the Periodic Health Examination. Screening for cervical cancer. In: *The Canadian Guide to Clinical Preventive Health Care.* Ottawa, Canada: Minister of Supply and Services; 1994: chap 73.

Crouse BS, Elliott BA, Nesin N. Clinical follow-up of cervical sampling with the Ayre spatula and Zelsmyr cytobrush. *Arch Fam Med.* 1993;2:145-148.

Eddy DM. Screening for cervical cancer. In: Eddy DM, ed. *Common Screening Tests.* Philadelphia, Pa: American College of Physicians; 1991: chap 10.

Hawkes AP, Kronenberger CB, MacKenzie TD, et al. Cervical cancer screening: American College of Preventive Medicine practice policy statement. *Am J Prev Med.* 1996;12(5):342-344.

Herbst AL. The Bethesda System for cervical/vaginal cytologic diagnoses: a note of caution. *Obstet Gynecol.* 1990;449-450.

Kruman RJ, Solomon D. *The Bethesda System for Reporting Cervical/Vaginal Cytologic Diagnoses. Definitions, Criteria, and Explanatory Notes for Terminology and Specimen Adequacy.* New York, NY: Springer-Verlag; 1994.

Lai-Goldman M, Nieberg RK, Mulcahy D, Wiesmeier. The cytobrush for evaluating routine cervicovaginal-endocervical smears. *J Repro Med.* 1990;35;959-963.

McCord ML, Stovall TG, Meric JL, Summitt RL, Coleman SA. Cervical cytology: a randomized comparison of four sampling methods. *Am J Obstet Gynecol.* 1992;166:1772-1779.

Mandelblatt J, Gogaul I, Wistreich M. Gynecological care of elderly women: another look at Papanicolaou testing. *JAMA.* 1986;256:367-371.

Miller AB, Anderson G, Brisson J, et al. Report of a national workshop on screening for cancer of the cervix. *Can Med Assoc J.* 1991;145:1301-1325.

National Cancer Institute Workshop. The 1988 Bethesda System for reporting cervical/vaginal cytologic diagnoses. *JAMA.* 1989;262:931-934.

National Cancer Institute Workshop. The revised Bethesda System for reporting cervical/vaginal cytologic diagnoses: report of the 1991 Bethesda workshop. *Acta Cytol.* 1992;36:273-275.

Neinstein JS, Church J, Akiyoshi T. Comparison of cytobrush with cervix-brush for endocervical cytologic sampling. *J Adoles Health.* 1992;13:520-523.

Ruffin MT, Van Noord GR. Improving the yield of endocervical elements in a Pap smear with the use of the cytology brush. *Fam Med.* 1991;23:365-369.

Schumann JL, O'Connor DM, Covell JL, Greening SE. Pap smear collection devices: technical, clinical, diagnostic, and legal considerations associated with their use. *Diagn Cytopathol.* 1992;8:492-502.

US Preventive Services Task Force. Screening for cervical cancer. In: *Guide to Clinical Preventive Services.* 2nd ed. Washington, DC: US Department of Health and Human Services; 1996: chap 9.

38

PLASMA GLUCOSE

An estimated 16 million Americans suffer from diabetes mellitus (DM), and approximately half of these cases are undiagnosed. Diabetes mellitus is the seventh leading cause of death in the United States. Approximately 5% of all persons with diabetes have type 1 DM, an absolute insulin deficiency, and require insulin for survival. Onset of type 1 DM is bi-modal, with the largest peak in the number of new cases occurring during childhood and a smaller peak occurring in early adulthood. Type 1 DM can occur as late as the eighth or ninth decade. Persons with type 1 DM tend to present with symptoms, and the disease is usually diagnosed soon after its clinical onset. The remaining 95% of individuals with diabetes have type 2 DM, a relative insulin deficiency and insulin resistance. As such, onset of their disease is insidious. They can be relatively symptom-free for years before diagnosis. Risk factors for type 2 DM include advancing age (older than age 45 years), obesity, family history, and a history of gestational DM.

Although DM affects approximately 6.2% of the US population, the prevalence of DM is significantly higher among certain ethnic groups, including Hispanics, African Americans, and American Indians. Diabetic complications are varied and serious. DM accounts for 30% of all cases of end-stage renal disease, and it is the leading cause of blindness and non-traumatic lower extremity amputations in adults. Other complications include neuropathy, cardiovascular disease, and peripheral vascular disease.

Screening can identify occult cases of type 2 DM. The most accurate method of screening is measurement of a fasting plasma glucose. Measurement of urine glucose has been used in the past but is much less accurate and is no longer recommended. Evidence indicates that early treatment of patients with established type 1 DM decreases the number of long-term, microvascular complications. This is also probably true of type 2 DM. Evidence also suggests that weight reduction, exercise, and diet change are beneficial for secondary prevention in type 2 DM. Primary prevention trials for both type 1 and 2 DM are presently underway. Most authorities recommend screening only those persons who are at increased risk for developing DM.

Screening for gestational DM, often performed as an aspect of prenatal care, is beyond the scope of this book.

Recommendations of Major Authorities

American College of Obstetricians and Gynecologists—Patients with one or more of the following risk factors should be screened for diabetes: family history in parents or siblings; obesity (body weight greater than 120% of ideal); high-risk ethnicity (American Indian, Hispanic, African American); history of glucose intolerance; hypertension or hyperlipidemia; history of gestational diabetes or macrosomia.

American College of Physicians—Screening for DM in healthy asymptomatic individuals is not recommended. Screening is reasonable in obese adults over the age of 40 years if a diagnosis of DM would motivate weight loss. Screening may also be indicated for women planning to become pregnant who are at increased risk of DM and in other people with one or more of the following risk factors: history of DM in a first-degree relative, age over 50 years, weight more than 25% over ideal body weight, personal history of gestational DM, and membership in an ethnic group with a high prevalence of DM.

American Diabetes Association—Screening for DM every 3 years should be considered for all adults age 45 and above. Testing should be considered at a younger age or more frequently in people with the following risk factors: history of DM in a first-degree relative; more than 20% over ideal body weight; American Indian, Hispanic, or African American heritage; on previous testing had impaired fasting glucose or impaired glucose tolerance; hypertension, HDL cholesterol at or below 35 mg/dL and/or a triglyceride level at or above 250 mg/dL; personal history of gestational DM or of one or more infants weighing more than 9 lb at birth.

Canadian Task Force on the Periodic Health Examination—Screening for diabetes mellitus in asymptomatic nonpregnant adults is not recommended. Selective case-finding (screening patients seen for other reasons) may be considered for adults with the following risk factors: obesity, older age, family history of diabetes, belonging to a high-risk ethnic group.

US Preventive Services Task Force—There is insufficient evidence to recommend for or against universal screening for type 2 diabetes in nonpregnant adults. Although evidence of a benefit of early detection is not available for any group, clinicians may decide to screen selected persons at high risk of type 2 DM on other grounds, including the increased predictive value of a positive test in individuals with risk factors and the potential (although unproven) benefits of reducing asymptomatic hyperglycemia through diet and exercise. Individuals at high risk of diabetes include obese men and women over 40, patients with a strong family history of diabetes, and members of certain ethnic groups (American Indians, Hispanics, African Americans).

Basics of Plasma Glucose Screening

1. Measurement of fasting plasma glucose is the principal method of screening in nonpregnant, asymptomatic adults.

2. Instruct patients not to ingest food or beverages (other than water) for at least 8 hours before the blood sample is collected. Performing the procedure in the morning is most convenient as patients will have fasted overnight. A venous blood sample is more accurate, but capillary samples may be more practical for office-based screening purposes.

3. A fasting plasma glucose level lower than 110 mg/dL is considered normal. According to the new guidelines from the Expert Committee on the Diagnosis and Classification of Diabetes Mellitus (Table 38.1), fasting blood glucose level greater than 126 mg/dL is considered elevated and fulfills the provisional diagnosis for diabetes. Fasting plasma glucose levels greater than 110 mg/dL and less than 126 mg/dL meet criteria for impaired fasting glucose (IFG) and require further monitoring according to these recent guidelines.

Table 38.1. Criteria for Diagnosing Diabetes in Nonpregnant Adults

Criteria for the diagnosis of diabetes (any one condition is sufficient).[1]	Classic symptoms of diabetes, including polydipsia, polyuria, polyphagia, and weight loss, accompanied by a random glucose >200 mg/dL OR Fasting plasma glucose (FPG) ≥ 126 mg/dL OR 2 hour plasma glucose (2hPG) ≥200 mg/dL during an oral glucose tolerance test[2] using the equivalent of 75g anhydrous glucose dissolved in water
Criteria for the diagnosis of impaired mg/dL glucose tolerance (IGT)	2 hour plasma glucose (2hPG) ≥140 but <200 mg/dL after a 75g glucose load
Criteria for the diagnosis of impaired mg/dL fasting glucose (IFG)	Fasting plasma glucose (FPG) ≥ 110 but <126 mg/dL

[1] In the absence of unequivocal hyperglycemia with metabolic decompensation, any one criterion should be confirmed by repeat testing on another day.

[2] The oral glucose tolerance test (OGTT) is no longer recommended for routine clinical use according to the new guidelines from the Expert Committee on the Diagnosis and Classification of Diabetes Mellitus. The 2hPG >200 mg/dL was previously identified as the point where the prevalence of microvascular complications increased dramatically. Several studies have shown the new lower limit of the diagnostic FPG of 126 mg/dL equally associated with these complications, and due to its lesser expense, reliability, and ease to perform, it has largely replaced the OGTT in these recent guidelines.

Adapted from: Expert Committee on the Diagnosis and Classification of Diabetes Mellitus. Report of the Expert Committee on the Diagnosis and Classification of Diabetes Mellitus. *Diabetes Care*. 1997;20(7): 1183-1197.

4. If a fasting sample is not available, random blood glucose levels can also be used in screening for DM. A random blood glucose level in excess of 200 mg/dL is considered elevated and an indicator for further assessment.

Patient Resources

Diagnosis Diabetes. To order this and other materials, contact the American Diabetes Association, 1660 Duke St, Alexandria, VA 22314; (800)232-3472.

The National Diabetes Information Clearinghouse has the following fact sheets and booklets available: *Diabetes in African Americans; Diabetes in Hispanics; Diabetes Research and Training Centers; Diabetic Neuropathy: The Nerve Damage of Diabetes; Diabetes Overview; Diabetes Control and Complications Trial; Diabetes Statistics; Hypoglycemia; Kidney Disease of Diabetes; Insulin-Dependent Diabetes; Noninsulin-Dependent Diabetes; The Diabetes Dictionary* (available in Spanish); *End-Stage Renal Disease: Choosing a Treatment That's Right for You; Directory of Diabetes Resources* (available in Spanish). 1 Information Way, Bethesda, MD 20892-3560, phone 301-654-3327. Internet address: http://www.niddk.nih.gov/DiabetesDocs.htm

Selected References

American College of Obstetricians and Gynecologists. *Guidelines for Women's Health Care.* Washington, DC: American College of Obstetricians and Gynecologists; 1996:84-85.

American College of Physicians. Guidelines. In: Eddy DM, ed. *Common Screening Tests.* Philadelphia, Pa: American College of Physicians; 1991:404-405.

Canadian Task Force on the Periodic Health Examination. Screening for diabetes mellitus in the non-pregnant adult. In: *The Canadian Guide to Clinical Preventive Health Care.* Ottawa, Canada: Minister of Supply and Services; 1994: chap 50.

Engelgau MM, Aubert RE, Thompson TH, Herman WH. Screening for NIDDM in nonpregnant adults. *Diabetes Care.* 1995;18:1606-1618.

Eriksson KF, Lindgarde F. Prevention of type 2 (noninsulin-dependent) diabetes mellitus by diet and physical exercise. *Diabetologia.* 1991;34:891-898.

Expert Committee on the Diagnosis and Classification of Diabetes Mellitus. Report of the Expert Committee on the Diagnosis and Classification of Diabetes Mellitus. *Diabetes Care.* 1997;20(7):1183-1197.

Gerken KM, Van Lente E. Effectiveness of screening for diabetes. *Arch Pathol Lab Med.* 1990; 114:201-203.

Harris, MI, Eastman, RC. Early detection of undiagnosed non-insulin-dependent diabetes mellitus. *JAMA.* 1996; 276:1261-2.

Howard BV, Abbott WGH, Swinburn BA. Evaluation of metabolic effects of substitution of complex carbohydrates for saturated fat in individuals with obesity and NIDDM. *Diabetes Care.* 1991;14:786-795.

Manson JE, Nathan DM, Krolewski AS, Stampfer MJ, Willett WC, Hennekens CH. A prospective study of exercise and incidence of diabetes among US male physicians. *JAMA.* 1992;268: 63-67.

Manson JE, Rimm EB, Stampfer MJ, et al. Physical activity and incidence of noninsulin-dependent diabetes mellitus in women. *Lancet*. 1991;338:774-778.

Marshall JA, Hamman RF, Baxter J. High-fat, low-carbohydrate diet and the etiology of non-insulin-dependent diabetes mellitus: The San Luis Valley diabetes study. *Am J Epidemiol*. 1991;134:590-603.

Schwartz MK. The role of the laboratory in the prevention and detection of chronic disease. *Clin Chem*. 1992;38:1539-1546.

Singer DE, Samet JH, Coley CM, Nathan DM. Screening for diabetes mellitus. *Ann Intern Med*. 1988;109:639-649.

US Preventive Services Task Force. Screening for diabetes mellitus. In: *Guide to Clinical Preventive Services*. 2nd ed. Washington, DC: US Department of Health and Human Services; 1996: chap 19.

World Health Organization Expert Committee on Diabetes Mellitus. *Third Report on Diabetes Mellitus*. Geneva, Switzerland: World Health Organization; 1985. WHO Technical Report Series 727.

39

PROSTATE-SPECIFIC ANTIGEN

Prostate cancer is the most frequently diagnosed cancer in men in the United States, with 209,900 new cases estimated for 1997 and 41,800 deaths. Prostate cancer is the second leading cause of cancer death in men. Risk factors for prostate cancer include increasing age (80% of prostate cancers are diagnosed in men over 65), African American race, family history, and (perhaps) increased dietary fat intake. Although prostate cancer is common, its course is extremely variable. Some prostate cancers grow rapidly, metastasize, and quickly lead to death. Many other prostate cancers, however, are clinically silent and found only incidentally at autopsy. Autopsy studies indicate that approximately 30% of men over age 50 have histologic evidence of prostate cancer, yet carry only a 3% lifetime risk for death from this disease.

The principal screening tests for prostate cancer are the digital rectal examination (DRE) (chapter 30) and elevated levels of certain tumor markers (eg, prostate-specific antigen (PSA) and prostatic acid phosphatase). PSA is a glycoprotein that is specific to the prostate but not to prostate cancer. Thus, it is produced by all types of prostate tissue, whether normal, hyperplastic, or malignant. Incomplete information regarding true- and false-negative results makes accurate calculations of the sensitivity and specificity of PSA screening impossible. The positive predictive value of a positive PSA test (values greater than 4 ng/dL) are reported in the range of 20% to 30%. Many men with benign prostatic hyperplasia will have an elevated PSA level, and some men with prostate cancer will have PSA tests in the normal range. Prostatic acid phosphatase has a much lower sensitivity and positive predictive value than PSA; thus, PSA has largely replaced it in screening.

Whether to screen asymptomatic men for prostate cancer with PSA testing is controversial. Unlike the use of Pap smears and mammograms, there are no data indicating that PSA screening decreases mortality from prostate cancer. Definitive evidence is lacking that treatments such as radical prostatectomy are superior to "watchful waiting" for localized prostate cancer.

See chapter 30 for information about digital rectal examination to detect prostate cancer.

Recommendations of Major Authorities

American Academy of Family Physicians—Clinicians should counsel men ages 50 to 65 years about the known risks and uncertain benefits of screening for prostate cancer.

American Cancer Society—Annual PSA testing in combination with annual digital rectal exam should be offered annually beginning at age 50 to all men who have a life expectancy of at least 10 years, or earlier to men at high risk for prostate cancer.

American College of Physicians—Rather than screening all men for prostate cancer as a matter of routine, physicians should describe the potential benefits and known harms of screening, diagnosis, and treatment; listen to the patient's concerns; and then individualize the decision to screen. The College strongly recommends that physicians help enroll eligible men in ongoing clinical studies.

American College of Radiology—Annual PSA testing is recommended for all men aged 50 years and older. Annual PSA testing beginning at age 40 is recommended for African American men and men with a family history of prostate cancer.

American Urological Association—Annual PSA testing in combination with annual digital rectal examination should be offered to all men aged 50 years and older with a life expectancy of ten years or more. Annual screening should be offered at age 40 to men at high risk for prostate cancer.

Canadian Task Force on the Periodic Health Examination—Routine use of PSA testing as part of the periodic health examination is not recommended.

US Preventive Services Task Force—Routine screening for prostate cancer with serum tumor markers (eg, PSA), digital rectal examination, or transrectal ultrasound is not recommended.

Basics of Prostate-Specific Antigen Screening

1. Many experts recommend that men 50 years of age and over receive individualized counseling about the known risks and possible benefits of PSA testing. Patients should be informed that:

   ■ Prostate cancer is an important health problem.

   ■ The benefits of one-time or repeated screening and aggressive treatment of prostate cancer have not yet been proven. The potential benefit of

PSA screening is decreased mortality from prostate cancer that is discovered early, but there are no data to show that PSA testing decreases mortality from prostate cancer.

■ DRE and PSA can both have false-positive and false-negative results.

■ The probability that further invasive evaluation will be required as a result of testing is relatively high. Aggressive therapy is necessary to realize any benefit from the discovery of a tumor. Prostate cancer treatments have serious side effects that can include impotence, incontinence, and surgical mortality ranging from 15% to 2%. Radical prostatectomy, radiation therapy, or both in combination have not been proven to be superior to watchful waiting for localized disease.

■ Early detection may save lives and may avert future cancer-related illness.

2. Concerns had been raised that PSA results, like prostatic acid phosphatase levels, would be falsely elevated by the compression of the prostate occurring during a DRE. A recent study by Crawford, et al, reported that the variations in PSA levels due to digital rectal examinations had little clinical significance (Selected References).

3. Although there is debate about the upper limits of normal for PSA testing, manufacturers recommend using 4.0 ng/mL for monoclonal PSA tests and 2.5 ng/mL for polyclonal PSA tests. Some authorities recommend varying the strategy for follow-up of a positive PSA depending on the degree of elevation. Thus, patients with levels of 10 ng/mL or more may all get a biopsy to determine if cancer is present, but those with levels greater than 4 and less than 10 ng/mL may first receive a rectal examination, a transrectal ultrasound of the prostate, or both to help determine whether a biopsy is needed.

4. Four methods have been proposed to improve the accuracy of PSA testing. PSA density (PSA concentration divided by the gland volume as measured by transrectal ultrasound) has been proposed as a more accurate marker for cancer because malignant tissue results in a higher level of PSA per unit weight than does normal or hypertrophied prostate tissue. PSA velocity is the annual calculation of the rate of change of PSA. Age-adjusted PSA cutoffs have also been advanced to address mean PSA increases with age. Percent free PSA is the proportion of free PSA, a particular molecular form of PSA, to the total PSA. Prostate cancer has been associated with a lower percent free PSA. These references are reviewed in Vashi (Selected References). Most authorities recommending the test advocate combining it with other modalities, such as digital rectal examination or transrectal ultrasound, to increase the positive predictive value.

Patient Resources

Prostate Disease: What Every Man Over 40 Should Know, and other patient materials on prostate cancer and PSA testing. Prostate Health Council. American Foundation for Urologic Disease, 1128 N. Charles Street, Baltimore, MD 21201.

The Prostate Puzzle. *Consumer Report.* 1993; 58(7):459-465.

Provider Resource

PDQ: The Physician Data Query System for Cancer Information. PDQ is the National Cancer Institute's computerized database providing the most up-to-date cancer information available. Access to the system can be gained 24 hours a day, 7 days a week, using a personal computer and standard telephone line, or through medical libraries. Ask a medical librarian or call 1-800 4-CANCER (option 3). In Hawaii, on Oahu, call 524-1234.

Selected References

American Academy of Family Physicians. *Summary of Policy Recommendations for Periodic Health Examination.* Kansas City, Mo: American Academy of Family Physicians; 1997.

American Cancer Society. *Cancer Facts and Figures-1997.* Atlanta, Ga: American Cancer Society; 1997.

American Cancer Society. *Summary of American Cancer Society Recommendations for the Early Detection of Cancer in Asymptomatic People.* Atlanta, Ga: American Cancer Society; 1992.

American Cancer Society. *Cancer Information Database.* Atlanta, Ga: American Cancer Society; June 1997.

American College of Physicians. Screening for prostate cancer. *Ann Intern Med.* 1997;126: 480-484.

American Urological Association. *Early Detection of Prostate Cancer.* Baltimore, Md: American Urological Association; 1995.

Benson MC, Whang IS, Olsson CA, et al. The use of prostate-specific antigen density to enhance the predictive value of intermediate levels of serum prostate-specific antigen. *J Urol.* 1992;147:817-21.

Canadian Task Force on the Periodic Health Examination. Screening for prostate cancer. In: *The Canadian Guide to Clinical Preventive Health Care.* Ottawa, Canada: Minister of Supply and Services; 1994: chap 67.

Carter HB, Pearson JD, Metter EJ, et al. Longitudinal evaluation of prostate-specific antigen levels in men with and without prostate disease. *JAMA.* 1992;267:2215-20.

Catalona WJ, Smith DS, Ratliff TL. Measurement of prostate-specific antigen in serum as a screening test for prostate cancer. *N Engl J Med.* 1991;324:1156-61.

Crawford ED, Schutz MJ, Clejan S. The effect of digital rectal examination on prostate-specific antigen levels. *JAMA.* 1992;267:2227-2228.

Coley CM, Barry MJ, Fleming C and Mulley AG. Early detection of prostate cancer—part I: prior probability and effectiveness of tests. *Ann Intern Med.* 1997;126:394-406.

Coley CM, Barry MH, Fleming C et al. Early detection of prostate cancer—part II: estimating the risks, benefits, and costs. *Ann Intern Med.* 1997; 126:468-479.

Fleming C, Wasson JH, Albertsen PC, Barry MJ, Wennberg JE. A decision analysis of alternative treatment strategies for clinically localized prostate cancer. *JAMA.* 1993;269:2650-2658.

Kramer BS, Brown ML, Prorok PC, Potosky AL, Hohagan JK. Prostate cancer screening: what we know and what we need to know. *Ann Intern Med.* 1993: 119:914-923.

Littrup PJ, Lee F, Mettlin C. Prostate cancer screening: current trends and future implications. *CA.* 1992;42:198-212.

Lu-Yao GL, McLerran D, Wasson J, Wennberg JE. An assessment of radical prostatectomy: time trends, geographic variation, and outcomes. *JAMA.* 1993;269:2633-2636.

Mettlin C, Jones G, Averette H, et al. Defining and updating the American Cancer Society guidelines for the cancer-related checkup: prostate and endometrial cancers. *CA.* 1993;43:42-46.

Stuart ME, Handley MA, Thompson RS, Conger M, Timlin D. Clinical practice and new technology: prostate-specific antigen (PSA). *HMO Practice.* 1993;6(4):5-11.

US Preventive Services Task Force. Screening for prostate cancer. In: *Guide to Clinical Preventive Services.* 2nd ed. Washington, DC: US Department of Health and Human Services; 1996: chap 10.

Vashi AR, Oesterling JE. Percent free prostate-specific antigen: entering a new era in the detection of prostate cancer. *Mayo Clinic Proceedings.* 1997;72:337-344.

Wingo PA, Landis S, Ries LAG. An adjustment to the 1997 estimate for new prostate cancer cases. *CA.* 1997;239-242.

40

SEXUALLY TRANSMITTED DISEASES AND HIV INFECTION

Sexually transmitted diseases (STDs) are common and damaging communicable diseases. Chlamydial infection, gonorrhea, and syphilis are easily treated when diagnosed early. If these conditions are not detected and treated, serious complications can result. Although no cure for HIV infection currently exists, early diagnosis and treatment can delay onset of acquired immunodeficiency syndrome (AIDS) and permit persons who are infected to avoid transmitting the virus. Groups at particularly high risk for STDs and HIV infection include sexually active persons younger than age 25 years, those who have multiple sexual partners, persons with a prior history of an STD, persons who practice anal intercourse, prostitutes and their sex partners, users of illicit drugs, and inmates of detention centers.

Prevention and control of STDs and HIV infection depend on four major activities: (1) educating persons who are at risk about means of reducing transmission; (2) detecting untreated cases, both symptomatic and asymptomatic; (3) effectively diagnosing and treating infection and counseling infected individuals; and (4) evaluating, counseling, and treating the sex partners of infected persons. Screening—along with early diagnosis, counseling, and treatment—plays an essential role in preventing STDs and HIV infection.

Many sexually transmitted diseases (AIDS; chancroid; *Chlamydia trachomatis* [genital infections only]; gonorrhea; hepatitis B; hepatitis C/non-A, non-B; HIV infection [pediatric cases only]; and syphilis) are currently designated as infectious diseases notifiable at the national level. Refer to Appendix C for further information on nationally notifiable diseases.

See chapters 23 and 59 for information on STD and HIV prevention counseling in adolescents and adults, respectively; chapters 14 and 48 for information on hepatitis B immunization and prophylaxis in children/adolescents and adults, respectively; chapters 25 and 61 for information about counseling on preventing unintended pregnancy in adolescents and adults, respectively. Screening for and treatment of STDs during pregnancy is an important component of prenatal care, but this topic is beyond the scope of this book.

SYPHILIS

The reported incidence of syphilis (all stages) increased dramatically between 1985 and 1990, from 28.5 to 54.3 cases per 100,000 population. The incidence decreased to 32.0 cases per 100,000 population in 1994. The incidence of congenital syphilis increased from 7 cases per 100,000 live births in 1985 to 107.2 cases per 100,000 live births in 1991, and decreased to 94.3 cases per 100,000 live births in 1992. More than 30,000 new cases of primary and secondary syphilis occur annually, and the prevalence of HIV infection among syphilis-infected persons is increasing.

The usual presentation of primary syphilis is a single painless ulcer or chancre on the genitalia. The ulcer usually heals spontaneously in 4 to 6 weeks without antibiotic therapy. Primary syphilis may not manifest at all, however, and may go unrecognized. Most untreated cases of primary syphilis progress to secondary syphilis. Clinical manifestations of secondary syphilis, which include skin lesions and generalized nontender lymphadenopathy, appear approximately 6 weeks after the healing of the chancre. These lesions subside in 2 to 6 weeks, and untreated patients enter the latent stage of the disease. About one third of untreated cases of latent syphilis eventually manifest as neurosyphilis or other late complications, such as gummatous lesions of bone, tissue, and skin, as well as cardiovascular problems (aortic valve lesions and aneurysms). Neurosyphilis can occur at any point in the course of untreated syphilis and may consist of meningitis, meningovascular lesions, psychiatric illnesses, and tabes dorsalis. Early diagnosis and treatment can prevent these grave complications.

Recommendations of Major Authorities

All major authorities, including the **American Academy of Family Physicians (AAFP), American Academy of Pediatrics (AAP), American College of Obstetricians and Gynecologists, American College of Physicians (ACP), American Medical Association (AMA), Canadian Task Force on the Periodic Health Examination, Centers for Disease Control and Prevention, and US Preventive Services Task Force (USPSTF)**—Syphilis screening should be performed on individuals at high risk of developing syphilis, sexual partners of known syphilis cases, and individuals with multiple sexual partners—especially in areas where syphilis prevalence is high. **AAP, AMA,** and **ACP** also recommend that males who engage in sex with other males be routinely screened; **AAFP, AAP, AMA,** and **USPSTF** also suggest screening prostitutes and persons who trade sex for drugs. **AAFP** also recommends syphilis screening for individuals seeking treatment for other sexually transmitted diseases.

American Academy of Family Physicians—Syphilis screening should be performed on sexual contacts of syphilis cases and prostitutes and on individuals seeking treatment for other sexually transmitted diseases.

Basics of Syphilis Screening

1. Because the causative agent of syphilis cannot be cultured, screening relies on serology. A nontreponemal test—usually either the Venereal Disease Research Laboratory (VDRL) test or the Rapid Plasma Reagin (RPR) test—is recommended for initial screening.

2. Occasionally, uninfected individuals may have reactive tests. If a sample is RPR- or VDRL-reactive, a treponemal test, such as the fluorescent treponemal antibody absorption (FTA-ABS) test, should be obtained to confirm the diagnosis. It is very uncommon for an individual to test falsely reactive to both treponemal and nontreponemal tests. Some causes of falsely reactive syphilis serologies are listed in Table 40.1.

3. Early in the course of syphilis, serology may be nonreactive. As many as 25% of all patients with primary syphilis may have nonreactive RPR and VDRL tests. Patients who have had recent contact with an individual who has documented syphilis (or is suspected of having primary syphilis) should be treated, even if serologic tests are nonreactive.

Table 40.1. Conditions That May Cause Falsely Reactive Syphilis Tests

Falsely Reactive RPR and VDRL	Falsely Reactive FTA-ABS
Viral infections	Infections
Measles	Infectious mononucleosis
Chicken pox	Lyme disease
Infectious mononucleosis	Malaria
Viral hepatitis	Leptospirosis
Nonviral infections	Other
Tuberculosis	Systemic lupus erythematosus
Scarlet fever	
Chancroid	
Pneumococcal pneumonia	
Other	
Pregnancy	
Injection drug use	
Connective tissue disease (including systemic lupus erythematosus)	
Malignancy	

4. RPR and VDRL test titers correlate with disease activity, usually becoming nonreactive after therapy; however, even in untreated patients, tests can revert to nonreactive after many years. FTA-ABS tests usually remain reactive for life. A reactive FTA-ABS test may not necessarily indicate the need for therapy if the patient was adequately treated for syphilis previously. If a patient's test is reactive, an accurate history and thorough search for previous syphilis tests or treatment are essential to determine the duration of infection and to plan appropriate therapy.

5. Screen patients with known exposure to syphilis and those with proven or suspected infection for other STDs; counsel patients to practice safe sex, including the use of latex condoms; and advise patients to seek HIV and hepatitis B counseling and testing.

CHLAMYDIA AND GONORRHEA

Chlamydial infection is the most common sexually transmitted disease in the United States, causing more than 4 million infections each year since 1992. Gonorrhea is the second most common sexually transmitted disease, with an estimated 1.1 million infections reported in 1992. These two infections usually cause urethritis in men and cervicitis in women. The clinical presentation of gonococcal infection is usually swifter and more dramatic than that of chlamydial infection, but the two conditions cannot be distinguished solely by history and physical findings. Often the two causative organisms are transmitted together; thus, the infections must be treated simultaneously. Usual symptoms in men include penile discharge and dysuria. Occasionally these infections can lead to epididymitis. Women may experience vaginal discharge and symptoms of pelvic inflammatory disease (PID). PID can result in infertility. Unlike chlamydial infection, gonorrhea may also cause pharyngitis, proctitis, and a disseminated infection involving dermatitis, tenosynovitis, and arthritis; rarely, it may cause meningitis and endocarditis. Both chlamydial infection and gonorrhea may cause only subtle symptoms, or infection may occur entirely without symptoms, particularly in females. Therefore, screening to detect asymptomatic carriers is important for preventing complicated infections and for controlling the spread of infection in the community.

Recommendations of Major Authorities

American Academy of Family Physicians—High-risk women, including those who exchange sex for money or drugs, have multiple or new sexual partners, have a history of sexually transmitted disease, and/or nonuse or inconsistent use of barrier contraceptives should be screened for gonorrhea and chlamydia.

American Academy of Pediatrics and American Medical Association—All sexually active adolescents should be screened annually for chlamydia and gonorrhea. Screening for boys can be performed with the use of a dipstick urinalysis test for leukocyte esterase.

American College of Obstetricians and Gynecologists, Centers for Disease Control and Prevention, and **US Preventive Services Task Force**—Asymptomatic individuals attending STD, family planning, or adolescent health clinics should be screened for chlamydia and gonorrhea. Those who have multiple sexual partners and sexually active individuals less than 20 years of age should also be screened. Prostitutes and individuals with a history of STDs should also be screened. Recent sexual partners of individuals with a documented gonococcal or chlamydial infection should be tested and treated.

Canadian Task Force on the Periodic Health Examination—Persons at high risk should be screened for gonorrhea and chlamydia. For gonorrhea, those at high risk are: males or females under 30 years of age who have had at least two sexual partners in the previous year, had first intercourse at less than 16 years of age, prostitutes, and sexual contacts of individuals known to have a sexually transmitted disease. There is fair evidence to support screening and treatment of pregnant women for chlamydia during the first trimester as well as annual screening and treatment of high-risk groups (sexually active females less than 25 years of age, men and women with a new partner or mulitple sexual partners in the preceding year, women who use nonbarrier contraceptive methods, women with symptoms of chlamydial infection: cervical friability, mucopurulent discharge, or intermenstrual bleeding). There is fair evidence to exclude routine screening for chlamydia in the general population.

US Preventive Services Task Force—Females at risk should be routinely screened for chlamydia and gonorrhea. For chlamydia, all sexually active adolescents should be screened and other women at risk due to: a history of prior STDs, a new partner or multiple sex partners, age under 25 years, inconsistent barrier contraceptive use, cervical ectopy, or being unmarried. In areas of high prevalence, screening of all women for chlamydia is justified. For gonorrhea, women at risk are: commercial sex workers, those with repeated episodes of gonorrhea, and women under 25 years of age with two or more sex partners in last year. In settings where prevalence is high, broader screening for gonorrhea may be justified. There is insufficient evidence to recommend for or against screening asymptomatic men for chlamydia and gonorrhea. In settings where prevalence is high, such as urban adolescent clinics, screening of males for chlamydia and gonorrhea may be justified on other grounds, including the potential benefits of early treatment for preventing transmission to uninfected sex partners. Screening of males with a dipstick urinalysis for leukocyte esterase is convenient and inexpensive, but is less sensitive and specific for asymptomatic chlamydial infections than more expensive urine assays and also requires confirmation of positive results.

Basics of Chlamydia and Gonorrhea Screening

1. Because chlamydial infection and gonorrhea cause similar symptoms and often occur simultaneously, diagnostic and screening tests for the two infections are usually performed together.

2. Collect specimens from the urethra in males and from the endocervix in females. In women who have had a hysterectomy, obtain urethral specimens. If spontaneous discharge from the urethra or cervix is apparent, perform diagnostic studies, including a Gram stain.

3. *Gonorrhea:* Gonorrhea culture remains the gold standard for screening and diagnosis of gonococcal infections. For routine screening and diagnosis of males, however, Gram staining is nearly as specific and sensitive as the culture. Performing a Gram stain in addition to a culture may be preferable because results can be obtained immediately. Perform specimen collection, Gram stain, and inoculation for gonorrhea culture as follows:

   ■ *For male patients:* Instruct patients to refrain from urinating for at least 2 hours before testing to minimize the possibility of a false-negative test result. An adequate sample can often be obtained by milking the penis from the base of the shaft to the glans, expressing exudate, and collecting it with a swab. If no exudate is apparent, insert a small calcium alginate or dacron swab into the urethral meatus, advance it into the canal 2 to 3 cm, and gently rotate it.

   ■ *For female patients:* Unless the need for urethral samples is anticipated, instruct the patient to void before the examination. Obtain the specimen by gently inserting a calcium alginate or dacron swab into the endocervical canal and rotating it. Also perform a bimanual and rectal examination, with careful attention to signs of PID: cervical motion tenderness, fundal or adnexal tenderness, or masses. Sample any endocervical discharge for microscopic examination.

   ■ Gram staining:
      1. Apply a thin film of exudate or discharge from the swab to a clean glass slide.
      2. Air-dry and fix the slide by passing it several times through a flame.
      3. Flood slide with crystal or gentian violet for 10 seconds, then rinse with running water.
      4. Flood with Gram's iodine for 10 seconds, then rinse with running water.
      5. Decolorize with 95% ethanol until thin areas of the smear are colorless. Rinse with running water.
      6. Flood with safranin for 10 seconds, then rinse with water. Air- or blot-dry.

- Cultures: Z-streak the swab onto a Thayer-Martin (chocolate agar) or Martin-Lewis plate that has been brought to room temperature, and transport inoculated culture plates to the laboratory in a candle jar or other CO_2-enriched environment.

4. *Chlamydia:* Culture and nonculture methods (such as enzyme immunoassay [EIA], direct fluorescent antibody, DNA probe, polymerase chain reaction, or solid-phase colorimetric assays) are available to detect chlamydial infection, but all available methods frequently give false-negative results. Although nonculture antigen detection methods are somewhat less sensitive and specific than culture, they have the advantages of being more economical and less technically demanding. Therefore, nonculture tests are more appropriate for screening purposes.

The objective of good specimen collection to detect chlamydial infection is to obtain columnar epithelial cells from the endocervix or the urethra. Collect specimens as follows:

- *Endocervical specimens:* Obtain specimens for chlamydial testing after collecting any specimens for Gram's staining, gonorrhea culture, and Papanicolaou smear. Before taking a specimen for a chlamydial test, remove all secretions and discharge from the cervical os with a sponge or a proctology or other large swab. Insert the appropriate swab or endocervical brush 1 to 2 cm into the endocervical canal (past the squamocolumnar junction). Rotate the swab against the wall of the endocervical canal several times during a 10- to 30-second period, then withdraw it without touching any vaginal surfaces, and place it in the appropriate transport medium (if it will be used for culture, EIA, or DNA probe testing), or use it to prepare a slide for direct fluorescent antibody (DFA) testing.

- *Urethral specimens:* If possible, delay taking specimens until at least 2 hours after the patient has voided. Obtain specimens for chlamydial tests after obtaining any specimens for Gram's staining or gonorrhea culture. Gently insert the appropriate urogenital swab into the urethra (1 to 2 cm in females, 2 to 4 cm in males). Rotate the swab in one direction for at least one revolution for approximately 5 seconds, then withdraw it, and place it in the appropriate transport medium (if it will be used for culture, EIA, or DNA probe testing), or use it to prepare a slide for DFA testing.

- *Swabs to use for chlamydia screening:* For nonculture chlamydia tests, use the swab and transport media supplied or specified by the manufacturer of the test.

For culture specimens, swabs with plastic or wire shafts are usually satisfactory. Swab tips can be made of cotton, rayon, dacron, or calcium alginate, although certain manufacturers' lots of calcium alginate swabs have been shown to be toxic for chlamydia. Do not use swabs with wooden shafts, because the wood may contain substances that are toxic to chlamydia. As part of routine quality control, labs offering chlamydia culture services should provide clinicians with prescreened swabs.

■ *Specimen transport:* Insert the specimen into chlamydia transport medium, and break off the tip to leave it immersed in the medium. The container should be sealed and transported to the laboratory. If specimens cannot be processed within 24 hours, they should be frozen at −70°C. For nonculture tests, follow the manufacturers' instructions.

5. Negative culture or nonculture screening test results do not completely rule out infection. Patients who have had sexual contact with a person having a documented gonorrheal or chlamydial infection should be treated immediately after cultures are taken, before the results are reported back.

6. Positive nonculture screening tests in patients from communities with a low prevalence of infection may be false-positives, and a second confirmatory test should be considered.

7. Some authorities have recently recommended using dipstick urinalysis to screen young males for chlamydial and gonorrheal infection. See chapter 10 for further information.

8. In areas with a high prevalence of syphilis, all patients with gonorrhea or chlamydial infection should have a serologic test for syphilis and should be offered confidential counseling and testing for HIV and hepatitis B infection.

9. Test and treat all recent sexual contacts of patients with gonorrhea or chlamydial infection.

HIV INFECTION

From 1981 through 1996, a total of 573,800 cases of AIDS in persons aged 13 years or older were reported to the Centers for Disease Control and Prevention. In 1995, approximately 50,000 deaths were attributed to AIDS. Although the number of deaths due to AIDS during the first 6 months of 1996 decreased for the first time since monitoring began, HIV infection remained the leading cause of death among persons aged 25 to 44 years in 1995. Seroprevalence studies show that HIV infection is present in 0.2% to 8.9% of patients visiting emergency departments and in 0.1% to 7.8% of patients admitted to acute-care hospitals. Groups at high risk of contracting HIV are identified in Recommendations of Major Authorities.

Many HIV-infected individuals are unaware of their status, since the characteristic symptoms of AIDS usually do not develop until years after infection. Early knowledge of HIV infection allows infected individuals to seek early treatment, which has been shown to delay the onset of AIDS, and to change high-risk behavior. Counseling and screening are, therefore, essential strategies for preventing the spread of HIV infection and the progression of symptoms. Screening high-risk individuals may be useful even when their test results are negative. The related counseling may change their behavior and thus may keep them free of disease.

Recommendations of Major Authorities

All major authorities including **American College of Obstetricians and Gynecologists, American Medical Association (AMA), Canadian Task Force on the Periodic Health Examination (CTFPHE), Centers for Disease Control and Prevention (CDC), and US Preventive Services Task Force (USPSTF)**—HIV screening should be offered to patients with another STD; homosexual and bisexual men; past or present injection drug users; individuals with a history of prostitution or multiple sexual partners; individuals whose past (or present) sexual partners are HIV-infected or injection drug users; patients with a history of blood transfusion between 1978 and 1985; and individuals born in or with long-term residence in a community where HIV is prevalent. **AMA** also recommends offering testing and counseling to high-risk individuals receiving family planning services or undergoing surgery. CDC recommends that health facilities with an HIV seroprevalence rate of at least 1% or an AIDS diagnosis rate of one or more per 1000 discharges should consider a policy of routine counseling and voluntary HIV testing for patients aged 15 to 54 years. The **CDC** recommends informing all new mothers who have not been screened for HIV of the potential benefits of screening for their infants. The **CTFPHE** recommends HIV antibody screening for neonates of HIV-positive women. The **USPSTF** recommends screening of infants born to high-risk mothers whose antibody status is not known.

American Academy of Family Physicians—HIV screening should be offered to the following individuals: men who had sex with men after 1975; past or present injection drug users; persons who exchange sex for money or drugs and their sex partners; those with current or past sex partners who were injection drug users, bisexual, or HIV-positive; persons seeking treatment for STDs; and infants born to high-risk mothers (as described above) whose HIV status is unknown.

Types of HIV Tests: Blood Screening

Serologic studies for the presence of antibodies to HIV-1 are the standard method of screening for HIV infection. Enzyme immunoassay (EIA) is the most widely used screening test for HIV-1 infection. Because any screening test can result in a false-positive reaction, positive results are validated with confirmatory testing, usually a Western blot test. HIV culture and polymerase chain reaction (PCR) testing are currently not used for screening.

Basics of HIV Blood Screening

1. A single serum or plasma specimen is tested first by EIA. If the test result is positive (reactive), multiple samples from the initial specimen are retested. If at least two of three retests are reactive, the specimen is considered repeatedly reactive, and the result must be verified with a supplemental test such as the Western blot.

2. The percentage of repeatedly reactive samples found positive with additional, more specific, tests varies according to the true antibody prevalence in the tested population. It has been estimated that when an EIA is properly performed, the average specificity is greater than 99.8%. In populations with a low prevalence of HIV-1 infection, the positive predictive value remains low (8-10%) despite this high level of specificity. The problem of low positive predictive value is addressed by further testing of repeatedly reactive EIAs with supplemental tests such as the Western blot, yielding positive predictive values approaching 100% for the complete testing algorithm.

3. Western blot tests may be interpreted as positive, negative, or indeterminate. In low-risk populations, it is estimated that the false-positive rate of combined EIA and Western blot testing is less than one in 100,000. Indeterminate Western blot patterns, which can occur in up to 15% of samples tested, require careful interpretation. Current experience suggests that indeterminate Western blot patterns that are persistent for 6 months or more indicate a lack of HIV infection. Persons presenting with indeterminate Western blots should be counseled that they should continue to be monitored for their band pattern by Western blot for at least 6 months. If no additional bands develop by that time and the patient has not engaged in any high-risk behavior, he or she can be considered negative for HIV-1 infection and so advised.

4. A time interval exists between infection with HIV and the development of detectable antibodies to HIV (seroconversion). The interval between infection and seroconversion is called the "window" period. At least 95% of infected persons seroconvert within 6 months. Individuals who test negative should be reminded that their test may have been taken during the "window period," and that they may be infected despite the initial negative test. Counsel all persons to stop engaging in high-risk behaviors and to return for retesting in 6 months or earlier, to make sure they have not converted to a positive test result. Patients who continue practicing high-risk behavior should be counseled and retested periodically.

5. HIV screening must always include pre- and post-test counseling. Individualized patient-centered counseling is recommended. Specially trained clinicians or counselors should provide patients with accurate, clear, understandable information regarding HIV testing at both pre- and post-test counseling sessions. Table 40.2 includes guidelines for information that should be provided in pre- and post-test counseling sessions. Also see chapter 59 for information about HIV counseling.

Table 40.2. Pre- and Post-test Information for HIV Testing

Counseling should include a review of the risk factors for acquiring HIV infection along with a focused and tailored risk assessment.

Counselors should review strategies for HIV prevention and assist the patient in developing a plan to reduce his/her risk of HIV infection or transmission.

Patients should understand the difference between a positive test for antibodies to HIV and development of clinical AIDS. The median duration between development of HIV antibodies and onset of clinical disease is approximately 10 years. Detection of antibodies can occur at any time between development of antibodies and clinical disease.

All patients must be informed that a negative antibody test does not conclusively exclude the possibility of HIV infection. Typically, it takes 3 to 6 months following infection before the test (ELISA) reliably detects HIV antibodies; it is important to inform the patient that a false-negative test may occur during this early period.

The importance of post-test counseling should be stressed. At the completion of the initial post-test counseling session, the counselor should assess the patient's need for additional sessions.

Patients who continue to engage in high-risk behavior should be counseled and retested periodically.

Adapted from: Centers for Disease Control and Prevention. Recommendations for HIV testing services for inpatients and outpatients in acute-care hospital settings and technical guidance on HIV counseling. *MMWR.* 1993;42:1–17.

Types of HIV Tests: Oral Fluid Test

On December 23, 1994, the FDA approved the first HIV oral test system in the United States, intended for use in subjects 13 years of age or older. This test is not as accurate as the approved HIV-antibody tests used on blood. Studies show that for every 100 persons infected with HIV, the oral-fluid-based test will miss one or two, and for every 100 persons who are not infected, test results will be incorrectly positive in approximately two. The test system includes a specially treated cotton pad on a stick and a preservative solution in a plastic container. A trained collector instructs the subject to place the pad between the lower gum and cheek to obtain a sample of oral fluid. The pad is then stored in the preservative until the sample is processed and analyzed by a qualified laboratory using an enzyme-linked immunosorbent assay (ELISA) specifically licensed for testing oral fluid samples. FDA approved this HIV test system with the following restrictions:

- The test system is available for purchase and distribution only through physicians.

- The test system may be administered only by individuals properly trained in its use.

- The test must not be provided to subjects for home use.

- Testing of the oral fluid samples for HIV antibodies may be carried out only with the Oral Fluid Vironostika HIV-1 Microelisa® System, manufactured by Organon Teknika Corporation of Durham, NC.

- The test may be used for diagnosis only and must not be used to screen blood donors.

- Before the oral fluid specimen is collected, subjects must be given information on HIV prevention and transmission, as well as technical information regarding the oral test. Because there are no confirmatory tests that use oral fluid samples, subjects must be informed that in the event of a positive oral fluid sample, they should have blood samples drawn and tested to verify their HIV status.

Types of HIV Tests: Urine-Based HIV Test

On August 6, 1996, the FDA approved the first HIV test that uses urine samples to detect the presence of antibodies to HIV-1 using an enzyme-linked immunosorbent assay (ELISA) method. This test will be available under two brand names: Calypte HIV-1 Urine EIA™ and Seradyn Sentinel™ HIV-1 Urine EIA. The test can be ordered only by a physician, and samples will be analyzed in certified medical laboratories. Any initially reactive sample will be retested twice. If either of the second tests is reactive, the screening test will be considered positive. A positive screening test must be followed by a blood test to confirm the results.

A patient information sheet provided with the new test will outline the limitations of urine HIV-1 testing in addition to HIV/AIDS information. After reading the information sheet, the person being tested will initial a statement confirming the receipt of the pretest counseling, peel off the sample label, and apply it to the urine collection cup.

The urine-based ELISA test is not approved to screen blood donors. In clinical studies, urine and blood samples were taken from 298 patients diagnosed with AIDS and tested with both the Calypte HIV-1 Urine EIA and a licensed ELISA test using a blood specimen. The urine test was positive as an initial screening test 99.3% of the time in persons known to have AIDS. In asymptomatic HIV-1-infected patients, the test would be expected to miss one or two persons out of every 100. Other studies showed that the urine-based test would give a falsely positive result in one or two persons of 100 without HIV-1 antibodies in their blood, compared to one in 1000 with a blood-based ELISA test.

Patient Resources

How to Prevent Sexually Transmitted Diseases; Genital Herpes, Gonorrhea and Chlamydia Infections, Pelvic Inflammatory Disease. American College of Obstetricians and Gynecologists, 409 12th St SW, Washington, DC 20024; (800)762-2264. Internet address: http://www.acog.com

National STD Hotline. (800)227-8922.

AIDS: How To Reduce Your Risk of Catching It. American Academy of Family Physicians, 8880 Ward Pkwy, Kansas City, MO 64114-2797; (800)944-0000. Internet address: http://www.aafp.org

Surgeon General's Report to the American Public on HIV Infection and AIDS; Condoms and Sexually Transmitted Diseases... Especially AIDS. CDC National AIDS Information Hot Line; 1-800-342-AIDS (English speaking); 1-800-344-SIDA (Spanish speaking); 1-800- AIDS-TTY (hearing impaired). All phone calls are confidential.

HIV in America: A Profile of the Challenges Facing Americans Living With HIV. National Association of People Living with AIDS, 1413 K St, NW, Washington, DC 20005; (202)898-0435.

Hemophilia and AIDS Network for the Dissemination of Information, 110 Green St, New York, NY 10012; (800)424-2634.

National AIDS Information Clearinghouse, PO Box 6003, Rockville, MD 20850; (800)458-5231 (English and Spanish).

Provider Resources

Gonorrhea and Chlamydial Infections (technical bulletin #190), 1994. American College of Obstetricians and Gynecologists, 409 12th St, SW, Washington, DC 20024; (800)762-2264. Internet address: http://www.acog.com

Gynecologic Herpes Simplex Virus Infection (technical bulletin #119). American College of Obstetricians and Gynecologists, 409 12th St, SW, Washington, DC 20024; (800)762-2264. Internet address: http://www.acog.com

HIV Infection and Physician Emotions (videotape and discussion guide). American Academy of Family Physicians, 8880 Ward Pkwy, Kansas City, MO 64114-2797; (800)944-0000. Internet address: http://www.aafp.org

Selected References

American Academy of Family Physicians. *Summary of Policy Recommendations for Periodic Health Examination.* Kansas City, Mo: American Academy of Family Physicians; 1997.

American College of Obstetricians and Gynecologists. *Guidelines for Women's Health Care.* Washington, DC: American College of Obstetricians and Gynecologists; 1996.

American Academy of Pediatrics, Committee on Infectious Diseases. *1994 Red Book: Report of the Committee on Infectious Diseases.* Elk Grove Village, Ill: American Academy of Pediatrics; 1994.

American Academy of Pediatrics, Committee on Practice and Ambulatory Medicine. Recommendations for pediatric preventive health care. *Pediatrics.* 1995;96:373-374.

American Medical Association. Rationale and recommendations: infectious diseases. In: *AMA Guidelines for Adolescent Preventive Services (GAPS): Recommendations and Rationale.* Chicago, Ill: American Medical Association; 1994: chap 15.

Canadian Task Force on the Periodic Health Examination. Prevention of gonorrhea. In: *The Canadian Guide to Clinical Preventive Health Care.* Ottawa, Canada: Minister of Supply and Services; 1994: chap 59.

Canadian Task Force on the Periodic Health Examination. Screening for HIV antibody. In: *The Canadian Guide to Clinical Preventive Health Care.* Ottawa, Canada: Minister of Supply and Services; 1994: chap 58.

Center for Health Statistics. *Health, United States, 1995.* Hyattsville, Md: Public Health Service; 1996

Centers for Disease Control and Prevention. Trends in AIDS incidence, deaths, and prevalence—United States, 1996. *MMWR.* 1997;46(8):165-173.

Centers for Disease Control. CDC estimates of HIV prevalence and projected AIDS cases: summary of a workshop, October 31-November 1, 1989. *MMWR.* 1990;39:110-112,117-119.

Centers for Disease Control. CDC Public health service guidelines for counseling and antibody testing to prevent HIV infection and AIDS. *MMWR.* 1987;36:509-515.

Centers for Disease Control. Sexually transmitted diseases treatment guidelines. *MMWR.* 1993;42 (No. RR-14).

Centers for Disease Control. Primary and secondary syphilis—United States, 1981-1990. *MMWR.* 1991;40:314-323.

Centers for Disease Control and Prevention. Recommendations for HIV testing services for inpatients and outpatients in acute-care hospital settings and technical guidance on HIV counseling. *MMWR.* 1993;42:1-17.

Centers for Disease Control and Prevention. Recommendations for the prevention and management of *Chlamydia trachomatis* infections. *MMWR.* 1993;42(No. RR-12):1-39.

Centers for Disease Control and Prevention. US Public Health Service recommendations for human immunodeficiency virus counseling and voluntary testing for pregnant women. *MMWR*. 1995;44(No. RR-7):1-15.

Davies HD, Wang EL. Periodic Health Examination, 1996 Update: 2. Screening for chlamydial infections. *Can Med Assoc J*. 1996;154(11):1631-1777.

Food and Drug Administration. FDA approves first urine-based HIV test. *FDA Talk Paper*. 1996; T96-55; http://www.fda.gov/bbs/topics/ANSWERS/ANS00752.html

Hardy AM. AIDS knowledge and attitudes for January-March 1991: provisional data from the National Health Interview Survey. *Advance Data*. August 21, 1992:216.

Hashimoto T. Gram Stain Technique. *Gram Stain*. Updated April 30, 1996. http://www.meddean.luc.edu/lumen/Dept Webs/micrbio/med/gram/tech.htm

Higgins DL, Galavotti C, O'Reilly KR, et al. Evidence for the effects of HIV antibody counseling and testing on risk behaviors. *JAMA*. 1991;266:2419-2429.

Hook EW, Marra CM. Acquired syphilis in adults. *N Engl J Med*. 1992;326:1060-1069.

Larson SA. Syphilis. *Clin Lab Med*. 1989;9:545-557.

Sellors JW, Pickard L, Gafini A, et al. Effectiveness and efficiency of selective vs. universal screening for chlamydia infection in sexually active young women. *Arch Intern Med*. 1992; 152(9):1837-1844.

Swango PA, Kleinman DV, Konzelman JL. HIV and periodontal health. *J Am Dent Assoc*. 1991;122:49-54.

US Preventive Services Task Force. Screening for chlamydial infection (including ocular prophylaxis in newborns). In: *Guide to Clinical Preventive Services*. 2nd ed. Washington, DC: US Department of Health and Human Services; 1996: chap 29.

US Preventive Services Task Force. Screening for infection with human immunodeficiency virus. In: *Guide to Clinical Preventive Services*. 2nd ed. Washington, DC: US Department of Health and Human Services; 1996: chap 28.

US Preventive Services Task Force. Screening for gonorrhea (including ocular prophylaxis in newborns). In: *Guide to Clinical Preventive Services*. 2nd ed. Washington, DC: US Department of Health and Human Services; 1996: chap 27.

US Preventive Services Task Force. Screening for syphilis. In: *Guide to Clinical Preventive Services*. 2nd ed. Washington, DC: US Department of Health and Human Services; 1996: chap 26.

41

SIGMOIDOSCOPY

Colorectal cancer is the third leading cause of death from cancer in the United States. The disease most often afflicts persons older than age 40 years. Of the three widely used methods of screening for colorectal cancer (digital rectal examination, sigmoidoscopy, and fecal occult blood testing), examination using a sigmoidoscope is the most specific and sensitive. The specificity of sigmoidoscopy approaches 100%, because this procedure enables the examiner to perform a biopsy during the procedure. The sensitivity of sigmoidoscopy is largely determined by the skill of the examiner and the length of the instrument. Approximately 30% of colorectal cancers are within reach of the 25-cm rigid sigmoidoscope. The 35-cm flexible sigmoidoscope can reach 45% to 50% of cancers, and the 60-cm flexible sigmoidoscope can reach 50% to 60% of cancers.

Screening with sigmoidoscopy has been limited by costs, patient and provider compliance, and earlier controversies about the effectiveness of this approach. Patient compliance problems have been somewhat diminished by development of the more comfortable flexible instruments. The 35-cm sigmoidoscope is particularly well accepted by patients, and the 60-cm sigmoidoscope is relatively well accepted. The controversy about effectiveness had stemmed from a lack of evidence that screening with sigmoidoscopy decreases mortality from colorectal cancer. Two recent case-control studies (Selby et al, 1992; Newcomb et al, 1992) demonstrated significant decreases (59% and 79%, respectively) in the risk of death from colorectal cancer among screened patients. In the Selby study, a significant benefit of rigid sigmoidoscopy was suggested even if screening was performed as infrequently as every 10 years.

See chapters 30 and 34 for information about colorectal cancer and other methods of screening for it.

Recommendations of Major Authorities

Normal Risk

American Academy of Family Physicians—Individuals aged 50 years and older and those aged 40 years and older with a family history of early colorectal cancer should be screened for colorectal cancer with fecal occult blood tests, sigmoidoscopy, colonoscopy, or barium enema.

American Cancer Society (ACS) and American Gastroenterological Association—Patients at normal risk should be screened with sigmoidoscopy every 5 years in combination with yearly fecal occult blood testing beginning at 50 years of age. Other recommended screening options beginning at age 50 include: colonoscopy every 10 years or double contrast barium enema every 5 to 10 years. The **ACS** further advises that digital rectal examination be performed along with the endoscopic or radiological procedure.

American College of Obstetricians and Gynecologists—Patients at normal risk should be screened with sigmoidoscopy every 3 to 5 years beginning at 50 years of age.

American College of Physicians—Men and women should be offered flexible sigmoidoscopies every 10 years from 50 to 70 years of age. In most settings and for most people, this strategy will provide the best balance of benefits and harms, logistic feasibility, and costs. In settings where it is logistically feasible and cost is reasonable, persons who want to achieve the maximum protection against colorectal cancer should be offered colonoscopy every 10 years from 50 to 70 years of age. In some settings, air-contrast barium enemas every 10 years from 50 to 70 years of age might be logistically preferable to colonoscopies, and some patients might prefer that procedure. For persons who decline these options, annual fecal occult blood testing should be offered.

Canadian Task Force on the Periodic Health Examination—There is insufficient evidence to support the inclusion or exclusion of sigmoidoscopic or colonoscopic screening of asymptomatic individuals over 40 years of age in the periodic health examination.

US Preventive Services Task Force—Screening for colorectal cancer is recommended for all persons 50 years of age or over. Sigmoidoscopy and fecal occult blood testing are effective methods of screening. There is insufficient evidence to determine which of these methods is preferable or whether the combination of both methods produces greater benefit than either method alone. There is insufficient evidence to recommend a periodicity for sigmoidoscopy screening.

Increased Risk

All major authorities—Patients at increased risk of colorectal cancer should consider more intensive screening. What constitutes increased risk and the nature and frequency of recommended screening differs slightly among the authorities.

American Cancer Society—For patients having a first-degree relative with a history of colorectal cancer at 55 years of age or younger, the entire colon and rectum should be examined with colonoscopy or air-contrast barium enema every 5 years beginning at 35 to 40 years of age. Members of families with a history of familial adenomatous polyposis should receive earlier screening utilizing flexible sigmoidoscopy. Members of families with a history of hereditary nonpolyposis colorectal cancer require earlier and more intense surveillance utilizing colonoscopy. Individuals with inflammatory bowel disease are at exceptionally high risk and require individualized treatment. Patients under age 55 years with a first-degree family member with a history of colorectal cancer are at increased risk and may need earlier and more frequent examinations. People with a history of breast, ovarian, or endometrial cancer are at some increased risk but should follow screening recommendations for normal-risk patients.

American College of Obstetricians and Gynecologists—
Colonoscopy should be a part of primary preventive care for individuals with a personal history of inflammatory bowel disease or colonic polyps, or a family history of familial polyposis coli, colorectal cancer, or cancer family syndrome.

American College of Physicians—Individuals who have one or more first-degree relatives with colorectal cancer should be offered colonoscopy at 40 years of age and at least every 10 years thereafter.

American Gastroenterological Association—Individuals with a first-degree relative who has had colorectal cancer or an adenomatous polyp should be screened beginning at age 40 years. Gene carriers for familial adenomatous polyposis (FAP) or people with a family history of FAP whose gene carrier status is indeterminate should be offered yearly flexible sigmoidoscopy beginning at puberty to see if they are expressing the gene. If polyposis is present, they should begin to consider when they should have colectomy. People with a family history of hereditary nonpolyposis colorectal cancer should be offered an examination of the entire colon (via colonoscopy or double contrast barium enema, preferably with sigmoidoscopy) every 1 to 2 years starting between the ages 20 and 30 years and every year after age 40 years. In patients with long-standing, extensive inflammatory bowel disease, surveillance colonoscopy should be considered, along with the extent and duration of the disease, as a guide to when or if colectomy should be considered. A common practice is to perform surveillance colonoscopy every 1 to 2 years beginning after 8 years of disease in patients with pancolitis or after 15 years in those with colitis involving only the left colon.

Canadian Task Force on the Periodic Health Examination—
There is insufficient evidence to recommend for or against the inclusion or exclusion of sigmoidoscopy in the periodic health examination of asymptomatic individuals over 40 years old (including those with a fam-

ily history of one or two relatives with colorectal cancer). There is fair evidence to exclude sigmoidoscopy from the periodic health examination of individuals with true cancer family syndrome; however, there is fair evidence for the inclusion of colonoscopy in the periodic health examination of individuals with true cancer family syndrome.

US Preventive Services Task Force—In high-risk groups, there is insufficient evidence to recommend for or against early or frequent screening or the use of colonoscopy rather than sigmoidoscopy. However, early and frequent colonoscopy screening of patients with a family history of familial polyposis coli or cancer family syndrome or with personal histories of previous adenomatous polyps or colorectal cancer may be recommended on other grounds, including the increased risk of colorectal cancer and of lesions in the proximal colon.

Basics of Sigmoidoscopy Screening

Performing sigmoidoscopies requires technical training and practice. It is beyond the scope of this book to explain the performance of this procedure; only very basic aspects will be addressed.

1. *Training*: Sigmoidoscopy should be performed only by or under the supervision of a trained examiner. Training should be obtained from an experienced endoscopist. Training may consist of diagnostic instruction with audiovisual materials, endoscopic models, and photo atlases, followed by patient demonstrations and successful completion of a number of supervised examinations.

2. *Sigmoidoscope type*: Most authorities recommend use of a flexible sigmoidoscope (preferably 60 cm in length) rather than a rigid sigmoidoscope because of better patient acceptance and the ability to visualize lesions higher in the sigmoid colon.

3. *Patient preparation*: Proper bowel preparation is essential for performance of an adequate screening examination. Recommendations for bowel preparation differ somewhat. The minimum preparation consists of administration of two enemas a few hours before examination.

4. *Follow-up of abnormal results*: All authorities agree that patients found to have adenomatous polyps of 1 cm or larger need colonoscopic examination of the entire colon. Approximately 10% of individuals screened will have small tubular adenomas less than 1 cm in diameter. Controversy exists about whether patients with these lesions need colonoscopic follow-up in view of their low potential for malignancy.

5. *Maintenance of competence*: Clinicians need to perform sigmoidoscopy routinely to maintain competence. Performing procedures only occasionally

may lead to missed or inappropriate diagnoses and a high rate of complications.

Patient Resources

Colorectal Cancer: Questions & Answers; Colonoscopy: Questions and Answers; Polyps of the Colon and Rectum: Questions and Answers. American Society of Colon and Rectal Surgeons, 800 E Northwest Hwy, Suite 1080, Palatine, IL 60067; (708)359-9184.

What You Need to Know about Cancer of the Colon and Rectum. Office of Cancer Communications, National Cancer Institute, Bethesda, MD 20892; (800)4-CANCER. Internet address: http://wwwicic.nci.nih.gov

Selected References

American Academy of Family Physicians. *Summary of Policy Recommendations for Periodic Health Examination.* Kansas City, Mo: American Academy of Family Physicians; 1997.

American Cancer Society. *Cancer Facts & Figures-1997.* Atlanta, Ga: American Cancer Society; 1997.

American Cancer Society. *Cancer Information Database.* Atlanta, Ga: American Cancer Society; June 1997.

American College of Obstetricians and Gynecologists. *Guidelines for Women's Health Care.* Washington, DC: American College of Obstetricians and Gynecologists; 1996.

American College of Physicians, Health and Public Policy Committee. Clinical competence in the use of flexible sigmoidoscopy for screening purposes. *Ann Intern Med.* 1987;107:589-591.

American College of Physicians. Guidelines. In: Eddy DM, ed. *Common Screening Tests.* Philadelphia, Pa: American College of Physicians; 1991:415-416.

Canadian Task Force on the Periodic Health Examination. Screening for colorectal cancer. In: *The Canadian Guide to Clinical Preventive Health Care.* Ottawa, Canada: Minister of Supply and Services; 1994: chap 66.

Eddy DM. Screening for colorectal cancer. *Ann Intern Med.* 1990;113:373-384.

Eddy DM, Ferioli C, Anderson DS. Screening for colorectal cancer. *Ann Intern Med.* In press.

Fleischer DE, Goldberg SB, Browning TH, et al. Detection and surveillance of colorectal cancer. *JAMA.* 1989;261:580-585.

Gorse GJ, Messner RL. Infection control practices in gastrointestinal endoscopy in the United States: a national survey. *Infect Control Hosp Epidemiol.* 1991;12:289-296.

Newcomb PA, Norfleet RG, Storer B, Surawicz, Marcus PM. Screening sigmoidoscopy and colorectal cancer mortality. *J Natl Cancer Inst.* 1992;84:1572-1575.

Ransohoff DF, Lang CA. Sigmoidoscopic screening in the 1990s. *JAMA.* 1993;269:1278-1281.

Selby JV, Friedman GD. Sigmoidoscopy in the periodic examination of asymptomatic adults. *JAMA.* 1989;261:595-601.

Selby JV, Friedman GD, Quesenberry CP, Weiss NS. A case-control study of screening sigmoidoscopy and mortality from colorectal cancer. *N Engl J Med.* 1992;326:653-657.

US Preventive Services Task Force. Screening for colorectal cancer. In: *Guide to Clinical Preventive Services*. 2nd ed. Washington, DC: US Department of Health and Human Services; 1996: chap 8.

Wigton RS, Bland LL, Monsour H, Nicolas JA. Procedural skills of practicing gastroenterologists. *Ann Intern Med.* 1990;113:540-546.

Winawer SJ, Fletcher RH, Miller L, et al. Colorectal cancer screening: clinical guidelines and rationale. *Gastroenterology.* 1997;112:594-642.

42

THYROID FUNCTION

Thyroid dysfunction affects 1% to 4% of adults in the United States. The annual incidence of hypothyroidism is 0.08%. The estimated annual incidence of hyperthyroidism is 0.05%. Both forms of thyroid dysfunction are more common in women, older adults, and persons with a family history of thyroid disease. Laboratory evidence of hypothyroidism is found in up to 10% of women and 2% of men aged 60 years and older. Other risk factors for thyroid hypofunction include prior autoimmune conditions, history of head or neck surgery or radiation exposure, Down's syndrome, and the postpartum state. In most affected persons, symptoms typically develop shortly after the onset of thyroid dysfunction. Lethargy, weight gain, confusion, cold intolerance, constipation, alopecia, dyspnea, myalgias, and paresthesias are common features of hypothyroidism. Restlessness, emotional lability, insomnia, heat intolerance, dyspnea, palpitations, ophthalmopathy, diarrhea, muscle atrophy, weakness, tremors, and tachycardia are symptoms of hyperthyroidism.

Some individuals, particularly older adults, can experience an insidious onset of thyroid disease. Apathetic hyperthyroidism occurs without the usual goiter, ophthalmopathy, and signs of sympathetic nervous system hyperactivity. Symptoms of hypothyroidism, such as fatigue, constipation, dry skin, and poor concentration may be attributed to the aging process or may be less frequent in older populations. Because hypothyroidism can cause secondary dyslipidemia, patients with subclinical hypothyroidism may first present with high cholesterol levels. Studies suggest that some patients with subclinical disease or mild alterations in thyroid function tests may benefit from early treatment if they are identified through screening. For this reason, some authorities recommend screening of certain high-risk populations for thyroid dysfunction.

See chapters 8 and 30 for information about screening for congenital hypothyroidism and thyroid cancer, respectively.

Recommendations of Major Authorities

High-risk Populations

American College of Obstetricians and Gynecologists—Thyroid-stimulating hormone (TSH) levels should be obtained every 3 to 5 years from all women aged 65 years and older and from younger women with an autoimmune condition or strong family history of thyroid disease.

American College of Physicians—Routine screening for thyroid disease is not indicated in asymptomatic individuals nor in patients admitted to the hospital for acute medical or psychiatric illnesses; testing may be indicated to identify unsuspected disease in women over 50 years of age who have general symptoms that could be caused by thyroid disease.

American Thyroid Association—Tests of thyroid function should not be a part of multiphasic screening for patients who are not suspected of having thyroid disease except in certain high-risk populations. Suspect populations include individuals with a strong family history of thyroid disease, elderly patients, postpartum women 4 to 8 weeks after delivery, and patients with autoimmune diseases.

Canadian Task Force on the Periodic Health Examination—There is insufficient evidence to support screening for hyperthyroidism and hypothyroidism among asymptomatic adults. The high prevalence of hypothyroidism among perimenopausal and postmenopausal women warrants a high index of suspicion and liberal use of the sensitive thyroid stimulating hormone (TSH) assay in the presence of even vague and subtle complaints.

Expert Panel on Detection, Evaluation, and Treatment of High Blood Cholesterol in Adults—Because hypothyroid states can raise LDL-cholesterol levels, any patient with LDL-cholesterol exceeding 190 mg/dL should be tested for hypothyroidism.

US Preventive Services Task Force—Routine screening for thyroid disorders is not warranted in asymptomatic adults. There is insufficient evidence to recommend for or against screening for thyroid disease with thyroid function tests in high-risk patients, including the elderly, postpartum women, and persons with Down's syndrome, but recommendations for such screening may be made on other grounds, such as the high prevalence of disease and the increased likelihood that symptoms of thyroid disease will be overlooked in these patients. Clinicians should remain alert for subtle or nonspecific symptoms of thyroid dysfunction when examining such patients, and maintain a low threshold for diagnostic evaluation of thyroid function.

Basics of Thyroid Function Screening

1. Many authorities now recommend performing a TSH level using a "sensitive" TSH assay as the initial screen and obtaining a free thyroxine (FT_4) or free thyroxine index (FT_4I) level only if the TSH level is abnormal. In unselected populations, these TSH assays have sensitivities of 85% to 95% and specificities of 90% to 96% for thyroid dysfunction. Determination of total thyroxine (TT_4) and FT_4I levels, while less expensive, is less sensitive and less specific compared with use of the "sensitive" TSH assays.

2. An elevated TSH value (>7 mU/L) and a suppressed FT_4 level (<0.8 ng/dL) suggest primary thyroid failure necessitating therapy. (Normal values may vary with each laboratory.) Whether asymptomatic patients with an elevated TSH level but a normal FT_4 or FT_4I level will benefit from treatment is unclear. Some evidence suggests that thyroid replacement may diminish the potential for developing long-term complications of subclinical thyroid hypofunction. Because overt disease develops in only a small number of these individuals, some authorities recommend serial testing of these patients rather than immediate use of replacement therapy.

3. A depressed TSH level (<0.4 mU/L) usually, but not always, indicates the presence of an elevated serum thyroxine (T_4) level. If clinical findings of hyperthyroidism are present, and the T_4 level is normal, measure serum total triiodothyronine (TT_3), because the patient may have T_3 thyrotoxicosis. In the absence of clinical findings, many authorities recommend following the patient closely and deferring treatment until symptoms develop.

4. Medications and clinical conditions can affect the interpretation of thyroid screening tests. TSH levels may be depressed in euthyroid patients who are taking large doses of glucocorticoids or dopamine. Also, the TSH level may be misleading in the presence of pituitary or hypothalamic hypothyroidism and during changes in thyroid status that occur in cases of subacute thyroiditis or after treatment of hyperthyroidism. In such cases, measurement of the FT_4 level is preferred. Phenytoin, carbamazepine, and rifampin can depress TT_4 levels. The effect of drugs on reported FT_4 levels varies with the laboratory method used. Increased levels of thyroid-binding globulin (TBG), resulting in elevated TT_4 levels, may occur with pregnancy, oral contraceptive or estrogen use, acute or chronic active hepatitis, acute intermittent porphyria, and certain inherited traits. Patients with cirrhosis, nephrotic syndrome, severe illness, and those using testosterone or corticosteroids may have slightly reduced TT_4 levels because of diminished TBG. Severe illnesses, such as those requiring treatment in an intensive-care unit, can also affect the production, secretion, distribution, and metabolism of thyroid hormone.

Patient Resources

Your Thyroid Gland: A Guide for the Patient. American Academy of Otolaryngology-Head and Neck Surgery, Order Department, 1 Prince St, Alexandria, VA 22314; (703)836-4444.

Provider Resources

Directory of Organizations for Endocrine and Metabolic Diseases; Thyroid Hormone Action and Nuclear Receptors; Attention Deficit Hyperactivity Disorder and Generalized Resistance to Thyroid Hormone. National Institute Diabetes and Digestive and Kidney Diseases, Bldg 31, Rm 9A04, Bethesda, MD 20892; (301)496-3583. Internet address: http://www.niddk.nih.gov/EndocrineDocs.htm

Selected References

American Academy of Family Physicians. *Summary of Policy Recommendations for Periodic Health Examination.* Kansas City, Mo: American Academy of Family Physicians; 1997.

American College of Obstetricians and Gynecologists. *Guidelines for Women's Health Care.* Washington, DC: American College of Obstetricians and Gynecologists; 1996.

American College of Physicians. Guidelines. In: Eddy DM, ed. *Common Screening Tests.* Philadelphia, Pa: American College of Physicians; 1991:406-408.

Becker DV, Bigos ST, Gaitan E, et al. Optimal use of blood tests for assessment of thyroid function. *JAMA.* 1993;269:2736-2737.

Canadian Task Force on the Periodic Health Examination. Screening for thyroid disorders and thyroid cancer in asymptomatic adults. In: *The Canadian Guide to Clinical Preventive Health Care.* Ottawa, Canada: Minister of Supply and Services; 1994: chap 51.

de los Santos ET, Starich GH, Mazzaferri EL. Sensitivity, specificity, and cost-effectiveness of the sensitive thyrotropin assay in the diagnosis of thyroid disease in ambulatory patients. *Arch Intern Med.* 1989;149:526-532.

Hay ID, Bayer MF, Kaplan MM, Klee GG, Larsen PR, Spencer CA. American Thyroid Association assessment of free thyroid hormone and thyrotropin measurements and guidelines for future clinical assays. *Clin Chem.* 1991;37:2002-2008.

Helfand M, Crapo LM. Screening for thyroid disease. *Ann Intern Med.* 1990;112:840-849.

National Cholesterol Education Program. *Second Report of the Expert Panel on Detection, Evaluation, and Treatment of High Blood Cholesterol in Adults (Adult Treatment Panel II).* Bethesda, Md: National Heart, Lung and Blood Institutes, National Institutes of Health, 1994. (NIH Publication no. 93-3095.)

Sawin CT, Geller A, Kaplan MM, Bacharach P, Wilson PWF, Hershman JM. Low serum thyrotropin (thyroid-stimulating hormone) in older persons without hyperthyroidism. *Arch Intern Med.* 1991;151:165-168.

Sawin CT. Thyroid dysfunction in older persons. *Advances Intern Med.* 1991;37:223-248.

Staub JJ, Althaus BU, Engler H, et al. Spectrum of subclinical and overt hypothyroidism: effect on thyrotropin, prolactin, and thyroid reserve, and metabolic impact on peripheral target tissues. *Am J Med.* 1992;92:631-642.

Surks MI, Chopra IJ, Mariash CN, Nicoloff JT, Solomon DH. American Thyroid Association guidelines for use of laboratory tests in thyroid disorders. *JAMA.* 1990;263:1529-1532.

US Preventive Services Task Force. Screening for thyroid disease. In: *Guide to Clinical Preventive Services.* 2nd ed. Washington, DC: US Department of Health and Human Services; 1996: chap 20.

43

TUBERCULOSIS (Including Prophylaxis and BCG Vaccination)

In 1995, a total of 22,860 new cases of active tuberculosis (TB) were reported in the United States. This marked the third consecutive year that the number of reported cases decreased and reflected the lowest rate of reported TB cases since national surveillance began in 1953. During the 1980s and early 1990s, the number of TB cases increased significantly. Factors that contributed to the increase included adverse social and economic conditions, the human immunodeficiency virus (HIV) epidemic, immigration of individuals with *Mycobacterium tuberculosis* infection, and clinician and patient noncompliance with recommended screening and treatment regimens. Efforts to control the spread of TB were also complicated by the emergence of strains of *M. tuberculosis* resistant to multiple drugs.

The more recent decline in the number of TB cases probably reflects a number of factors, according to the Centers for Disease Control and Prevention, including (1) improved laboratory methods to allow prompt identification of *M. tuberculosis*; (2) broader use of drug-susceptibility testing; (3) expanded use of preventive therapy in high-risk groups; (4) decreased transmission of *M. tuberculosis* in congregate settings (eg, hospital and correctional facilities) because of implementation of infection-control guidelines; and (5) improved follow-up of persons with TB.

In the United States, control of tuberculosis depends on screening high-risk populations and providing preventive therapy to persons in whom active disease is most likely to develop. Groups at high risk for TB infection include: (1) close contacts of persons known or suspected to have TB; (2) persons infected with HIV; (3) persons who inject illicit drugs or other locally identified high-risk substance abusers (eg, crack cocaine users); (4) persons who have medical risk factors known to increase the risk for TB disease if infection occurs; (5) residents and employees of high-risk congregate settings (eg, correctional institutions, nursing homes, mental institutions, other long-term residential facilities, and shelters for the homeless); (6) health care workers who serve high-risk clients; (7) foreign-born persons, including children, who have arrived within 5 years from countries with a high incidence or prevalence of TB; and (8) some medically underserved, low-income populations. Conditions and chronic diseases that predispose patients to development of TB disease include HIV infection, diabetes mellitus, end-stage renal disease, and hematologic and reticuloendothelial diseases; history of intestinal bypass or gastrectomy, chronic malabsorption syndromes, silicosis, cancers of the upper gastrointestinal tract or oropharynx, prolonged steroid use and immunosuppressive therapy; and being 10% or more below desirable body weight.

Prophylaxis with isoniazid is very effective in preventing the onset of clinical tuberculous disease. Use of isoniazid for 12 months in an at-risk population has been shown to reduce the occurrence of TB disease by 54% to 88%. Its efficacy is directly related to the length of prophylaxis, the extent of patient compliance with the prophylactic regimen, and the susceptibility of the infecting organism to isoniazid. The effectiveness of bacillus of Calmette and Guérin (BCG) vaccination is considerably less certain; effectiveness rates varied from 0% to 76% in major trials.

See chapter 9 for information on TB screening, preventive therapy, and BCG immunization in children and adolescents.

Tuberculosis is currently designated as an infectious disease notifiable at the national level. Refer to Appendix C for further information on nationally notifiable diseases.

Recommendations of Major Authorities

Screening

All major authorities, including **American Academy of Family Physicians, American College of Obstetricians and Gynecologists, American Thoracic Society, Canadian Task Force on the Periodic Health Examination, Centers for Disease Control and Prevention, and US Preventive Services Task Force**—Tuberculin skin testing should be performed on all individuals at high risk. The need for repeat skin testing should be determined by the likelihood of continuing exposure to infectious TB.

Prophylaxis

American Thoracic Society (ATS), Canadian Task Force on the Periodic Health Examination, Centers for Disease Control and Prevention (CDC), and US Preventive Services Task Force— Adults with a reactive skin test and no evidence of active disease should be considered for preventive therapy with isoniazid based on age and risk factors. **ATS** and **CDC** also recommend that anergic patients recently exposed to an active TB case or from populations where the prevalence of TB is greater than 10% (injection drug users, homeless individuals, migrant laborers, and first-generation immigrants from Asia, Africa, or Latin

America) should be considered for isoniazid prophylaxis even when their skin test is negative.

BCG Vaccination

American Thoracic Society, Centers for Disease Control and Prevention (CDC), and US Preventive Services Task Force—Vaccination with BCG is not recommended for adults in the United States. However, **CDC** recommends that BCG vaccination should be considered for health care workers who work in settings in which (a) a high percentage of TB patients are infected with *M. tuberculosis* resistant to both isoniazid and rifampin, (b) transmission of such drug-resistant *M. tuberculosis* strains is likely, and (c) comprehensive infection control precautions have been implemented and have not been successful.

Canadian Task Force on the Periodic Health Examination recommends BCG vaccination for tuberculin-negative contacts of persons with active TB in Canadian communities in which the infection rate is high.

Basics of Tuberculosis Screening

1. Use the Mantoux test exclusively in high-risk populations. The Mantoux test is the standard methods of testing. Multiple-puncture tests should not be used to determine whether a person is infected.

2. For the Mantoux test, administer 0.1 mL of purified protein derivative (PPD) containing 5 tuberculin units (TU) on the volar or ventral surface of the forearm. Administer the injection intradermally using a disposable tuberculin syringe with the bevel of the needle facing upward. The injection should produce a pale, discrete 6-mm to 10-mm weal on the skin.

3. Read the test results 48 to 72 hours after administration by palpating the margin of induration and measuring the diameter transverse to the long axis of the forearm. It may be helpful to outline the margin of induration with a ballpoint pen. Always record the actual millimeters of induration, not the erythema surrounding the induration. Simply recording "positive" or "negative" is not precise enough and may lead to improper treatment.

4. Absence of a tuberculin reaction does not exclude a diagnosis of TB infection, especially when symptoms suggest the presence of active disease. Induration of less than 5 mm may occur early in the course of TB infection or in individuals with altered immune function. Anergy testing with at least two other delayed-type hypersensitivity skin tests (eg, *Candida*, mumps, or tetanus toxoid) may be conducted in conjunction with PPD testing in adults at risk for decreased cell-mediated immune function (in-

cluding persons with HIV infection). The scientific basis for anergy testing is tenuous, however, and no standardization exists for most skin-test antigens used for anergy testing. Therefore, anergy testing is not part of routine screening for TB infection.

5. Reactions to PPD may wane with age but can be restored by repeat testing. Because of this "booster effect," patients (particularly those over age 55 years) who undergo repeat testing may be falsely classified as new converters and unnecessarily treated with isoniazid. Some authorities recommend initially screening adults in institutional and hospital settings using a two-step PPD testing procedure. If the first Mantoux test result is negative, perform a second test 1 to 2 weeks later. Reaction to the "booster" test usually indicates old—not new—TB infection. CDC recommends this two-step procedure for the initial screening of residents and employees of long-term care facilities, such as nursing homes, adult foster-care homes, and board and care homes.

6. A small percentage of tuberculin reactions may be caused by errors in administering the test or reading the result, cross-reaction with antigens shared between mycobacteria, and vaccination with BCG. The probability that a positive skin test results from infection with *M. tuberculosis* rather than from BCG vaccination increases: (1) as the size of the reaction increases; (2) when the patient is a contact of a person who has TB; (3) when the patient has a family history of TB or the incidence/prevalence of TB in their country of origin is high; and (4) as the interval between vaccination and tuberculin testing increases (vaccination-induced reactivity is unlikely to occur for 10 years after vaccination).

7. Live vaccines, such as measles-mumps-rubella (MMR) and oral polio vaccine (OPV), may interfere with the response to the Mantoux test. To avoid confusion, administer live vaccines and the TB test concurrently, or delay the TB test for 4 to 6 weeks.

Basics of Tuberculosis Prophylaxis

1. Indications

CDC has issued recommendations for preventive therapy in previously untreated adults without evidence of active TB (Table 43.1). Certain anergic patients should be considered for preventive therapy regardless of their skin test reaction. Other groups for whom prophylaxis is indicated include adults who have had close contact with a person with infectious TB in the past 3 months and individuals who are members of populations in which the prevalence of TB is greater than 10% (eg, injection drug users, homeless persons, migrant laborers, and persons born in Asia, Africa, or Latin America).

Table 43.1. Criteria for Determining Need for Preventive Therapy by Category and Age Group

Category	Age Group (Years)	
	<35	**≥35**
With risk factor*	Treat at all ages if reaction to 5 TU purified protein derivative ≥10 mm (or ≥5 mm and recent TB contact, HIV-infected, or has radiographic evidence of old TB)	
Without risk factor High-incidence group†	Treat if PPD ≥10 mm	Do not treat
Without risk factor Low-incidence group	Consider treating if PPD ≥15 mm‡	Do not treat

*Risk factors include: HIV infection; recent (within past 3 months) contact with infectious person; radiograph other than entirely normal; injection drug abuse; certain medical risk factors; and recent skin-test conversion. Recent converters are defined as: infants and children younger than 4 years of age with a 10-mm PPD; children and adults younger than 35 years of age with an increase in PPD reaction of ≥10 mm within a 2-year period; or adult ≥35 years of age with an increase in PPD reaction ≥15 mm within a 2-year period. Medical risk factors include: HIV infection, diabetes, end-stage renal disease, hematologic and reticuloendothelial diseases, prolonged steroid use, immunosuppressive therapy, and conditions associated with rapid weight loss (intestinal bypass surgery, gastrectomy, peptic ulcer disease, chronic malabsorption, chronic alcoholism, carcinomas of the oropharynx and upper gastrointestinal tract that prevent adequate nutrition).

†High-incidence groups include: foreign-born persons from high-prevalence countries; medically underserved low-income populations (including high-risk racial or ethnic minority populations, especially African Americans, Hispanics, and American Indians); and residents of long-term care facilities.

‡Consider treatment with isoniazid (INH) based on individual assessment of risks and benefits.

Adapted from: Centers for Disease Control. The use of preventive therapy for tuberculosis infection in the United States: recommendations of the Advisory Committee for the Elimination of Tuberculosis. *MMWR.* 1990;39:(No. RR-8):9–12.

Information also incorporated from: American Thoracic Society. Treatment of tuberculosis and tuberculosis infection in adults and children. *Am J Respir Crit Care Med.* 1994;149:1359–1374. Official journal of the American Thoracic Society. Copyright American Lung Association.

2. Dose and Administration

Initiate preventive therapy with isoniazid (INH). The correct daily dose of isoniazid for adults is 5 mg/kg (maximum, 300 mg) taken orally. For noncompliant adult patients, isoniazid may be administered by a health professional on a twice-weekly schedule of 15 mg/kg per dose (maximum, 900 mg). In general, continue isoniazid prophylaxis for at least 6 months, up to a maximum of 12 months. Patients who are HIV-positive or have evidence of prior untreated TB on chest X-ray should receive isoniazid prophylaxis for 12 months. If a patient has had contact with a person known to have infectious TB that is resistant to isoniazid, consider administering preventive therapy with rifampin (600 mg by mouth daily for 1 year).

3. Contraindications/Precautions

Contraindications to isoniazid prophylaxis include acute or active liver disease of any etiology or previous adverse reaction to isoniazid. Among adults over 35 years of age, the incidence of mild isoniazid-induced liver function test abnormalities is 10% to 20%. During the course of therapy, adults over age 35 years should undergo baseline and periodic (monthly) testing for transaminase (ALT or AST) levels. If the transaminase level is three to five times higher than the upper limit of the laboratory normal range, consider discontinuing isoniazid. Closely monitor individuals who use alcohol daily or in whom chronic liver disease is suspected for isoniazid-induced hepatitis. Supplementation with pyridoxine (vitamin B_6, 50 mg by mouth daily) may be helpful in preventing neuropathy in certain patients on isoniazid, such as those with diabetes, uremia, alcoholism, or malnutrition. Delay therapy for pregnant women who are candidates for preventive treatment until after delivery. If it is likely that the woman has been recently infected, therapy may be instituted after completion of the first trimester of pregnancy.

4. Adverse Reactions

While patients are taking isoniazid, monitor them monthly for signs and symptoms of adverse reactions. These include drug fever or rash, hypersensitivity reactions, peripheral neuritis, and hepatitis. Signs and symptoms of hepatitis include loss of appetite, nausea, vomiting, persistent dark urine, jaundice, fever, and abdominal tenderness—especially in the right upper quadrant. Patients who are taking other medications concurrently with isoniazid should be monitored for potential drug interactions.

Basics of BCG Vaccination

1. Indications

Routine BCG vaccination is not recommended for adults in the United States.

2. Dose and Administration

The Tice® strain is the only BCG preparation currently available in the United States. The dose and administration is the same for both adults and children (see chapter 9 for details).

3. Precautions

Do not administer BCG vaccine to individuals who may be immunocompromised or immunosuppressed, including those with known or suspected HIV infection.

4. Adverse Reactions

Side effects occur in 1% to 10% of vaccinated individuals and may include severe or prolonged ulceration at the vaccination site, lymphadenitis, and lupus vulgaris.

Patient Resources

Tuberculosis: Get the Facts; Tuberculosis: Connection between TB and HIV; Questions and Answers about TB. Centers for Disease Control and Prevention, Attn: Information, Technology and Services Office, NCHSTP, CDC, 1600 Clifton Rd NE, M/S E-06, Atlanta, GA 30333; or National Center for HIV, STD, and TB Prevention Voice Information System: (404)639-1819.

Facts About the TB Skin Test; Facts About Tuberculosis. American Lung Association, 1740 Broadway, New York, NY 10019-4374; (212)315-8700.

Provider Resources

Multidrug Resistant Tuberculosis; TB Care Guide; Core Curriculum on Tuberculosis; TB Treatment: A Clinical Care Guide; Improving Patient Adherence to Tuberculosis Treatment; Reported TB in the United States; Tuberculosis Control Laws-United States. To order these and other documents, contact the Centers for Disease Control and Prevention, Attn: Information, Technology and Services Office, NCHSTP, CDC, 1600 Clifton Rd, NE, M/S E-06, Atlanta, GA 30333; or the National Center for HIV, STD, and TB Prevention Voice Information System: (404)639-1819.

Selected References

American Academy of Family Physicians. *Summary of Policy Recommendations for Periodic Health Examination.* Kansas City, Mo: American Academy of Family Physicians; 1997.

American College of Obstetricians and Gynecologists. *Guidelines for Women's Health.* Washington, DC: American College of Obstetricians and Gynecologists; 1996.

American Thoracic Society. Control of tuberculosis in the United States. *Am Rev Respir Dis.* 1992;146:1623-1633.

American Thoracic Society. Treatment of tuberculosis and tuberculosis infection in adults and children. *Am J Respir Crit Care Med.* 1994;149:1359-1374.

American Thoracic Society/Centers for Disease Control. Diagnostic standards and classification of tuberculosis. *Am Rev Respir Dis.* 1990;142:725-735.

Canadian Task Force on the Periodic Health Examination. Screening and isoniazid prophylactic therapy for tuberculosis. In: *The Canadian Guide to Clinical Preventive Health Care.* Ottawa, Canada: Minister of Supply and Services; 1994: chap 62.

Centers for Disease Control and Prevention. Prevention and control of tuberculosis in correctional facilities: recommendations of the Advisory Council for the Elimination of Tuberculosis. *MMWR.* 1996;45(No. RR-8):1-27.

Centers for Disease Control and Prevention. Guidelines for preventing the transmission of *Mycobacterium tuberculosis* in health-care facilities, 1994. *MMWR*. 1994;43(No. RR-13):1-132.

Centers for Disease Control. Prevention and control of tuberculosis in facilities providing long-term care to the elderly: recommendations of the Advisory Committee for Elimination of Tuberculosis. *MMWR*. 1990;39(No. RR-10):7-20.

Centers for Disease Control. Prevention and control of tuberculosis in U.S. communities with at-risk minority populations and prevention and control of tuberculosis among homeless persons: recommendations of the Advisory Council for Elimination of Tuberculosis. *MMWR*. 1992;41(No. RR-5):1-23.

Centers for Disease Control. Purified protein derivative (PPD) tuberculin anergy and HIV infection: guidelines for anergy testing and management of anergic persons at risk of tuberculosis. *MMWR*. 1991;40(No. RR-5):27-33.

Centers for Disease Control and Prevention. Screening for tuberculosis and tuberculosis infection in high-risk populations: recommendations of the Advisory Committee for the Elimination of Tuberculosis. *MMWR*. 1995;44(No. RR-11):19-34.

Centers for Disease Control and Prevention. Tuberculosis morbidity, United States, 1995. *MMWR*. 1996;45:365-370.

Centers for Disease Control and Prevention. The role of BCG vaccines in the prevention of tuberculosis in the United States: a joint statement by the Advisory Committee for Immunization Practices and the Advisory Committee for Elimination of Tuberculosis. *MMWR*. 1996;45(No. RR-4):1-18.

Centers for Disease Control. The use of preventive therapy for tuberculous infection in the United States: recommendations of the Advisory Committee for the Elimination of Tuberculosis. *MMWR*. 1990;39(No. RR-8):9-12.

Frieden TR, Sterling T, Pablos-Mendez A. The emergence of drug-resistant tuberculosis in New York City. *N Engl J Med*. 1993;328:523-526.

Iseman MD, Cohn DL, Sbarbaro JA. Directly observed treatment of tuberculosis: we can't afford not to try it. *N Engl J Med*. 1993;328:576-578.

Physician's Desk Reference. Oradell, NJ: Medical Economics Company; 1993:898-899, 1689-1692.

Pust RE. Tuberculosis in the 1990's: resurgence, regimens, and resources. *South Med J*. 1992; 85:584-593.

US Preventive Services Task Force. Screening for tuberculosis infection (including BCG immunization). In: *Guide to Clinical Preventive Services*. 2nd ed. Washington, DC: US Department of Health and Human Services; 1996: chap 25.

44

URINALYSIS

Examination of urine for signs of occult disease has a long tradition in medical care. The development of modern "dipsticks" that can perform multiple tests in a matter of minutes has made urinalysis inexpensive and quick. Most of the abnormalities detected by screening adults with urinalysis are indicative of benign disorders, such as idiopathic proteinuria, or of conditions for which the value of treatment is unclear, such as occult bacteriuria. For this reason, most authorities recommend use of screening urinalysis only for certain conditions in specific high-risk populations.

OCCULT BACTERIURIA

Urinalysis is most often recommended to screen for occult bacteriuria. Urinary tract infections are a significant source of disease and morbidity in diabetic women, pregnant women, and older persons (particularly women). Table 44.1 shows the prevalence of asymptomatic bacteriuria in selected adult populations and the positive predictive value of nitrite and leukocyte esterase (LE) dipstick tests for detecting asymptomatic bacteriuria in these populations. The positive predictive value of urinalysis in these groups is relatively low, except in institutionalized older adults and women with diabetes.

Treatment of asymptomatic bacteriuria in institutionalized older adults has not been shown to decrease morbidity or mortality or even to lead to sustained periods without bacteriuria. Some evidence suggests that treating elderly women in the community leads to fewer symptomatic infections, but the significance of such an approach for long-term health is unknown. The theory that treatment of women with diabetes leads to fewer symptomatic urinary tract infections and decreased long-term morbidity is plausible but not proven. Treating asymptomatic bacteriuria in pregnant women is of definite proven benefit. For this reason, pregnant women are routinely screened with urine culture, which is more sensitive and specific than dipstick testing.

OCCULT HEMATURIA

Screening has also been advocated to detect occult hematuria, which can be indicative of urinary tract malignancies. The incidence of these malignancies

Table 44.1. Prevalence of Asymptomatic Bacteriuria in Adults and Estimated Positive Predictive Values of Nitrite and Leukocyte Esterase Dipstick Tests

Population	Estimated Prevalence (%)	Positive Predictive Value* (%)
Women age <60 years	3.0	8.1
Men age <60 years	0.3	0.8
Women age >60 years in the community	7.0	17.6
Men age >60 years in the community	2.2	6.0
Institutionalized elderly	22.0	44.4
Pregnant women	5.0	13.0
Diabetic women	15.0	33.3

*Proportion of persons in whom at least one of the two tests (nitrite or leukocyte esterase) is positive who will have bacteriuria.

Adapted from: Pels RJ, Bor DH, Woolhandler S, Himmelstein DU, Lawrence RS. Bacteriuria. In: Goldbloom RB, Lawrence RS, eds. *Preventing Disease: Beyond the Rhetoric.* New York, NY: Springer-Verlag; 1990; chap 8. Used with permission of Springer-Verlag New York and the authors; copyright © 1990.

increases significantly after age 40 years, and they occur twice as frequently in men as in women. Dipsticks are reasonably accurate for detecting hematuria, but microscopic hematuria is not specific for bladder cancer or other urologic cancers. The positive predictive value of a positive heme dipstick test for malignancy in older men has been found to be between 6% and 8%. Unnecessary evaluations for a potential urinary tract malignancy can be harmful. Intravenous pyelograms, for example, can lead to diminished renal function and, rarely, death.

PROTEINURIA

Screening for proteinuria in the general population is of little value, because most causes are either benign or untreatable. Screening for diabetes with urinalysis is very inaccurate and is better accomplished with plasma glucose measurements (chapter 38). See chapter 10 for a discussion of the use of screening urinalysis in children.

Recommendations of Major Authorities

All major authorities—Screening urinalysis is recommended in prenatal care for pregnant women.

American Academy of Family Physicians and US Preventive Services Task Force (USPSTF)—Routine screening of males and most females for asymptomatic bacteriuria is not recommended. In diabetic or elderly ambulatory women evidence is insufficient to recommend for or against screening for asymptomatic bacteriuria, but recommendations against such screening may be made on other grounds, including the high likelihood of recurrence and the potential adverse effects of antibiotic therapy. The **USPSTF** recommends screening for asymptomatic bacteriuria by urine culture in all pregnant women.

American College of Obstetricians and Gynecologists—Urinalysis for asymptomatic bacteriuria is recommended for women over 65 years of age or with diabetes mellitus as part of periodic evaluation visits, which should occur yearly or as appropriate.

American College of Physicians—Urinalysis and urine culture should not be routinely used to screen for asymptomatic bacteriuria.

Canadian Task Force on the Periodic Health Examination—Dipstick urinalysis for protein to prevent progressive renal disease is recommended for patients with insulin-dependent diabetes mellitus. Urinalysis to detect asymptomatic bacteriuria in the elderly is not recommended. However, for ambulatory elderly women the evidence is insufficient to recommend for or against screening for asymptomatic bacteriuria.

Basics of Urinalysis Screening

1. Urine collected early in the morning, at least 6 hours after previous voiding and after 8 hours of fasting, is most concentrated and most likely to reveal abnormalities. Do not perform routine screening urinalysis on menstruating women.

2. Obtain a specimen using the "clean catch" technique, which permits a follow-up culture if indicated. Instruct women to clean the vulvar region with lukewarm water, spreading the labia and washing the urethral meatus with a moistened cotton wad or pad several times from front to back. Use each wad or pad only once. Avoid use of soap or disinfectants because of possible effects on the sample. Instruct men to clean the glans and urethral meatus several times with a cotton wad or pad, using each only once. Instruct uncircumcised men to draw back their foreskins.

3. Provide patients with a clean container to collect a midstream "clean catch" sample of urine. Instruct uncircumcised men to retract the foreskin to avoid impingement of the urine flow. Instruct women to hold their labia open to avoid impingement of the urine flow. Patients should start to urinate in the toilet and switch to the specimen container. Fill the container half full and finish urinating in the toilet.

4. Perform urinalysis as soon as possible after collection, using any one of the many available types of urine dipsticks. No major authority recommends using urine cultures for routine screening of nonpregnant adults. Immediately refrigerate specimens that cannot be examined immediately.

5. When interpreting the test, keep in mind the possible causes of false-positive and false-negative results (Tables 44.2 and 44.3).

Table 44.2. Causes of Inaccurate Nitrite Dipstick Tests

False Positives	False Negatives
Specimen contamination	Presence of non-nitrate-reducing organisms (eg, many non-*Enterobacteriaceae* species)
	Presence of occasional organisms that further reduce nitrate to ammonia
	Failure to perform test on first voided specimen of the morning
	Frequent voiding
	Dilute urine
	High specific gravity
	Urine pH <6
	Presence of urobilinogen
	Large dietary intake of vitamin C

From: Pels RJ, Bor DH, Woolhandler S, Himmelstein DU, Lawrence RS, Bacteriuria. In: Goldbloom RB, Lawrence RS, eds. *Preventing Disease: Beyond the Rhetoric*. New York, NY: Springer-Verlag; 1990; chap 8. Used with permission of Springer-Verlag New York and the authors; copyright 1990.

Table 44.3. Causes of Inaccurate Leukocyte Esterase (LE) Dipstick Tests

False Positives	False Negatives
Contamination during collection	Increased specific gravity
	Glycosuria
	Presence of urobilinogen
	Therapy with phenazopyridine hydrochloride,
	nitrofurantoin, or rifampin
	Large dietary intake of vitamin C

Note: Use of the LE dipstick to detect the diverse conditions associated with sterile (culture-negative) pyuria is not considered here.

From: Pels RJ, Bor DH, Woolhandler S, Himmelstein DU, Lawrence RS. Bacteriuria. In: Goldbloom RB, Lawrence RS, eds. *Preventing Disease: Beyond the Rhetoric.* New York, NY: Springer-Verlag; 1990; chap 8. Used with permission of Springer-Verlag New York and the authors; copyright 1990.

Patient Resources

Urinary Tract Infections. American College of Obstetricians and Gynecologists. ACOG Patient Education Pamphlet AP050. American College of Obstetricians and Gynecologists, 409 12th St, SW, Washington, DC 20024; (800)762-2264. Internet address: http://www.acog.org

Urinary Tract Infection: A Common Problem for Some Women. American Academy of Family Physicians, 8880 Ward Parkway, Kansas City, MO 64114-2797; (800)944-0000. Internet address: http://www.aafp.org

Urinary Tract Infection in Adults. National Institute of Diabetes and Digestive and Kidney Diseases' National Kidney and Urologic Diseases Information Clearinghouse, 3 Information Way, Bethesda, MD 20892-3580; (301)654-4415. Internet address: http://www.niddk.nih.gov/UrologicDocs.htm

Selected References

American Academy of Family Physicians. *Summary of Policy Recommendations for Periodic Health Examination.* Kansas City, Mo: American Academy of Family Physicians; 1997.

American College of Obstetricians and Gynecologists. *Guidelines for Women's Health Care.* Washington, DC: American College of Obstetricians and Gynecologists; 1996.

Boscia JA, Kobasa WD, Knight RA, et al. Therapy vs no therapy for bacteriuria in elderly ambulatory nonhospitalized women. *JAMA.* 1987;257:1067-1071.

Canadian Task Force on the Periodic Health Examination. Dipstick proteinuria screening of asymptomatic adults to prevent progressive renal disease. In: *The Canadian Guide to Clinical Preventive Health Care.* Ottawa, Canada: Minister of Supply and Services; 1994: chap 38.

Canadian Task Force on the Periodic Health Examination. Screening for Asymptomatic bacteriuria in the elderly. In: *The Canadian Guide to Clinical Preventive Health Care.* Ottawa, Canada: Minister of Supply and Services; 1994: chap 81.

Canadian Task Force on the Periodic Health Examination. *Periodic Health Examination Monograph.* Hull, Quebec: Minister of Supply and Services; 1980.

Komaroff AL. Urinalysis and urine culture in women with dysuria. In: Sox HC Jr, ed. *Common Diagnostic Tests: Use and Interpretation.* 2nd ed. Philadelphia, Pa: American College of Physicians; 1990:286-301.

Pels RJ, Bor DH, Woolhandler S, Himmelstein DU, Lawrence RS. Bacteriuria. In: Goldbloom RB, Lawrence RS, eds. *Preventing Disease: Beyond the Rhetoric.* New York, NY: Springer-Verlag; 1990: chap 8.

US Preventive Services Task Force. Screening for asymptomatic bacteriuria. In: *Guide to Clinical Preventive Services.* 2nd ed. Washington, DC: US Department of Health and Human Services; 1996: chap 31.

Woolhandler S, Pels RJ, Bor DH, Himmelstein DU, Lawrence RS. Hematuria and proteinuria. In: Goldbloom RB, Lawrence RS, eds. *Preventing Disease: Beyond the Rhetoric.* New York, NY: Springer-Verlag; 1990: chap 37.

45

VISION

Vision loss is common in adults, and the prevalence of vision loss increases with advancing age. Approximately 13% of persons aged 65 years and older and 28% of those aged 85 years and older report some degree of visual impairment. More than 90% of older adults need corrective lenses at some time. Common visual disorders affecting adults include cataracts, macular degeneration, glaucoma, and diabetic retinopathy. Such disorders frequently contribute to trauma from falls, automobile crashes, and other types of accidental injuries. According to one study, 18% of hip fractures are attributable to impaired vision. Many older adults are unaware of decreases in their visual acuity, and up to 25% of such persons may have the wrong corrective lens prescription.

Surgical treatment of cataracts can lead to improved vision and quality of life. Medical and surgical treatment of glaucoma may help prevent visual loss. Early laser surgical treatment can help prevent visual loss attributable to diabetic retinopathy and (in some cases) macular degeneration. Visual acuity testing can be performed easily and accurately by primary care clinicians. Glaucoma screening, however, as usually practiced by primary care clinicians using a Schiotz tonometer, is relatively insensitive and nonspecific. The predictive value of a positive Schiotz test is only about 5%.

Recommendations of Major Authorities

American Academy of Family Physicians—Vision screening with Snellen acuity testing is recommended for the elderly.

American Academy of Ophthalmology—A comprehensive eye examination, including screening for visual acuity and glaucoma by an ophthalmologist, should be performed every 3 to 5 years in African Americans aged 20 to 39 years, and, regardless of race, every 2 to 4 years in individuals aged 40 to 64 years, and every 1 to 2 years beginning at age 65 years. Diabetic patients, at any age, should have exams at least yearly.

American College of Obstetricians and Gynecologists—Women 65 years of age and older should be evaluated for visual acuity yearly or as appropriate.

American Optometric Association—Comprehensive eye and vision examinations are recommended for normal-risk adults as follows: 19 to 40 years of age, every 2 to 3 years; 41 to 60 years of age, every 2 years; 61 years of age and older, yearly. Adults 19 to 60 years of age at increased risk for eye disease (eg, with diabetes, hypertension, family history of glaucoma, work in highly visually demanding or eye hazardous occupations, taking certain systemic medications with ocular side effects) should have examinations every 1 to 2 years or as recommended.

Canadian Task Force on the Periodic Health Examination—There is fair evidence to include in the periodic health examination visual acuity testing with a Snellen sight chart for adults aged 65 years or older. In addition, funduscopy or retinal photography is recommended for elderly patients (> 65 years) with diabetes of at least 5 years' duration. The place of funduscopy in the detection of age-related macular degeneration and glaucomatous changes is controversial. For patients at high risk for glaucoma (eg, positive family history, African American race, severe myopia, diabetes), a prudent recommendation would be to include periodic assessment by an ophthalmologist.

National Eye Institute—A comprehensive eye examination, including screening for visual acuity and glaucoma, should be performed by an eye care professional every 2 years beginning at age 40 years in African Americans and at age 60 years in all other individuals. Diabetic patients, at any age, should have yearly exams.

US Preventive Services Task Force—Routine vision screening with Snellen acuity testing is recommended among the elderly. The frequency is left to clinical discretion. Selected questions about vision may be helpful in detecting vision problems in the elderly, but do not appear to be as sensitive or specific as direct assessment of acuity. There is insufficient evidence to recommend for or against routine screening for diminished visual acuity among non-elderly adults. There is also insufficient evidence to recommend for or against routine screening by primary care clinicians for elevated intraocular pressure or early glaucoma. Effective screening for glaucoma is best performed by eye specialists who have access to specialized equipment to evaluate the optic disc and measure visual fields. Recommendations may be made on other grounds to refer patients at high risk for glaucoma for evaluation by eye specialists including: the substantial prevalence of unrecognized glaucoma in these populations, the progressive nature of untreated disease, and expert consensus that reducing intraocular pressure may slow the rate of visual loss with early glaucoma or severe intraocular hypertension. Patients at high risk for glaucoma include: African Americans over 40 years of age; Caucasians over 65 years of age; patients with diabetes, severe myopia, or a family history of glaucoma. The optimal frequency for glaucoma screening has not been determined.

Basics of Vision Screening

1. Refer older adults and individuals at high risk to eye-care professionals for periodic examinations. See Recommendations of Major Authorities.

2. Perform visual acuity screening using a standard Snellen wall chart at a distance of 20 feet. A tumbling "E" chart may be used for patients who are not familiar with the Western alphabet. Give a passing score for each line for which the patient gives a majority of correct responses. Test each eye separately. The patients should wear any corrective lenses during screening. If a patient is found to have significant changes in visual acuity or visual acuity of 20/40 or less when using corrective lenses, refer him or her to an eye-care specialist for further examination.

3. Risk factors for glaucoma include increasing age, family history of glaucoma, African American race, diabetes mellitus, and myopia. Evaluate each patient's risk factors for glaucoma and other ocular problems, and refer appropriate patients to eye-care professionals for screening.

4. Loss of vision can begin slowly and may go unnoticed for some time, particularly in older adults. Encourage patients to seek evaluation at the first sign of vision problems. Use of a standardized, self-administered questionnaire (Table 45.1) can help identify individuals needing evaluation of their vision. More extensive questionnaires have been developed (Mangione et al, 1992).

Table 45.1. Visual Impairment Questionnaire

Does your vision (with glasses if you wear them) make it difficult for you to— (place a check mark next to each question you answer yes)

_____ Feed yourself?

_____ Recognize your pills or read medication labels?

_____ Dress yourself (find fasteners, button buttons)?

_____ Groom yourself (shave and wash without missing areas)?

_____ Handle your money (make change, write checks)?

_____ Recognize people (nearby, across the street)?

_____ Avoid bumping into objects when moving about in your house?

_____ Find your way around in places outside your own home (stores, shopping malls)?

_____ Read ordinary newsprint?

Place a check mark next to each visual aid you now use

_____ Glasses

_____ Contact lenses

_____ Magnifying lenses

_____ Portable lights

_____ Large print books

_____ Writing guides

One or more "yes" answers indicates the need for further visual acuity testing. Use of one or more visual aids is an indication for review of the patient's last optometric or ophthalmologic examination.

Adapted from: Rubenstein LZ, Lohr KN. _Conceptualization and Measurement of Physiologic Health for Adults._ vol 12: Vision Impairments. Santa Monica, Ca: Rand Corporation; 1982. Publication R-2262/12-HHS. Used with permission of Rand Corporation; copyright © 1982.

Patient Resources

Your Vision, the Second Fifty Years; Do Adult Vision Problems Cause Reading Problems? and other publications. American Optometric Association, 243 N Lindbergh Blvd, St. Louis, MO 63141; (314)991-4100. Internet address: http://www.aoanet.org/aoanet

Age-Related Macular Degeneration; Cataracts; Diabetic Retinopathy; Don't Lose Sight of Diabetic Eye Disease; Don't Lose Sight of Glaucoma; Glaucoma. National Eye Health Education Program, National Institutes of Health, 2020 Vision Pl, Bethesda, MD 20892; (301)496-5248. Internet address: http://www.nei.nih.gov

Age Page—Aging and Your Eyes. National Institute on Aging, Bldg 31, Room 5C27, 31 Center Dr MSC 2922 Bethesda, MD 20892-2922; (301)496-1752. Internet address: http://www.nih.gov/nia

Provider Resources

Glaucoma; Cataracts; Strabismus in Adults; Cataract Surgery; Diabetic Retinopathy. American Academy of Ophthalmology, PO Box 7424, San Francisco, CA 94120. Send a business-size, self-addressed, stamped envelope with your request. Internet address: http://www.eyenet.org

Policy Statement: Frequency of Ocular Examinations; National Eyecare Project (for those who do not have an eye doctor); Glaucoma 2001 Project (for people at risk for glaucoma). American Academy of Ophthalmology, PO Box 7424, San Francisco, CA 94120. Send a business-size, self-addressed, stamped envelope with your request. Internet address: http://www.eyenet.org

Comprehensive Adult Eye and Vision Examination and other clinical practice guidelines. American Optometric Association, 243 N Lindbergh Blvd, St. Louis, MO 63141; (314)991-4100. Internet address: http://www.aoanet.org/aoanet/members

National Eye Institute Statement on Detection of Glaucoma; National Eye Institute Statement on Vision Screening in Adults. National Eye Health Education Program, National Institutes of Health, 2020 Vision Pl, Bethesda, MD 20892; (301)496-5248. Internet address: http://www.nei.nih.gov

Selected References

American Academy of Family Physicians, Summary of Policy Recommendations for Periodic Health Examination. Kansas City, Mo: American Academy of Family Physicians; 1997.

American Academy of Ophthalmology, Quality of Care Committee. *Comprehensive Adult Eye Examination*. San Francisco, Ca: American Academy of Ophthalmology; 1992.

American Academy of Ophthalmology. *Detection and Control of Diabetic Retinopathy*. San Francisco, Ca: American Academy of Ophthalmology; 1992.

American Optometric Association. *Comprehensive Adult Eye and Vision Examination*. St. Louis, Mo: American Optometric Association; 1994.

Canadian Task Force on the Periodic Health Examination. Screening for visual impairment in the elderly. In: *The Canadian Guide to Clinical Preventive Health Care*. Ottawa, Canada: Minister of Supply and Services; 1994: chap 78.

Leske MC. The epidemiology of open-angle glaucoma: a review. *Am J Epidemiol*. 1983;118: 166-169.

Mangione CM, Phillips RS, Seddon JM, et al. Development of the activities of daily vision scale: a measure of visual functional status. *Med Care*. 1992;30:1111-1126.

Nelson KA. Visual impairment among elderly Americans: statistics in transition. *J Vis Impair Blind*. 1987;81:331-334.

Podgor MJ, Leske MC, Ederer F. Incidence estimates for lens changes, macular changes, open angle glaucoma and diabetic retinopathy. *Am J Epidemiology*. 1983;118:206.

Reuben DB. Visual impairment. In: Beck JC, ed. *Geriatrics Review Syllabus: A Core Curriculum in Geriatric Medicine*. New York, NY: American Geriatrics Society; 1991.

Rubenstein LZ, Lohr KN. *Conceptualization and Measurement of Physiologic Health for Adults*. vol 12: Visual Impairments. Santa Monica, Ca: Rand Corporation; 1982. Publication R-2262/12-HHS.

US Preventive Services Task Force. Screening for glaucoma. In: *Guide to Clinical Preventive Services*. 2nd ed. Washington, DC: US Department of Health and Human Services; 1996: chap 34.

US Preventive Services Task Force. Screening for visual impairment. In: *Guide to Clinical Preventive Services*. 2nd ed. Washington, DC: US Department of Health and Human Services; 1996: chap 33.

Winograd CH, Gerety MB. *Geriatric assessment and concepts: visual and hearing assessment*. New York, NY: American Geriatrics Society; 1989. Abstract.

46

ASPIRIN

More than 13 million Americans have coronary heart disease, according to the Third National Health and Nutrition Examination Survey (NHANES III). Heart disease continues to be the leading cause of death in both men and women, and in 1993, nearly 490,000 Americans died of ischemic heart disease. Studies suggest that aspirin in low doses is beneficial in patients with ischemic cardiovascular disease. The Swedish Aspirin Low-Dose Trial (SALT) supports the indication that aspirin reduces the risk of death or stroke in subjects with transient ischemic attack (TIA) or ischemic stroke. The use of aspirin in the primary prevention of myocardial infarction (MI) in patients with stable angina is supported by the Swedish Angina Pectoris Trial (SAPAT). The use of aspirin is also supported in patients who have had a previous MI.

Evidence from the US Physicians' Health Study (a randomized controlled trial) and the Nurses' Health Study (a prospective cohort study) suggests that use of low-dose aspirin significantly decreases the incidence of first MI in middle-aged men and women. However, these studies did not document a decrease in total cardiovascular mortality with aspirin prophylaxis, and the risk of hemorrhagic stroke and sudden death may be increased with its use. A smaller British study of aspirin prophylaxis in physicians found no significant reduction in the incidence of MI. The Women's Health Study, a large randomized, controlled trial that includes aspirin prophylaxis, is in progress.

Aspirin use for the primary prevention of colon cancer is also being investigated. Observational studies have shown an association between aspirin use and a reduction in the incidence of colon cancer. Although this association is of interest, prospective confirmation (eg, in a randomized, controlled trial) is lacking.

Recommendations of Major Authorities

American Academy of Family Physicians—Men aged 40 to 84 years with risk factors for coronary artery disease should be counseled about the risks and benefits of aspirin prophylaxis.

American Heart Association—Care should be exercised before beginning a lifelong program of aspirin therapy. The decision to begin taking aspirin should be made only after consultation by each individual with his or her physician. The individual who begins a regular aspirin regimen should be aware of the side effects of the drug and should report symptoms to his or her physician. All risk factors for coronary heart disease and stroke should be determined and a concerted program to reduce those risk factors begun.

Canadian Task Force on the Periodic Health Examination—The evidence is not strong enough to support a recommendation that routine aspirin therapy be used or not be used for the primary prevention of cardiovascular disease in asymptomatic men and women. The decision on whether to prescribe aspirin should be made on an individual basis after the benefits of decreased risk of ischemic cardiovascular events have been balanced against the potential risks associated with prolonged aspirin use.

US Preventive Services Task Force—There is insufficient evidence to recommend for or against routine aspirin prophylaxis for the primary prevention of myocardial infarction in asymptomatic persons. Although aspirin reduces the risk of myocardial infarction in men 40 to 84 years of age, its use is associated with important adverse effects, and the balance of benefits and harms is uncertain. If aspirin prophylaxis is considered, clinicians and patients should discuss potential benefits and risks for the individual before beginning its use.

Basics of Aspirin Prophylaxis

1. Indications

Individuals should not take aspirin daily for cardiovascular uses without first consulting a physician. No major authority recommends routine universal aspirin prophylaxis. People who have had coronary heart disease, TIA, or ischemic stroke are most likely to benefit.

2. Dosage

The optimal dosage of aspirin for the primary, secondary, and tertiary prevention of heart disease is not clearly established. The dose regimens from clinical trials range from 50 mg to 325 mg taken by mouth daily. Doses greater than 325 mg daily confer no added protection but increase the incidence of side effects. It remains to be established whether doses of less than 325 mg every other day confer protection.

3. Contraindications/Precautions

The only contraindication to regular aspirin use is allergy to aspirin. Because of an increased risk of adverse events, individuals with liver or kidney disease, peptic ulcer disease, history of gastrointestinal bleeding, or bleeding disorder should specifically address this issue with their clinicians before starting aspirin prophylaxis. Because of the potential increased risk of hemorrhagic stroke, it is not advisable to use aspirin for prophylaxis in patients with poorly controlled hypertension. Patients using aspirin prophylaxis should inform their surgeon or dentist before undergoing even minor surgical or dental procedures. Prolonged bleeding can persist for up to 10 days after terminating use of aspirin.

4. Adverse Reactions

Side effects of aspirin prophylaxis are dose-related and include gastrointestinal upset and bleeding disorders (eg, easy bruising, epistaxis, hematemesis, melena), gout, and kidney stones. These events require medical attention, and clinicians must consider discontinuation of aspirin prophylaxis if any of these events occur.

Provider Resources

Aspirin: A New Look at an Old Drug. FDA Office of Consumer Affairs. HFE 88 Room 1675, 5600 Fishers Ln, Rockville, MD 20857; (800)532-4440.

Summary Minutes of the January 23, 1997, Joint Meeting of the Nonprescription Drugs Advisory Committee and the Cardiovascular and Renal Drugs Advisory Committee. A copy of the summary minutes can be obtained through a written request to the Freedom of Information Office (HFI-35), Food and Drug Administration, Rm 12A-16, 5600 Fishers Lane, Rockville, MD 20857.

Selected References

American Academy of Family Physicians. *Summary of Policy Recommendations for Periodic Health Examination.* Kansas City, Mo: American Academy of Family Physicians; 1997.

American Heart Association. *Heart and Stroke Facts: 1996 Statistical Supplement.* Dallas, Tex: American Heart Association; 1995.

American Heart Association. Physicians' Health Study report on aspirin. *Circulation.* 1988;77: 1447A.

Buring JE, Hennekens CH. The Women's Health Study: summary of the study design. *J Myocardial Ischemia.* 1992;4:27-29.

Canadian Task Force on the Periodic Health Examination. Acetylsalicylic acid and the primary prevention of cardiovascular disease. In: *The Canadian Guide to Clinical Preventive Health Care.* Ottawa, Canada: Minister of Supply and Services; 1994: chap 56.

Fuster V, Dyken ML, Vohonas PS, Hennekens C. AHA medical/scientific statement: Aspirin as a therapeutic agent in cardiovascular disease. *Circulation.* 1993;87:659-675.

Fuster V, Cohen M, Halperin J. Aspirin in the prevention of coronary disease. *N Engl J Med.* 1989;321:183-186.

Internal analgesic, antipyretic and antirheumatic drug products for over-the-counter human use; tentative final monograph. Notice of proposed rulemaking (CFR 343.10). *Federal Register.* November 16, 1988; 53:46204-46260.

Manson JE, Stampfer MJ, Colditz GA, et al. A prospective study of aspirin use and primary prevention of cardiovascular disease in women. *JAMA*. 1991;266:521-527.

Physicians' Health Study Research Group, Steering Committee. Final report from the aspirin component of the ongoing Physicians' Health Study. *N Engl J Med*. 1989;321:129-135.

Peto R, Gray R, Collins R, et al. A randomized trial of the effects of prophylactic daily aspirin among male British doctors. *Br Med J*. 1988;296:320-331.

SALT Collaborative Group. Swedish aspirin low-dose trial (SALT) of 75 mg aspirin as secondary prophylaxis after cerebrovascular ischaemic events. *Lancet*. 1991; 338:1345-1349.

Swedish Angina Pectoris Aspirin Trial (SAPAT) Group. Double-blind trial of aspirin in primary prevention of myocardial infarction in patients with stable chronic angina pectoris. *Lancet*. 1992; 340:1421-1425.

Thun MJ, Namboodiri MM, Heath CW. Aspirin use and reduced risk of fatal colon cancer. *N Engl J Med*. 1991;325:1593-1596.

US Preventive Services Task Force. Aspirin prophylaxis for the primary prevention of myocardial infarction. In: *Guide to Clinical Preventive Services*. 2nd ed. Washington, DC: US Department of Health and Human Services; 1996: chap 69.

Willard JE, Lange RA, Hillis LD. The use of aspirin in ischemic heart disease. *N Engl J Med*. 1992;327:175-181.

47

ESTROGEN AND PROGESTIN

In postmenopausal women, use of supplemental estrogen can reduce the risk of osteoporosis. Osteoporosis contributes to approximately 1.2 million fractures in the United States annually; about two thirds of these fractures occur in women. Women who are older, Caucasian, slender, and those who have had a bilateral oophorectomy or early menopause are at increased risk for developing osteoporosis-related fractures. Approximately 15% of Caucasian women older than age 50 years suffer hip fractures, and approximately 1.5% of women in this population die as a result. According to a recent meta-analysis, use of estrogen was associated with a 25% decrease in the relative risk of hip fracture in women over age 50 years. Numerous observational and non-randomized experimental studies suggest that the benefits of hormone replacement therapy (HRT) on bone mass and fracture risk wane after stopping estrogen. As a result, preventing fractures in older, postmenopausal women may require indefinite HRT. (See chapter 62 for information on osteoporosis.)

The use of estrogen to prevent coronary heart disease is currently being investigated in a multi-center prospective trial. Coronary heart disease causes approximately 30% of deaths of women over 50 years of age. A large case-control study was recently published that showed a reduced risk of mortality from all causes of 37% for women using post-menopausal HRT. According to Grodstein et al, the largest reduction in the risk of mortality was for coronary heart disease (53%); however, this protective effect was only statistically significant for women with one or more risk factors for cardiovascular disease. Other observational studies have shown that estrogen supplementation is associated with a 35% reduction in the relative risk of death from coronary heart disease. Estrogen supplementation also provides several benefits that improve climacteric symptoms, such as decreasing vasomotor symptoms (hot flushes or flashes) and alleviating genitourinary symptoms (dryness, urgency, incontinence, frequency).

Use of estrogen supplementation may, however, lead to significant adverse health outcomes. In women with an intact uterus who use estrogen for 10 to 20 years, the incidence of endometrial cancer increases eight-fold. Concomitant use of progestin decreases the risk of endometrial cancer to a level comparable to that of women not taking estrogen. Whether use of progestin will blunt any potential cardiovascular benefits of estrogen is unclear. Whether estrogen supplementation increases a woman's risk for breast cancer also remains controversial. This potential risk appears not to be associated with short-term estrogen use (fewer than 5 years), but may increase by approximately 25% with more than 10 years of estrogen use. Adding progestin to estrogen supplementation does not appear to protect against the risk of breast cancer. Estrogen increases the risk of venous thromboembolism.

Recommendations of Major Authorities

American Academy of Family Physicians—All perimenopausal women should be counseled about the benefits and risks of postmenopausal HRT.

American College of Obstetricians and Gynecologists, American College of Physicians (ACP), Canadian Task Force on the Periodic Health Examination, and **US Preventive Services Task Force (USPSTF)**—All perimenopausal and postmenopausal women should be counseled regarding the probable risks and benefits of HRT, so that they can participate fully with their health care provider in deciding whether to take preventive hormone therapy. According to the **USPSTF,** there is insufficient evidence to recommend for or against HRT in all postmenopausal women. According to the **ACP,** all women, regardless of race, should consider preventive hormone therapy. Women who have had a hysterectomy are likely to benefit from estrogen therapy. There is no reason to add progestin to the hormone regimen in such women. Women who have coronary heart disease or who are at increased risk for coronary heart disease are more likely to benefit from HRT. If such women have a uterus, progestin should be added to the estrogen therapy unless careful endometrial monitoring is performed. The risks of HRT may outweigh its benefits in women who are at increased risk for breast cancer.

Basics of Estrogen/Progestin Prophylaxis

1. Considerations

Table 47.1 presents the relative risk of selected conditions associated with long-term HRT. In addition, consider the following factors:

- Coronary heart disease risk factors, such as family history, blood pressure, weight, smoking status, cholesterol
- Osteoporosis risk factors, such as race, body build, physical activity level, bone mineral density
- Breast cancer risk factors, such as personal and family history, late parity (after age 30 years), early menarche (before age 12 years), and late menopause (after age 50 years)

Table 47.1. Relative Risk of Selected Conditions for a 50-Year-Old White Woman Treated with Long-Term Hormone Replacement

Condition	Relative Risk*	
	Estrogen Therapy	**Estrogen Plus Progestin**
Coronary Heart Disease	0.65	0.65–0.80
Stroke	0.96	0.96
Hip Fracture	0.75	0.75
Breast Cancer	1.25	1.25–2.00
Endometrial Cancer	8.22	1.00

*Best estimate of the relative risk for developing each condition in long-term hormone users compared with nonusers.

From: Grady D, Rubin SM, Petitti DB, et al. Hormone therapy to prevent disease and prolong life in postmenopausal women. *Ann Intern Med*. 1992;117:1016–1037. Reproduced by permission of the American College of Physicians; copyright 1992.

- Patient desire to decrease climacteric symptoms, such as decreased vasomotor and genitourinary tract symptoms

- Patient tolerance for side effects, such as endometrial bleeding and breast tenderness

- Patient willingness to participate in follow-up, such as endometrial sampling and mammography

2. Dosage and Administration

To prevent irreversible bone loss, begin estrogen replacement soon after the onset of menopause. An absolute upper age limit for estrogen replacement has not been established. Use of progestin or careful endometrial monitoring is recommended for women with intact uteri.

Several different regimens for hormone replacement have been developed. Oral preparations have been better evaluated for primary prevention than has transdermal or other routes of administration. The most common initial oral dosage in the United States is 0.625 mg of conjugated estrogen taken every day. For women who cannot tolerate this dosage, 0.3 mg of conjugated estrogen daily with 1500 mg of calcium daily may provide protection against bone loss. Cyclic regimens of estrogen have been widely used, but they provide no physiologic advantages and cause patient confusion. Progestin may be given cyclically or continuously. The usual dosage for cyclic administration is 5 mg to 10 mg of progesterone acetate (or equivalent) daily for the first 10 to 14 days of the month. The usual dosage for continuous administration of progesterone acetate is 2.5 mg daily.

3. Contraindications

Contraindications to estrogen replacement include:

- Unexplained vaginal bleeding
- Active liver disease
- Chronic impaired liver function
- Recent venous thrombosis (with or without emboli)
- Carcinoma of the breast
- Endometrial carcinoma, except in certain circumstances

Conditions that may be relative contraindications to estrogen replacement include:

- Seizure disorders
- Hypertension
- Uterine leiomyomas
- Familial hyperlipidemia
- Migraine headaches
- Thrombophlebitis
- Endometriosis
- Gallbladder disease

4. Adverse Reactions

The most common side effects of estrogen therapy include endometrial bleeding, breast tenderness, nausea, bloating, and headaches. Other risks include an increased risk of endometrial cancer and the potential risk of breast cancer and thromboembolic events. When a progestin is added to estrogen therapy, the most common side effects are bloating, weight gain, nausea, irritability, breast tenderness, and depression. These symptoms generally can be alleviated by decreasing the dose of progestin. If progestin is used in a continuous regimen, it causes unpredictable endometrial bleeding in 30% to 50% of women. Such bleeding abates after 6 to 8 months of use because of uterine atrophy.

5. Surveillance

The American College of Physicians (1992) has issued the following recommendations for surveillance of endometrial cancer in women taking estrogen:

For Women Taking Unopposed Estrogen

At onset of treatment:

■ Pelvic examination

■ Endometrial evaluation (endometrial biopsy, transvaginal ultrasound, or dilatation and curettage) to rule out hyperplasia or cancer

Evaluation of vaginal bleeding:

■ Any episode of vaginal bleeding should prompt evaluation by endometrial biopsy, transvaginal ultrasound, or dilatation and curettage unless the woman has had a normal evaluation in the previous 6 months

Frequency of screening while on treatment:

■ Probably yearly

For Women Taking Estrogen and Progestin

At onset of treatment:

■ Pelvic examination

■ No endometrial evaluation required

Evaluation of vaginal bleeding:

■ For women on cyclic estrogen-plus-progestin therapy: If bleeding occurs other than at the time of expected withdrawal bleeding (days 10 through 15 if the progestin is given on days 1 through 10), an endometrial biopsy, transvaginal ultrasound, or dilatation and curettage should be performed.

■ For women on continuous estrogen-plus-progestin therapy: If bleeding is heavy (heavier than a normal menstrual period), prolonged (more than 10 days), or frequent (more often than monthly), and if bleeding persists longer than 10 months after beginning therapy, an endometrial biopsy, transvaginal ultrasound, or dilatation and curettage should be performed.

Frequency of screening while on treatment:

■ No routine screening required

6. Breast Cancer Surveillance

Both the American College of Obstetricians and Gynecologists and the American College of Physicians recommend screening for breast cancer at the same frequency and with the same methods as those used for women who are not taking estrogen/progestin replacement.

Patient Resources

Hormone Replacement Therapy: Facts To Help You Decide; Action for a Healthier Life: A Guide for Mid-Life and Older Women. American Association of Retired Persons, Fulfillment Services, 601 E St, NW, Washington, DC 20049; (202)434-2277.

Osteoporosis in Women: Keeping Your Bones Healthy and Strong. American Academy of Family Physicians, 8880 Ward Parkway, Kansas City, MO 64114-2797; (800)944-0000. Internet address: http://www.aafp.org

Age Page—Osteoporosis: The Bone Thinner; Age Page—Should You Take Estrogen? National Institute on Aging, Bldg 31, Room 5C27, 31 Center Dr MSC 2922, Bethesda, MD 20892-2922; (301)496-1752. Internet address: http://www.nih.gov/nia/health/pubpub/pubpub.htm

Hormone Replacement Therapy; Preventing Osteoporosis. American College of Obstetricians and Gynecologists, 409 12th St SW, Washington, DC 20024; (800)762-2264. Internet address: http://www.acog.org

Selected References

American Academy of Family Physicians. *Summary of Policy Recommendations for Periodic Health Examination.* Kansas City, Mo: American Academy of Family Physicians; 1997.

American College of Obstetricians and Gynecologists, Committee on Technical Bulletins. *Hormone Replacement Therapy.* Washington, DC: American College of Obstetricians and Gynecologists; 1992. ACOG Technical Bulletin 166.

American College of Obstetricians and Gynecologists. *Guidelines for Women's Health Care.* Washington, DC: American College of Obstetricians and Gynecologists; 1996.

American College of Physicians. Guidelines for counseling postmenopausal women about preventive hormone therapy. *Ann Intern Med.* 1992;117:1038-1041.

Barrett-Connor E, Bush TL. Estrogen and coronary heart disease in women. *JAMA.* 1992;265:1861-1867.

Canadian Task Force on the Periodic Health Examination. Prevention of osteoporotic fractures in women by estrogen replacement therapy. In: *The Canadian Guide to Clinical Preventive Health Care.* Ottawa, Canada: Minister of Supply and Services; 1994: chap 52.

Grady D, Rubin SM, Petitti DB, et al. Hormone therapy to prevent disease and prolong life in postmenopausal women. *Ann Intern Med.* 1992;117:1016-1037.

Grodstein F, Stampfer MJ, Colditz GA, et al. Postmenopausal hormone therapy and mortality. *N Engl J Med.* 1997;336(25):1769-1775.

Henrich JB. The postmenopausal estrogen/breast cancer controversy. *JAMA.* 1992;268:1900-1902.

Mann KV, Wiese WH, Stachenko S. Postmenopausal osteoporosis and fractures. In: Goldbloom RB, Lawrence RS. *Preventing Disease: Beyond the Rhetoric.* New York, NY: Springer-Verlag; 1990: chap 24.

US Preventive Services Task Force. Postmenopausal hormone prophylaxis. In: *Guide to Clinical Preventive Services.* 2nd ed. Washington, DC: US Department of Health and Human Services; 1996: chap 68.

48

HEPATITIS B

At least 200,000 new hepatitis B virus (HBV) infections occur yearly in the United States. Most of these infections occur in young adults, primarily as a result of blood or sexual contact. (See Table 48.1 for a list of groups at high risk for infection.) HBV infection causes significant morbidity and mortality. Approximately 30% to 40% of infected persons become ill with jaundice, and each year approximately 15,000 hospitalizations and 350 to 450 deaths are attributable to acute HBV infection. Between 1% and 10% of adults with acute HBV infection become chronically infected. Chronic active HBV infection develops in an estimated 25% of individuals with chronic infection. Cirrhosis and liver failure ultimately develop in 3000 to 4000 of these persons annually. The risk of liver cancer is significantly increased in individuals with chronic HBV infection. HBV-related liver cancer leads to 1000 to 1500 deaths annually in the United States.

Hepatitis B vaccine is 95% effective in preventing HBV infection. Among vaccine recipients in whom adequate antibody levels develop, the effectiveness is virtually 100%. The antibody response to hepatitis B vaccination is decreased in patients with human immunodeficiency virus (HIV) infection, those undergoing hemodialysis, and persons aged 40 years and older. Furthermore, antibody levels decrease with time. After 7 years, antibody levels are low or undetectable in as many as 50% of vaccine recipients. However, patients with normal immune systems continue to be protected against infection.

For persons experiencing percutaneous or sexual contact with HBV, administration of hepatitis B immune globulin (HBIG) is approximately 75% effective for preventing infection.

Hepatitis B is currently designated as an infectious disease notifiable at the national level. Refer to Appendix C for further information on nationally notifiable diseases.

See chapter 14 for information on hepatitis B immunization and prophylaxis for children and adolescents.

Table 48.1. Groups at High Risk for Hepatitis B Virus Infection

Heterosexual individuals who have had more than one sex partner in the previous 6 months and/or those with a recent episode of a sexually transmitted disease

Sexually active homosexual or bisexual males

Household contacts and sex partners of HBsAG-positive persons

Injection drug users

Health care workers and others at occupational risk

Clients and staff of institutions for the developmentally disabled—including nonresidential day-care programs if attended by known HBV carriers

Hemodialysis patients

Hemophiliacs and other recipients of certain blood products

Household contacts of adoptees from hepatitis B-endemic, high-risk countries who are HBsAG-positive

International travelers who spend more than 6 months in areas with high HBV infection rates and have close contact with the local population; also short-term travelers who have contact with blood or sexual contact with residents in high- or intermediate-risk areas

Inmates of long-term correctional institutions

Adapted from: Advisor Committee on Immunization Practices (ACIP). Hepatitis B virus: a comprehensive strategy for eliminating transmission in the United States through universal childhood vaccination. *MMWR*. 1991;40:(No. RR-13): 1–25.

Recommendations of Major Authorities

Immunization

All major authorities, including **Advisory Committee on Immunization Practices, American Academy of Family Physicians (AAFP), American College of Obstetricians and Gynecologists, American College of Physicians,** and **US Preventive Services Task Force (USPSTF)**—Individuals in groups at increased risk for HBV infection (see Table 48.1) should be vaccinated with the hepatitis B vaccine. The **USPSTF** has also recommended routine immunization of all young adults not previously immunized. The **AAFP** recommends offering immunization to young adults to age 24 years who have no reliable history of HBV infection or previous immunization.

Prophylaxis

All major authorities, including **Advisory Committee on Immunization Practices, American College of Physicians (ACP), Canadian Task Force on the Periodic Health Examination,** and **US Preventive Services Task Force**—HBIG should be used for prophylaxis of unimmunized or inadequately immunized adults exposed to percutaneous or mucosal contact with hepatitis B surface antigen (HBsAg)-positive blood or sexual contact with a person with acute HBV infection. **ACP** has also recommended HBIG use after sexual contact with an asymptomatic person who is HBsAg-positive.

Basics of Hepatitis B Immunization

1. Vaccine Types

Two types of recombinant-derived hepatitis B vaccines are currently licensed for use in the United States—Recombivax HB® and Engerix-B®. These vaccines may be used interchangeably at any point in the vaccination schedule. Plasma-derived vaccine is no longer distributed in the United States.

2. Schedule

Both vaccines are given as a three-dose series, with the second and third doses administered 1 and 6 months after the first dose. If a three-dose series is interrupted after the first dose, administer the second dose as soon as possible. Separate administration of the second and third doses by at least 2 months. A four-dose series (at 0, 1, 2, and 12 months), which may induce immunity faster than a three-dose series, has been approved for Engerix-B® vaccine but has not been shown to be advantageous in clinical trials. Upon completion, both the three- and four-dose regimens confer essentially the same level of immunity. For hemodialysis patients, the fourth dose of Engerix-B® vaccine should be given 6 months (rather than 12 months) after the first dose. Patients in whom postvaccination testing shows inadequate antibody response after the initial vaccination series may receive one or more additional doses of vaccine.

3. Assessing Immunity

In adult populations at high risk for HBV infection, prevaccination antibody testing with hepatitis B core antibody (anti-HBc) and hepatitis B surface antibody (anti-HBs) may be cost-effective. The decision to undertake prevaccination testing should take into account the cost of vaccination, the cost of testing for susceptibility, and the expected number of immune individuals. Also consider the likelihood of patient follow-up and vaccine delivery after prevaccination testing.

Postvaccination testing is indicated for immunocompromised persons who are at continued risk of HBV infection (eg, dialysis patients), because their future medical management may depend on knowledge of their immune status. Persons at occupational risk with continued percutaneous/mucosal exposures (eg, sharp injuries, blood splashes) should be tested after vaccination, because knowledge of their antibody status is needed to determine proper postexposure prophylaxis. All health care workers who have contact with patients or blood (eg, physicians, nurses, operating room technicians, dentists, dental hygienists, emergency medical technicians, phlebotomists, laboratory technologists/technicians, physician assistants, nurse practitioners) should be tested. Health care personnel who were vaccinated as students should also undergo postvaccination testing. Postvaccination testing is not indicated for persons at low risk of continued mucosal or percutaneous exposures to blood (eg, public safety workers, health care workers without direct patient contact). Consider postvaccination testing of sexual partners of persons with chronic HBV infection. If such contacts are aware of their immune status, those who are vaccine nonresponders can use methods to prevent sexual transmission of HBV infection.

Perform postvaccination antibody testing between 1 and 2 months after completion of the vaccine series. Maximum antibody response occurs at approximately 6 weeks following the third dose of vaccine. Antibody has been shown to disappear within 6 months of vaccination in adults.

4. Dose and Administration

For adults older than 19 years of age, the recommended dose of both types of vaccine is 1 mL given intramuscularly. (See Table 14.2 for recommended doses of hepatitis B vaccine for individuals 19 years of age and younger.) The proper injection site is the deltoid muscle; injection into the buttock results in decreased antibody response because of deposition of vaccine into fat. Hepatitis B vaccine may be given concurrently with HBIG and other vaccines but at different sites. Increase the dose for hemodialysis patients and those who are immunocompromised. The Advisory Committee on Immunization Practices recommends using either 1 mL of a special formulation of Recombivax HB® containing 40 μg or two 1-mL doses of Engerix-B® given at the same site.

5. Contraindications/Precautions

The only contraindication to hepatitis B vaccination is prior anaphylaxis or severe hypersensitivity to the vaccine or its components. Pregnancy and lactation are not contraindications to vaccination.

6. Adverse Reactions

The side effects of hepatitis B vaccination are relatively minor and include pain at the injection site (3% to 29% of patients) and temperature higher than 37.7°C (100°F) (1% to 6% of patients). The reported rate of occurrence of Guillain-Barré syndrome is very low (0.5 cases per 100,000 population) among adults receiving plasma-derived HBV vaccine. No such association has been found with the use of recombinant hepatitis vaccines, although insufficient data are available from which to draw firm conclusions on this issue. The estimated incidence of anaphylaxis is low (one case per 600,000 doses distributed). Very rarely hepatitis B vaccine may cause a life-threatening hypersensitivity reaction in certain individuals.

Any adverse side effects should be reported to the Vaccine Adverse Events Reporting System (VAERS). See Table B.4 for a detailed listing of adverse events. VAERS forms and instructions are available in the *FDA Drug Bulletin* (Food and Drug Administration) and the *Physician's Desk Reference* or by calling the 24-hour VAERS information recording at (800)822-7967. Refer to Appendix B for details.

7. Patient Education

The US Department of Health and Human Services has developed vaccine information statements about hepatitis B vaccination (see Patient Resources). These statements must be available to patients in facilities where federally purchased vaccines are used, and their availability in other settings is encouraged.

8. Vaccine Storage and Handling

Store vaccine at 2° to 8°C (36° to 46°F); freezing the vaccine will destroy its potency. Do not use vaccine that has been frozen. Handle all vaccine preparations according to manufacturers' instructions.

Basics of Hepatitis B Postexposure Prophylaxis

1. Indications

According to the Advisory Committee on Immunization Practices (ACIP), all susceptible sexual partners of persons with acute HBV infection should receive a dose of HBIG if prophylaxis can begin within 14 days of the last sexual exposure; the HBV vaccine series should also be started. HBIG is not recommended for sexual contacts of persons with chronic HBV infection. For postexposure prophylaxis of persons not previously vaccinated, ACIP recommends use of hepatitis B vaccine in addition to HBIG. An alternative treatment for exposed individuals who would not routinely be considered at high risk and in need of vaccination is to administer one dose of HBIG (without vaccine) and retest the sex partner's HBsAg status 3 months later. If the sex partner has become HBsAg-negative, no further treatment is needed. If the sex partner is still HBsAg-positive, a second dose of HBIG should be given and a vaccination series begun. Adult household contacts of individuals with acute HBV infection do not need prophylaxis with HBIG unless they have had identifiable blood exposure, such as that which occurs by sharing a toothbrush or razor with the infected individual. Patients with such exposures should be treated in the same manner as patients with sexual exposure. If the index patient becomes a HBV carrier, all household contacts should receive hepatitis B vaccine. The recommendations of ACIP for HBV prophylaxis

Table 48.2. Recommendations for Hepatitis B Prophylaxis Following Percutaneous Exposure

Exposed Person	Treatment When Source Is Found To Be:		
	HBsAG-Positive	HBsAG-Negative	Unknown or Not Tested
Unvaccinated	Administer HBIG x 1 and initiate vaccine	Initiate vaccine	Initiate vaccine
Previously vaccinated, adequate anti-HBs*	No treatment	No treatment	No treatment
Previously vaccinated, inadequate anti-HBs*	HBIG x 2 or HBIG x 1 and initiate revaccination	No treatment	If known high-risk source, may treat as if source were HBsAg-positive
Previously vaccinated, response unknown	Test exposed person for anti-HBs*: 1. If inadequate, HBIG x 1, plus vaccine booster dose 2. If adequate, no treatment	No treatment	Test exposed person for anti-HBs*: 1. If inadequate, initiate revaccination 2. If adequate, no treatment

*Adequate anti-HBs level is ≥10 mIU/mL

Adapted from: Advisory Committee on Immunization Practices (ACIP). Hepatitis B virus infection: a comprehensive strategy for eliminating transmission in the United States through universal childhood vaccination. *MMWR.* 1991;40:(No. RR-13):22.

following percutaneous or mucosal exposure to blood and for sexual contacts of persons with acute HBV infection are given in Table 48.2.

2. Schedule

Administer HBIG as soon as possible after exposure to infection. HBIG may be given as late as 14 days after exposure, but the effectiveness of HBIG is uncertain if it is given 7 days or more after exposure. If the patient is known to have been nonresponsive to a primary HBV vaccination series (by anti-HBsAg level), give a second injection of HBIG 1 month later in lieu of a vaccine booster dose.

3. Dose and Administration

The recommended dose of HBIG is 0.06 mL/kg given intramuscularly. The preferred site for administration in adults is the deltoid muscle. If the gluteal region is used, administer the vaccine only to the upper, outer quadrant. Before injection, draw back the plunger to verify that injection into a vein or artery will not occur. HBIG and hepatitis B vaccine may be given concurrently but at different sites.

4. Contraindications/Precautions

Use HBIG with caution in patients with a history of hypersensitivity to human immune globulin (IG) preparations or thimerosal.

5. Adverse Reactions

The main side effects of HBIG injection are pain and swelling at the injection site. Urticaria, angioedema, and very rarely, anaphylaxis can occur. HIV is not known to be transmitted by HBIG injection.

Patient Resources

Hepatitis B: What Patients Need To Know. US Department of Health and Human Services. Available from state and local health departments.

Provider Resources

Resource Guide for Adult Immunization, 2nd ed. Provides a comprehensive listing of materials relevant to adolescent and adult immunization. To receive a free, single copy write to National Center for Adult Immunization Resource Guide, 4733 Bethesda Ave, Suite 750, Bethesda, MD 20814-5228; fax: (301)907-0878. Internet address: adultimm@aol.com

Hepatitis B Fact Sheets (set of three: adolescents, high risk adults, and health care providers). To receive a free sample set, write to National Center for Adult Immunization Resource Guide, 4733 Bethesda Ave, Suite 750, Bethesda, MD 20814-5228; fax: (301)907-0878. Internet address: adultimm@aol.com

Selected References

American Academy of Family Physicians. *Recommendations for Hepatitis B Preexposure Vaccination and Postexposure Prophylaxis.* Kansas City, Mo: American Academy of Family Physicians; 1992.

American College of Obstetricians and Gynecologists. *Guidelines for Women's Health Care.* Washington, DC: American College of Obstetricians and Gynecologists; 1996.

American College of Physicians Task Force on Adult Immunization and Infectious Diseases Society of America. Clinical issues regarding specific vaccines: hepatitis B. In: *Guide for Adult Immunization.* 3rd ed. Philadelphia, Pa: American College of Physicians; 1994:74-83.

Canadian Task Force on the Periodic Health Examination. The periodic health examination: 2. 1984 update. *Can Med Assoc J.* 1984;130:1278-1285.

Centers for Disease Control. Hepatitis B virus: a comprehensive strategy for eliminating transmission in the United States through universal childhood vaccination: Recommendations of the Advisory Committee on Immunization Practices (ACIP). *MMWR.* 1991;40(No. RR-13):1-25.

Centers for Disease Control. Protection against viral hepatitis: Recommendations of the Advisory Committee on Immunization Practices (ACIP). *MMWR* 1990;39(No. RR-2):1-26.

Centers for Disease Control and Prevention. Update: Recommendations to prevent Hepatitis B virus transmission—United States. *MMWR.* 1995;44:574-575.

US Preventive Services Task Force. Adult immunizations. In: *Guide to Clinical Preventive Services.* 2nd ed. Washington, DC: US Department of Health and Human Services; 1996: chap 66.

49

INFLUENZA (Including Childhood Immunization)

Influenza is a significant cause of mortality and morbidity in the United States. Between 1972 and 1992, at least 10,000 deaths occurred in each of nine separate influenza epidemics in the United States. In four of these epidemics, more than 40,000 deaths occurred. Approximately 90% of influenza-related deaths occur in persons aged 65 years and older. Older adults with underlying health problems, such as pulmonary or cardiovascular disorders, are at particularly high risk of death and serious illness from influenza. Nonelderly adults and children with certain chronic medical problems are also at increased risk for influenza-related complications (Table 49.1).

Influenza vaccine is approximately 50% to 60% effective in preventing hospitalizations and pneumonia and 80% effective in preventing death in older adults. Approximately 55% of noninstitutionalized older adults receive immunization annually. The antiviral agents amantadine and rimantadine are 70% to 90% effective for preventing influenza type A illness in adults, but these medications do not prevent influenza type B.

Recommendations of Major Authorities

Immunization

Advisory Committee on Immunization Practices, American Academy of Family Physicians, American College of Physicians, American Geriatrics Society, Canadian Task Force on the Periodic Health Examination, and **US Preventive Services Task Force**—Influenza immunization should be provided annually to all individuals 65 years of age or older. Immunization should also be provided to adults and children at least 6 months of age who are at increased risk for influenza-related complications due to certain medical conditions, such as chronic pulmonary and cardiovascular disorders (Table 49.1), or who may transmit influenza to individuals at increased risk, such as health care workers and household members (Table 49.2).

American College of Obstetricians and Gynecologists—All women 60 years of age and older should receive immunization against influenza yearly.

Prophylaxis

Advisory Committee on Immunization Practices (ACIP), American College of Physicians, and US Preventive Services Task Force—Amantadine and rimantidine may be used prophylactically in the following situations: (1) for high-risk persons who have not yet received the vaccine or are vaccinated after influenza type A activity in the community has already begun, (2) for unimmunized persons who provide care for high-risk persons, (3) for immunocompromised patients and others expected to have a suboptimal response to immunization or (4) for high-risk persons in whom the vaccine is contraindicated (eg, those with anaphylactic hypersensitivity to egg protein). **ACIP** stipulates that use is only appropriate in persons older than 1 year of age.

Canadian Task Force on the Periodic Health Examination— There is good evidence that early daily administration of amantadine to high-risk persons and to unvaccinated persons exposed to influenza type A during an outbreak of influenza reduces the spread of the infection.

Table 49.1. Groups at Increased Risk for Influenza-Related Complications

---

Persons ≥65 years of age

Residents of nursing homes and other chronic-care facilities housing persons of any age with chronic medical conditions

---

Adults and children with chronic disorders of the pulmonary or cardiovascular systems, including children with asthma

---

Adults and children who needed regular medical follow-up or hospitalization during the preceding year because of chronic metabolic diseases (including diabetes mellitus), renal dysfunction, hemoglobinopathies, or immunosuppression (including immunosuppression caused by medications)

Children and teenagers (6 months to 18 years of age) who are receiving long-term aspirin therapy and therefore may be at risk of developing Reye's syndrome after influenza

---

Women who will be beyond the first trimester of pregnancy during the influenza season

---

From: Centers for Disease Control and Prevention. Prevention and control of influenza: recommendations of the Advisory Committee on Immunization Practices (ACIP). *MMWR*. 1997;46(No. RR-9):1–25.

Table 49.2. Groups That Can Transmit Influenza to Persons at High Risk

Physicians, nurses, and other personnel in both hospital and outpatient-care settings

Employees of nursing homes and chronic-care facilities who have contact with patients or residents

Providers of home care to persons at high risk (eg, visiting nurses, volunteer workers)

Household members (including children) of persons in high-risk groups

From: Centers for Disease Control and Prevention. Prevention and control of influenza: recommendations of the Advisory Committee on Immunization Practices (ACIP). *MMWR*. 1997;46(No. RR-9):1–25.

Basics of Influenza Immunization

1. Vaccine Types

Two basic types of influenza vaccine are available; one is prepared from whole-virus particles, and the other is prepared from split-virus particles. Either type of vaccine is equally appropriate for use in adults and children older than age 12 years. Use only the split-virus preparation in children aged 12 years or younger. The vaccines are trivalent—containing viruses or virus particles from three strains: two type A and one type B. The mixture of viruses used is updated annually according to antigenic change in the viruses causing infection.

2. Schedule

Administer influenza vaccine annually, preferably shortly before the onset of the influenza season. Because antibody levels decline with time, do not give immunizations too early in the season. Because the influenza season in the United States usually begins in December, the period between October and mid November is usually the optimal time for immunization campaigns. Take advantage, however, of the opportunity to begin immunizing all high-risk patients, including older adults, who are seen for health care beginning in September. Immunization programs may begin as soon as the current vaccine is available if regional influenza activity is expected to begin earlier than December. Offer immunization up to and even after the time that influenza virus activity is documented in a community. In some years, this activity may occur as late as April.

3. Dose and Administration

The recommended dose in adults and children aged 3 years and older is 0.5 mL, administered intramuscularly. The recommended dose for children aged 6 to 35 months is 0.25 mL. Use only split-virus vaccine for children aged 12 years and younger. Administer two doses of vaccine, at least 1 month apart, to children younger than age 9 years who have not previously been vaccinated; this approach maximizes the chance of a satisfactory antibody response. Administer the second dose before December, if possible. The vaccine may be given concurrently with pneumococcal vaccine and all routine childhood vaccines, including diphtheria-tetanus-pertussis vaccines (DTaP/DTP). Because the influenza vaccine can cause fever when administered to young children, DTaP (which is less frequently associated with fever and other adverse reactions) is preferable to DTP.

4. Contraindications/Precautions

Do not routinely administer inactivated influenza vaccine to persons known to have anaphylactic hypersensitivity to eggs or other components of the influenza vaccine. Use of an antiviral agent (eg, amantadine or rimantadine) is an option for preventing influenza type A in such persons. Persons who have a history of anaphylactic hypersensitivity to vaccine components but who are also at high risk for complications of influenza may benefit from vaccination after appropriate allergy evaluation and desensitization. Specific information about vaccine components can be found in package inserts for each manufacturer. Do not vaccinate adults with acute febrile illness until their symptoms have abated. The presence of minor illness, with or without fever, is not a contraindication to use of influenza vaccine, particularly in children with mild upper respiratory tract infection or allergic rhinitis.

5. Adverse Reactions

Because influenza vaccine contains only noninfectious viruses, it cannot cause influenza. Respiratory disease that occurs after vaccination represents coincidental illness unrelated to influenza vaccination. Adverse reactions to vaccination generally are mild. Soreness at the site of injection persisting up to 2 days is the most common side effect. Fever, malaise, myalgia, and other systemic symptoms occur infrequently; these symptoms may occur as early as 6 hours after immunization and can persist for as long as 48 hours. Rarely, an immediate allergic reaction can occur. Guillain-Barré syndrome was associated with swine flu immunization in 1976, but has not subsequently been clearly associated with influenza immunization.

Any adverse side effects should be reported to the Vaccine Adverse Event Reporting System (VAERS). See Table B.4 for a detailed listing of adverse events. VAERS forms and instructions are available in the *FDA Drug Bulletin* (Food and Drug Administration) and the *Physician's Desk Reference* or by calling the

24-hour VAERS information recording at (800)822-7967. Refer to Appendix B for details.

6. Patient Education

Educational efforts and outreach to older adults are necessary to attain better rates of influenza immunization. Distribution of informational brochures, use of posters in office waiting rooms, and mailing of reminder postcards are useful interventions to improve immunization rates.

The US Department of Health and Human Services has developed vaccine information statements about influenza vaccination (Patient Resources). These statements must be available to patients in facilities where federally purchased vaccines are used, and their availability in other settings is encouraged.

7. Vaccine Storage and Handling

Discard all unused vaccine from the previous year. Store vaccine at 2° to 8°C (36° to 46°F), and do not freeze. Handle all vaccine preparations according to manufacturers' instructions.

Basics of Influenza Prophylaxis

1. Schedule

Amantadine or rimantadine may be administered daily for 2 weeks following immunization during a community outbreak of influenza type A. For immunodeficient patients and patients for whom influenza vaccine is contraindicated, amantadine or rimantadine may be administered daily for the duration of a community outbreak. When used for control of institutional outbreaks, amantadine and rimantadine should be administered for at least 1 week after the outbreak is terminated.

2. Dosage and Administration

See Table 49.3.

3. Contraindications/Precautions

Use amantadine or rimantadine with caution in patients who have reduced renal function or a history of seizures or neuropsychiatric disorders. Use amantadine with caution in patients who take psychotropic medication.

4. Adverse Reactions

Side effects occur in 5% to 10% of patients receiving amantadine. These reactions mainly affect the central nervous system (nervousness, anxiety, insom-

Table 49.3. Recommended Dosage for Amantadine and Rimantadine Prophylaxis

	Age			
Antiviral Agent	**1–9 yrs**	**10–13 yrs**	**14–64 yrs**	**≥65 yrs**
Amantadine[1]	5 mg/kg/day up to 150 mg in two divided doses[2]	100 mg twice daily[3]	100 mg twice daily	≤100 mg/day
Rimantadine[4]	5 mg/kg/day up to 150 mg in two divided doses[2]	100 mg twice daily[3]	100 mg twice daily	100 or 200 mg/day[5]

1. Consult the drug insert for dosage recommendations about administering amantadine to persons with creatinine clearance <50 mL/min.
2. 5 mg/kg of amantadine or rimantadine syrup = 1 tsp/22 lbs.
3. Administer amantadine or rimantadine at a dose of 5 mg/kg/day to children ≥10 years of age who weigh <40 kg.
4. Reduce the dose of rimantadine to 100 mg/day for persons with severe hepatic dysfunction or those with creatinine clearance of ≤10 mL/min. Closely observe other persons with less severe hepatic or renal dysfunction who are taking >100 mg/day of rimantadine; reduce the dosage or discontinue the drug if necessary.
5. Administer only 100 mg/day of rimantadine to elderly nursing home residents. Consider reducing the dose to 100 mg/day for all persons ≥65 years of age who experience side effects when taking 200 mg/day.

From: Centers for Disease Control and Prevention. Prevention and control of influenza: recommendations of the Advisory Committee on Immunization Practices (ACIP). *MMWR.* 1997;46(No. RR-9):1–25.

nia, difficulty concentrating, lightheadedness) and gastrointestinal tract (anorexia or nausea). More serious but less common central nervous system side effects (seizures, confusion) associated with amantadine use have affected older people, those with renal failure, and those with seizure, mental, or behavioral disorders. Rimantadine may also cause central nervous system side effects but less frequently than amantadine. Side effects tend to diminish or resolve after 1 week of continuous use of either drug and cease after discontinuation.

Because rimantadine has only recently been approved for marketing, its safety in certain patient populations (eg, chronically ill and elderly persons) has not been thoroughly evaluated. Be aware that more than 90% of amantadine is excreted unchanged, whereas approximately 75% of rimantadine is metabolized by the liver. Both drugs and their metabolites are excreted by the kidney.

Patient Resources

Age Page—What to Do About Flu; Age Page—"Shots" for Safety; Age Page—Pneumonia Prevention: Its Worth a Shot. National Institute on Aging, Bldg 31, Room 5C27, 31 Center Dr MSC 2922, Bethesda, MD 20892-2922; (301)496-1752; Internet address: http://www.nih.gov/nia/health/pubpub/pubpub.htm

Flu. National Institute of Allergy and Infectious Diseases, 31 Center Dr, Bldg 31, Room 7A50, Bethesda, MD 20892; (301)496-5717.

Vaccine Information Statement—*Influenza Vaccine: What you need to know before you or your child gets the vaccine*, #I1904. National Immunization Program, M/S E-34, Centers for Disease Control and Prevention, 1600 Clifton Rd, NE, Atlanta, GA 30333; (404)639-8225; fax (404)639-8828. Other sources of this information are state and local health departments and the American Academy of Pediatrics, Division of Publications, PO Box 927, Elk Grove Village, IL 69990-0927; (800)433-9016. Internet address: http://www.aap.org

Provider Resources

Prevention and control of influenza, #I1829; *Six common misconceptions about vaccination and how to respond to them*, #00-6561. National Immunization Program, M/S E-34, Centers for Disease Control and Prevention, 1600 Clifton Rd, NE, Atlanta, GA 30333; (404)639-8225. Fax (404)639-8828.

Selected References

American Academy of Pediatrics, Committee on Infectious Diseases. Influenza. In: *Report of the Committee on Infectious Diseases*. 23rd ed. Elk Grove Village, Ill: American Academy of Pediatrics; 1994:275-283.

American Academy of Family Physicians. *Summary of Policy Recommendations for Periodic Health Examination*. Kansas City, Mo: American Academy of Family Physicians; 1997.

American College of Physicians Task Force on Adult Immunization and Infectious Diseases Society of America. Influenza. In: *Guide for Adult Immunization*. 3rd ed. Philadelphia, Pa: American College of Physicians; 1994:91-94.

American Geriatrics Society, Clinical Practices Committee. *Prevention and Treatment of Influenza in the Elderly*. New York, NY: American Geriatrics Society; 1988.

Canadian Task Force on the Periodic Health Examination. Prevention of influenza. In: *The Canadian Guide to Clinical Preventive Health Care*. Ottawa, Canada: Minister of Supply and Services; 1994: chap 61 and Appendix B.

Centers for Disease Control and Prevention. Prevention and control of influenza: recommendations of the Advisory Committee on Immunization Practices (ACIP). *MMWR*. 1996; 45(No. RR-5):1-24.

Centers for Disease Control and Prevention. Prevention and control of influenza: recommendations of the Advisory Committee on Immunization Practices (ACIP). *MMWR*. 1997; 46(No. RR-9):1-25.

Murphy KR, Strunk RC. Safe administration of influenza vaccine in asthmatic children hypersensitive to egg proteins. *J Pediatr*. 1985;106:931-933.

US Preventive Services Task Force. Adult immunizations. In: *Guide to Clinical Preventive Services*. 2nd ed. Washington, DC: US Department of Health and Human Services; 1996: chap 66.

50

PNEUMOCOCCUS (Including Childhood Immunization)

Streptococcus pneumoniae infections are a major cause of morbidity and mortality in the United States, causing up to 36% of cases of community-acquired pneumonia in adults and approximately 40,000 deaths annually. Bacteremia develops in up to 30% of patients with pneumococcal pneumonia. The risk of mortality from pneumococcal infection is particularly high in older adults; mortality from pneumococcal bacteremia may be as high as 40% among persons aged 84 years and older. Other groups at increased risk include the very young and persons with chronic cardiovascular and pulmonary conditions, organ transplants, diabetes mellitus, alcoholism, cirrhosis, functional or anatomic asplenia (eg, sickle cell disease or splenectomy), Hodgkin's and non-Hodgkin's lymphomas, multiple myeloma, renal failure, nephrotic syndrome, and human immunodeficiency virus (HIV) infection (Table 50.1).

The currently available 23-valent pneumococcal vaccine, which replaced a 14-valent vaccine in 1983, contains antigens for at least 85% to 90% of the serotypes of *S. pneumoniae* causing bacteremia in the United States. The 23-valent vaccine has a protective efficacy of approximately 60% (for included serotypes) for all patients. Efficacy of the vaccine may decrease with increasing age and as the period of time since vaccination increases. In immunocompromised patients and those with certain chronic illnesses, the initial antibody response to pneumococcal vaccine is lower and declines more rapidly.

Compliance with recommendations for immunization with pneumococcal vaccine has been poor. According to data from the 1994 Behavioral Risk Factor Survillance System, only 37% of persons aged 65 years and older report being vaccinated. Many opportunities for vaccination, such as during hospitalization or at discharge, are missed. Data suggest that two thirds of patients with serious pneumonia were hospitalized at least once during the preceding 3 to 5 years. Recent research indicates that predischarge vaccination of patients hospitalized for pneumonia of any etiology decreases the rate of subsequent hospitalization for pneumococcal disease in this group. The emergence of drug-resistant strains of *S. pneumoniae* emphasizes the need for preventing pneumococcal infections by improving vaccine coverage.

Table 50.1. Groups at Increased Risk for Pneumococcal Disease

---

Persons ≥65 years of age

Adults and children with chronic illness—cardiovascular disease, pulmonary disease, diabetes mellitus, alcoholism, cirrhosis, or cerebrospinal fluid leaks. This does not include recurrent upper respiratory tract infections such as otitis media and sinusitis.

Immunocompromised individuals—those with splenic dysfunction (eg, sickle cell anemia) or anatomic asplenia, Hodgkin's or non-Hodgkin's lymphoma, multiple myeloma, chronic renal failure, nephrotic syndrome, organ transplantation, or other conditions associated with immunosuppression

---

Persons with HIV infection (asymptomatic or symptomatic)

Residents of special environments or social settings who have an identified increased risk of pneumococcal disease or its complications (eg, certain American Indian populations)

Adapted from: Centers for Disease Control. Update an adult immunization: recommendations of the Advisory Committee on Immunization Practices (ACIP). *MMWR.* 1991;40:(No. RR-12);1–94.

S. pneumoniae infection (drug-resistant invasive disease only) is currently designated as an infectious disease notifiable at the national level. Refer to Appendix C for further information on nationally notifiable diseases.

Recommendations of Major Authorities

Immunocompetent Persons

> **Advisory Committee on Immunization Practices (ACIP), American Academy of Family Physicians, American College of Obstetricians and Gynecologists, American College of Physicians (ACP), and US Preventive Services Task Force (USPSTF)**—All immunocompetent persons 65 years of age or older should be immunized once with pneumococcal vaccine. Immunization is also indicated for persons younger than age 65 years with medical or living conditions that put them at risk for invasive pneumococcal disease.
>
> **ACP, USPSTF, and ACIP**—Routine revaccination is not recommended. **ACP** recommends that persons older than 65 years of age receive a second dose of vaccine if they received the vaccine more than 6 years previously and were less than 65 years of age at the time of primary vaccination. **ACIP** recommends a second dose of vaccine only in persons 65 years of age or older who received the vaccine more than 5 years previously and were less than 65 years of age at the time of primary vaccination. According to **USPSTF,** revaccination may be appropriate in im-

munocompetent persons at highest risk for morbidity and mortality from pneumococcal disease (eg, persons older than 75 years of age or with severe chronic disease) who were vaccinated more than 5 years previously.

American College of Obstetricians and Gynecologists—All immunocompetent women 65 years of age or older should be offered immunization against pneumococcal disease. In addition, immunizations should be offered to immunocompetent women aged 19 to 64 years who have chronic conditions (eg, cardiopulmonary disorders, diabetes mellitus, renal dysfunction, alcoholism, cirrhosis) or who live in a chronic care facility.

Canadian Task Force on the Periodic Health Examination— There is insufficient evidence to include vaccination or exclude it from the periodic health examination of immunocompetent persons 55 years of age or older living independently. There is good evidence to include vaccination in the periodic health examination of immunocompetent persons 55 years of age or older living in institutions and patients with sickle cell disease or a history of splenectomy.

Immunocompromised Persons

Advisory Committee on Immunization Practices (ACIP) and American Academy of Pediatrics (AAP)—Immunocompromised persons older than age 2 years should receive immunization. **ACIP** recommends a one-time revaccination for persons over 2 years of age who are at highest risk for serious pneumococcal infection and those who are likely to have a rapid decline in pneumococcal antibody levels, provided that at least 5 years have passed since receipt of a previous dose of pneumococcal vaccine. According to the **American College of Physicians,** revaccination is recommended for immunocompromised adults who were vaccinated 6 or more years previously. **AAP** recommends considering revaccination in 3 to 5 years for immunocompromised children who will be 10 years of age or younger at the time of revaccination.

American Academy of Family Physicians—Children over age 2 years and adolescents and adults with chronic cardiac or pulmonary disease, diabetes mellitus, or anatomic asplenia, as well as any person over age 2 years who lives in a special environment or social setting with an increased risk of pneumococcal disease should be vaccinated.

American College of Obstetricians and Gynecologists—Women 19 years of age and older who are immunocompromised should be offered immunization against pneumococcal disease.

Canadian Task Force on the Periodic Health Examination— There is fair evidence to exclude pneumococcal vaccination from the periodic health examination of immunosuppressed patients.

US Preventive Services Task Force—There is insufficient evidence to recommend for or against pneumococcal vaccine as an efficacious vaccine for immunocompromised individuals, but recommendations for vaccinating these persons may be made on other grounds, including the high incidence and case-fatality rates of pneumococcal disease and minimal adverse effects from the vaccine. It may be appropriate to consider periodic revaccination in these high-risk immunocompromised patients, who are likely to have poor initial antibody response and rapid decline of antibodies after vaccination.

Basics of Pneumococcal Immunization

1. Vaccine Types

Only 23-valent vaccine is currently available in the United States. A protein-polysaccharide conjugate vaccine, which is immunogenic in infants, is currently under development; however, these vaccines are likely to contain fewer than 23 pneumococcal serotypes.

2. Schedule

Some disagreement among authorities exists regarding the indications for vaccination and revaccination (see Recommendations of Major Authorities). Consider health-care contacts of all types, including hospitalizations, as opportunities to provide immunization to appropriate patients. If possible, vaccinate patients who are undergoing splenectomy at least 2 weeks before surgery.

3. Dose and Administration

The recommended dose for adults and children is 0.5 mL given intramuscularly or subcutaneously. Pneumococcal vaccine and influenza vaccine may be given concurrently but at different sites.

4. Contraindications/Precautions

Known hypersensitivity to any of the vaccine components is a contraindication to vaccination. Revaccination may lead to an increased incidence of adverse reactions, particularly if revaccination is performed at intervals of 3 years or less.

5. Adverse Reactions

Mild, local side effects, such as erythema and pain at the injection site, develop in approximately 50% of patients. Fever, myalgia, and severe local reactions are reported in fewer than 1% of persons vaccinated. Anaphylactic reactions are rare (approximately five reactions per 1 million doses of vaccine).

Any adverse side effects should be reported to the Vaccine Adverse Event Reporting System (VAERS). See Table B.4 for a detailed listing of adverse events. VAERS forms and instructions are available in the *FDA Drug Bulletin* (Food and Drug Administration) and the *Physician's Desk Reference* or by calling the 24-hour VAERS information recording at (800)822-7967. Refer to Appendix B for details.

6. Patient Education

Educational efforts and outreach to older adults are necessary to attain better rates of pneumococcal immunization. The National Institute on Aging has developed patient education materials on pneumococcal vaccination (see Patient Resources).

7. Vaccine Storage and Handling

Store vaccine at 2° to 8°C (36° to 46°F). Handle all vaccine preparations according to manufacturers' instructions.

Patient Resources

Age Page—"Shots" for Safety; Age Page—Pneumonia Prevention: It's Worth a Shot. National Institute on Aging, Bldg 31, Rm 5C27, 31 Center Dr MSC 2922, Bethesda, MD 20892-2922; (301)496-1752. Internet address: http://www.nih.gov/nia/health/pubpub/pubpub.htm

Provider Resources

Pneumococcal Polysaccharide Vaccine (MMWR 1997 Reprint); *Immunization Is a Family Affair: Adults Need Them Too* (Poster); *Immunization of Adults: a Call to Action; Today's Health: Immunization 1995* (Videotape Segment on Vaccine Misconceptions); *Six Common Misconceptions about Vaccination and How to Respond to Them.* To order these and other materials, contact the National Immunization Program, M/S E-34, Centers for Disease Control and Prevention, 1600 Clifton Rd, NE, Atlanta, GA 30333; (404)639-8225; fax (404)639-8828.

Selected References

American Academy of Family Physicians. *Summary of Policy Recommendations for Periodic Health Examination.* Kansas City, Mo: American Academy of Family Physicians; 1997.

American Academy of Pediatrics, Committee on Infectious Diseases. Pneumococcal infections. In: *Report of the Committee on Infectious Diseases.* 23rd ed. Elk Grove Village, Ill: American Academy of Pediatrics; 1994.

American College of Obstetricians and Gynecologists. *Guidelines for Women's Health Care.* Washington, DC: American College of Obstetricians and Gynecologists; 1996.

American College of Physicians Task Force on Adult Immunization and Infectious Diseases Society of America. Immunization for healthy adults. In: *Guide for Adult Immunization*. 3rd ed. Philadelphia, Pa: American College of Physicians; 1994: chap. 3.

Atkinson W, Furphy L, Gantt J, et al, eds. *Epidemiology and Prevention of Vaccine-Preventable Diseases*. Washington DC: Department of Health and Human Services-Public Health Service; 1996: chap 12.

Broome CV, Breiman RF. Pneumococcal vaccine—past, present, and future. *N Engl J Med.* 1991;325:1506-1508.

Butler JC, Breiman RF, Campbell JF, Lipman HB, Broome CV, Facklam RR. Pneumococcal polysaccharide vaccine efficacy. *JAMA.* 1993;270:1826-1831.

Butler JC, Hofmann J, Cetron MS, Elliott JA, Facklam RR, Breiman RF. The continued emergence of drug-resistant *Streptococcus pneumoniae* in the United States: an update from the Centers for Disease Control and Prevention's Pneumococcal Sentinel Surveillance System. *J Infect Dis.* 1996;174:986-993.

Canadian Task Force on the Periodic Health Examination. Administration of pneumococcal vaccine. In: *The Canadian Guide to Clinical Preventive Health Care*. Ottawa, Canada: Minister of Supply and Services; 1994: chap 34.

Centers for Disease Control and Prevention. Prevention of pneumococcal disease: recommendations of the Advisory Committee on Immunizations Practices (ACIP). *MMWR.* 1997; 46(No. RR-8):1-24.

Centers for Disease Control. Update on adult immunization: Recommendations of the Advisory Committee on Immunization Practices (ACIP). *MMWR.* 1991;40(No. RR-12):1-94.

Centers for Disease Control and Prevention. CDC Surveillance Summaries, August 1, 1997. *MMWR.* 1997;45(No. SS-3).

Fedson DS, Harward MP, Reid RA, Kaiser DL. Hospital-based pneumococcal immunization: epidemiologic rationale from the Shenandoah study. *JAMA.* 1990;264:1117-1122.

Gable CB, Holzer SS, Engelhart L, et al. Pneumococcal vaccine: efficacy and associated cost savings. *JAMA.* 1990;264:2910-2915.

Hofmann J, Cetron MS, Farley MM, et al. The prevalence of drug resistant *Streptococcus pneumoniae* in Atlanta. *N Engl J Med.* 1995;333:481-486.

Plouffe JF, Breiman RF, Facklam RR; for The Franklin County Pneumonia Study Group. Bacteremia with *Streptococcus pneumoniae* in adults: implications for therapy and prevention. *JAMA.* 1996;275:194-198.

Shapiro ED, Berg AT, Austrian R, et al. The protective efficacy of polyvalent pneumococcal polysaccharide vaccine. *N Engl J Med.* 1991;325:1453-1460.

US Preventive Services Task Force. Adult immunizations. In: *Guide to Clinical Preventive Services*. 2nd ed. Washington, DC: US Department of Health and Human Services; 1996: chap 66.

51

RUBELLA

The incidence of rubella has decreased markedly since the rubella vaccine was introduced in 1969. However, in the adult population, rubella continues to be a concern for nonimmunized women of child-bearing age. When rubella is contracted during pregnancy, especially during the first trimester, it can result in miscarriage, stillbirth, or the development of congenital rubella syndrome (CRS). CRS develops in an estimated 85% of infants born to women who acquire rubella during the first trimester of pregnancy. The most frequently occurring clinical manifestations of CRS are deafness, low birth weight, hepatomegaly, splenomegaly, ocular defects, psychomotor retardation, congenital heart disease, and petechiae. In 1995, approximately 128 cases of rubella and 6 cases of CRS were reported.

Rubella vaccine is approximately 95% effective at conferring immunity, which is probably lifelong. Screening and subsequent immunization of susceptible women of childbearing age have been shown to decrease the incidence of CRS.

Rubella is currently designated as an infectious disease notifiable at the national level. Refer to Appendix C for further information on nationally notifiable diseases.

See chapter 15 for information on immunization of children and adolescents against measles, mumps, and rubella.

Recommendations of Major Authorities

Advisory Committee on Immunization Practices (ACIP), American Academy of Pediatrics (AAP), American College of Obstetricians and Gynecologists, American College of Physicians (ACP), Canadian Task Force on the Periodic Health Examination (CTFPHE), and US Preventive Services Task Force (USPSTF)—Women of childbearing age who lack documented evidence of immunity or prior immunization should be immunized. The **CTFPHE** and **USPSTF** state that an acceptable alternative is to offer immunization to all women of childbearing age without consideration of immunity or prior immunization. Some authorities (**ACIP, AAP,** and **ACP**) recommend immunization of susceptible males as well. The **CTFPHE** and **USP-STF** state that there is insufficient evidence to recommend for or against vaccination of young men in settings where large numbers of susceptible adults of both sexes congregate, such as military bases or colleges, and that men in other settings should not be routinely vaccinated.

American College of Physicians—All health care workers should have documented serologic immunity or be vaccinated.

American Academy of Family Physicians—Clinicians should assure the immunity of women of childbearing potential by history, serology, or vaccination. All persons needing immunization should be given a single-dose vaccination. Adolescents and young adults in settings where such individuals congregate (eg, high schools, technical schools, and colleges) should be given a second dose at least 1 month after the first dose if they have not previously received a second dose.

Basics of Rubella Immunization

1. Vaccine Types

Rubella vaccine is made from a live virus. The currently available vaccine is designated RA 27/3 and is available in either a monovalent form (rubella only) or in combinations: measles-rubella (MR), rubella-mumps, and measles-mumps-rubella (MMR). Any of these vaccines may be used in adults, but authorities recommend using MMR, unless it is contraindicated.

2. Assessing Immunity

Screen all women of childbearing age for immunity to rubella. Immunize those who have neither documentation of prior immunization after 12 months of age nor documented immunity by antibody testing. Do not accept a reported history of infection as evidence of immunity. Antibody testing may be offered to persons suspected of lacking immunity, but authorities agree that immunization may be provided without such testing. Screening and vaccination may be considered for other adults, especially those living in high-risk settings (eg, colleges, military bases).

3. Dose and Administration

Administer a 0.5-mL dose of reconstituted vaccine (any type) subcutaneously, using a 5/8 in to 3/4 in, 23- to 25-gauge needle.

4. Contraindications/Precautions

Do not administer rubella vaccine to pregnant women, and advise all women receiving the vaccine not to become pregnant for 3 months after vaccination.

Counsel women who do become pregnant within 3 months of vaccination that concerns for the fetus exist but that generally interruption of the pregnancy is not necessary. Do not immunize patients who are immunocompromised (except those who are HIV-positive).

Immune globulin-containing preparations, such as immune globulin (IG), hepatitis B immune globulin (HBIG), varicella zoster immune globulin (VZIG), packed red blood cells, whole blood, or plasma, may interfere with the immune response to MMR vaccination. Therefore, do not administer MMR 2 weeks before or 3 to 11 months after such preparations are given (depending on the immune globulin content of the preparation). Repeat vaccination after the window of immune globulin interference has expired, or perform antibody testing to determine the patient's immunity status. The Advisory Committee on Immunization Practices provides detailed information regarding this issue in their general recommendations on immunization (see Selected References).

Do not delay administration of rubella or MMR vaccine to rubella-susceptible postpartum women even if they are receiving treatment for D (formerly Rh) sensitization with anti-Rh_o(D)IG (human) or any other blood product containing IG. Women who received anti-Rh_o(D)IG (human) during the last trimester of pregnancy or at the time of delivery and received postpartum rubella immunization should have their immunity confirmed by antibody level testing 3 months after immunization.

Delay immunizing adults who have a febrile illnesses. Use caution when administering rubella vaccine in the form of MMR to adults with a history of allergy to eggs. Do not administer rubella vaccine to adults who have experienced anaphylactic reactions to topically or systemically administered neomycin.

5. Adverse Reactions

Arthralgia develops in approximately 25% of adults immunized with rubella vaccine, and 13% to 15% of immunized adults report arthritis-like symptoms. Such symptoms generally develop 1 to 3 weeks after vaccination, persist for 1 day to 3 weeks, and seldom recur. Rarely, recurrent arthralgia and sometimes arthritis persist for an extended length of time. Paresthesias and pain in the arms and legs may also rarely develop and follow the same course as arthralgias. These adverse reactions seem to occur more often in patients who are nonimmune after vaccination. Other adverse reactions include low-grade fever, rash, and lymphadenopathy.

Any adverse side effects should be reported to the Vaccine Adverse Event Reporting System (VAERS). Refer to Table B.4 for a detailed listing of adverse events. VAERS forms and instructions are available in the *FDA Drug Bulletin* (Food and Drug Administration) and the *Physician's Desk Reference* or by calling the 24-hour VAERS information recording at (800)822-7967. Refer to Appendix B for details.

6. Patient Education

The National Childhood Vaccine Injury Act requires health care providers to provide the following information to patients prior to administering MMR: (1) a concise description of the benefits of the vaccine, (2) a concise description of the risks associated with the vaccine, (3) notice of the availability of the National Vaccine Injury Compensation Program. See Appendix B for details. For additional information about this requirement, contact the Training Coordinator, National Immunization Program, Centers for Disease Control and Prevention: (404)639-8226.

7. Vaccine Storage and Handling

Discard reconstituted vaccine that is not used within 8 hours. Store unreconstituted vaccine at 2° to 8°C (36° to 46°F) or colder; protect it from light. Handle all vaccine preparations according to manufacturers' instructions.

Patient Resource

Measles, Mumps, and Rubella: What You Need to Know. US Department of Health and Human Services. This material is available from State and local health departments and from the American Academy of Pediatrics, Division of Publications, PO Box 927, Elk Grove Village, IL 60009-0927, (800)433-9016. Internet address: http://www.aap.org

Selected References

Advisory Committee on Immunization Practices (ACIP). General recommendations on immunization. *MMWR.* 1994;43(No. RR-1):1-38.

Advisory Committee on Immunization Practices (ACIP). Rubella prevention. *MMWR.* 1990; 39(No. RR-15):1-18.

American Academy of Family Physicians. *Summary of Policy Recommendations for Periodic Health Examination.* Kansas City, Mo: American Academy of Family Physicians; 1997.

American Academy of Pediatrics, Committee on Infectious Diseases. Rubella. In: *Report of the Committee on Infectious Diseases.* 23rd ed. Elk Grove Village, Ill: American Academy of Pediatrics; 1994.

American College of Obstetricians and Gynecologists. *Guidelines for Women's Health Care.* Washington, DC: American College of Obstetricians and Gynecologists; 1996.

American College of Physicians. *Guide for Adult Immunization.* 3rd ed. Philadelphia, Pa: American College of Physicians; 1994:36.

American College of Physicians Task Force on Adult Immunization and Infectious Diseases Society of America. Rubella. In: *Guide for Adult Immunization.* 3rd ed. Philadelphia, Pa: American College of Physicians; 1994:125-129.

Atkinson W, Furphy L, Gantt J, et al, eds. *Epidemiology and Prevention of Vaccine-Preventable Diseases*. Washington DC: US Dept of Health and Human Services, Public Health Service; 1996: chap 8.

Canadian Task Force on the Periodic Health Examination. Screening and vaccinating adolescents and adults to prevent congenital rubella syndrome. In: *The Canadian Guide to Clinical Preventive Health Care*. Ottawa, Canada: Minister of Supply and Services; 1994: chap 12.

Canadian Task Force on the Periodic Health Examination. The periodic health examination 1979. *Can Med Assoc J*. 1979;121:1193-1254.

Centers for Disease Control and Prevention. General recommendations on immunization: recommendations of the Advisory Committee on Immunization Practices (ACIP). *MMWR*. 1994;43(No. RR-1):1-38.

Centers for Disease Control. Rubella prevention: recommendations of the Advisory Committee on Immunization Practices (ACIP). *MMWR*. 1990;39(No. RR-15):1-13.

US Preventive Services Task Force. Screening for vaccinating adolescents and adults to prevent congenital rubella syndrome. In: *Guide to Clinical Preventive Services*. 2nd ed. Washington, DC: US Department of Health and Human Services; 1996: chap 32.

52

TETANUS AND DIPHTHERIA

Tetanus occurs almost exclusively in unvaccinated or inadequately vaccinated persons. Approximately 50 cases are reported each year in the United States. Sixty-seven percent of cases occur in adults over age 50 years. The overall case fatality rate is approximately 25%, but mortality is considerably higher among older adults than among groups of other ages. Serologic studies have demonstrated that approximately 30% of adults over 70 years of age lack protective levels of antitoxin antibodies. Immunization with tetanus toxoid is almost 100% effective for preventing illness. Tetanus immune globulin (TIG) is highly protective when given prophylactically for wound management.

Diphtheria immunization of children has reduced the incidence of this disease in the United States to fewer than 10 cases yearly; these cases occur primarily in adults. As with tetanus, most cases of diphtheria occur in unimmunized or incompletely immunized persons. The overall case fatality rate is 5% to 10%; death rates are higher (up to 20%) among children younger than age 5 years and adults older than age 40 years. Diphtheria immunization has resulted in serologic evidence of immunity in most children, but up to 60% of adults lack protective levels of antitoxin antibodies. Administration of a complete vaccination series substantially reduces the risk of developing diphtheria, and vaccinated individuals in whom disease develops have milder illness. Vaccination does not prevent carriage of the causative agent (*Clostridium diphtheriae*).

Tetanus and diphtheria are currently designated as infectious diseases notifiable at the national level. Refer to Appendix C for further information on nationally notifiable diseases.

See chapter 12 for information on the general clinical presentations of diphtheria, tetanus, and pertussis and for immunization and prophylaxis information for children and adolescents.

Recommendations of Major Authorities

Advisory Committee on Immunization Practices, American College of Obstetricians and Gynecologists, and **American College of Physicians (ACP)**—Adults should receive a tetanus-diphtheria (Td) booster vaccination every 10 years. **ACP** also recommends an alternative strategy of a single booster at 50 years of age for persons who have completed the full primary series, including the teenage and young-adult boosters.

American Academy of Family Physicians—A tetanus-diphtheria (Td) vaccine series should be completed for adults who have not received the primary series. Booster vaccination should be given every 10 years or at least at age 50 years.

Canadian Task Force on the Periodic Health Examination—Adults in good health should receive a tetanus booster vaccination every 10 years. Concomitant booster vaccination against diphtheria is optional.

US Preventive Services Task Force—The series of combined tetanus-diphtheria (Td) toxoids should be completed for patients who have not received the primary series, and all adults should receive periodic Td boosters. The optimal interval for booster doses is not established. The standard regimen is to provide Td at least once every 10 years, but in the US, intervals of 15 to 30 years between boosters are likely to be adequate in persons who received a complete five-dose series in childhood.

Basics of Tetanus and Diphtheria Immunization

1. Vaccine Types

There are three basic types of toxoid available for immunization of adults: tetanus and diphtheria toxoids adsorbed for adult use (Td), tetanus toxoid (TT), and tetanus toxoid fluid. Use Td unless immunization against diphtheria is not desired. US authorities recommend giving combined tetanus-diphtheria booster immunizations to adults because of the prevalence of low levels of diphtheria antitoxin antibodies in adults. Of the two single-antigen preparations available for tetanus immunization, TT is preferable because it is more immunogenic than the fluid preparation. Diphtheria and tetanus toxoids and pertussis vaccine adsorbed (DTP) and diphtheria and tetanus toxoids adsorbed (DT) are for use in children under 7 years of age. Do not use these preparations in adults.

2. Schedule

The standard regimen is to provide booster vaccinations every 10 years, although some authorities have recently stated that boosters may be given less frequently (see Recommendations of Major Authorities). If childhood immunizations have been received according to the usual schedule, with a booster dose at 14 to 16 years of age, the first adult vaccination will be needed at about 25 years of age. Administer three vaccinations to adults who have not received a primary series; give the second vaccination 4 to 8 weeks after the first, and give the third vaccination 6 to 12 months after the second. After administering this series, give booster vaccinations every 10 years.

A primary series may be completed without restarting with the first vaccination, regardless of how much time has elapsed between vaccinations. Because immunosuppressive therapies may reduce the immune response, defer vaccination for 1 month after discontinuation of immunosuppressive therapy.

For management of certain wounds, administration of a tetanus booster may be indicated if the patient has completed a primary series and 5 years have elapsed since the last vaccination (Table 52.1). Td booster should always be given as part of wound management when vaccination history is unknown or fewer than 3 doses have been received.

3. Dose and Administration

The recommended dose for all adult tetanus and diphtheria vaccines is 0.5 mL given intramuscularly, preferably in the deltoid muscle using a 1- to 1 1/2-inch, 20- to 25-gauge needle. Tetanus toxoid fluid may be given subcutaneously. Td, TT, or tetanus toxoid (fluid) may be administered concurrently with TIGs but different sites of delivery and separate syringes must be used.

4. Contraindications/Precautions

A history of a neurologic or a severe hypersensitivity reaction (eg, anaphylaxis) following a previous dose is a contraindication to receiving diphtheria and tetanus toxoids.

If an anaphylactic reaction to a previous dose is suspected, perform intradermal skin testing to document immediate hypersensitivity before discontinuing tetanus toxoid vaccinations. Mild, nonspecific skin-test reactivity is common. Avoid administering vaccinations more frequently than every 10 years (except for management of certain wounds), because induction of high serum tetanus antitoxin antibody levels may lead to Arthus hypersensitivity reactions (severe local reactions starting 2 to 8 hours after a vaccination and often associated with fever and malaise). Patients who have experienced an Arthus reaction should not receive booster vaccinations more frequently than every 10 years, even for wound treatment. Do not vaccinate women during the first trimester of pregnancy.

5. Adverse Reactions

Local reactions (usually erythema and induration, with or without tenderness) can occur after vaccination with Td or other preparations. Fever and other systemic reactions can occur but are less common. Arthus reactions can occur (as discussed above), particularly among patients who have received multiple tetanus boosters using the adsorbed preparations. Severe reactions (eg, anaphylaxis and neurologic complications) have been reported rarely.

Any adverse side effects should be reported to the Vaccine Adverse Event Reporting System (VAERS). Refer to Table B.4 for a detailed listing of adverse events. VAERS forms and instructions are available in the *FDA Drug Bulletin* (Food and Drug Administration) and the *Physician's Desk Reference* or by calling the 24-hour VAERS information recording at (800)822-7967. Refer to Appendix B for details.

6. Patient Education

The National Childhood Vaccine Injury Act requires health care providers to provide the following information to patients prior to administering MMR: (1) a concise description of the benefits of the vaccine, (2) a concise description of the risks associated with the vaccine, (3) notice of the availability of the National Vaccine Injury Compensation Program. See Appendix B for details. For additional information about this requirement, contact the Training Coordinator, National Immunization Program, Centers for Disease Control and Prevention: (404)639-8226.

7. Storage and Handling

Store toxoids at 2° to 8°C (36° to 46°F); do not freeze. Do not use vaccine that has been frozen. Handle all vaccine preparations according to manufacturers' instructions.

Basics of Tetanus Postexposure Prophylaxis

1. Indications

Patients who may have been exposed to tetanus because of wounds may need prophylaxis via immediate passive immunization with tetanus immune globulin (TIG), active immunization with tetanus toxoid (preferably Td), or both. See Table 52.1 for guidelines on passive and active immunization according to the nature of the wound and the patient's immunization status.

2. Dose and Administration

The recommended adult dose of TIG is 250 units injected intramuscularly, preferably in the deltoid muscle. It can be given concurrently with tetanus toxoid, but it should be given at a different site and with a different syringe.

3. Contraindications/Precautions

Avoid intravenous injection, which can cause an anaphylactic reaction.

4. Adverse Reactions

The side effects of TIG are relatively minor (site soreness and mild temperature elevation), but a few cases of more serious side effects (anaphylaxis, angioneurotic edema, nephrotic syndrome) have been reported.

Table 52.1. Summary Guide to Tetanus Prophylaxis in Routine Wound Management

Number of previous tetanus vaccinations	Clean, minor wounds		All other wounds[1]	
	Give Td[2]	Give TIG	Give Td	Give TIG
Unknown, uncertain, or fewer than 3	Yes	No	Yes	Yes
3 or more[3]	No[4]	No	No[5]	No

1. Such as, but not limited to: wounds contaminated with dirt, feces, and saliva; puncture wounds; avulsions; and wounds resulting from missiles, crushing, burns, and frostbite

2. For children ≤7 years of age DTaP or DTP (DT if pertussis vaccine is contraindicated) is preferred to tetanus toxoid alone. For persons ≥7 years of age, Td (tetanus-diphtheria toxoid for adult use) is preferred to tetanus toxoid alone.

3. If only 3 doses of fluid toxoid have been received, then a fourth dose of toxoid, preferably an adsorbed toxoid, should be given

4. Administer a booster if more than 10 years have elapsed since the last dose

5. Administer a booster if more than 5 years have elapsed since the last dose. (More frequent boosters are not needed and can accentuate side effects).

Adapted from: Diphtheria, tetanus, and pertussis: recommendations for vaccine use and other preventive measures. *MMWR*. 1991;40(No. RR-10):1–28.

Patient Resources

Age Page—"Shots" for Safety. National Institute on Aging, Bldg 31, Room 5C27, 31 Center Dr MSC 2922, Bethesda, MD 20892-2922; (301) 496-1752. Internet address: http://www.nih.gov/nia/health/pubpub/pubpub.htm

Selected References

American Academy of Family Physicians. *Summary of Policy Recommendations for Periodic Health Examination*. Kansas City, Mo: American Academy of Family Physicians; 1997.

American College of Obstetricians and Gynecologists. *Guidelines for Women's Health Care*. Washington, DC: American College of Obstetricians and Gynecologists; 1996.

American College of Physicians Task Force on Adult Immunization and Infectious Diseases Society of America. Tetanus and diphtheria. In: *Guide for Adult Immunization*. 3rd ed. Philadelphia, Pa: American College of Physicians; 1994:130-133.

Atkinson W, Furphy L, Gantt J, et al, eds. *Epidemiology and Prevention of Vaccine-Preventable Diseases*. Washington DC: US Department of Health and Human Services, Public Health Service; 1996: chap 2-3.

Canadian Task Force on the Periodic Health Examination. The periodic health examination 1979. *Can Med Assoc J*. 1979;121:1193-1254.

Centers for Disease Control. Diphtheria, tetanus, and pertussis: guidelines for vaccine prophylaxis and other preventive measures. *MMWR*. 1985;34:405-426.

Centers for Disease Control. Diphtheria, tetanus, and pertussis: recommendations for vaccine use and other preventive measures: recommendations of the Advisory Committee on Immunization Practices (ACIP). *MMWR*. 1991;40(No. RR-10):1-28.

Centers for Disease Control and Prevention. General recommendations on immunization: recommendations of the Advisory Committee on Immunization Practices (ACIP). *MMWR*. 1994;43(No. RR-1):1-38.

Centers for Disease Control. Update on adult immunization: recommendations of the Advisory Committee on Immunization Practices (ACIP). *MMWR*. 1991;40(No. RR-12):1-94.

Gergen PJ, McQuillan GM, Kiely M, Ezzati-Rice TM, Sutter RW, Virella G. A population-based serologic survey of immunity to tetanus in the United States. *N Engl J Med*. 1995; 332: 761-6.

US Preventive Services Task Force. Adult immunizations. In: *Guide to Clinical Preventive Services*. 2nd ed. Washington, DC: US Department of Health and Human Services; 1996: chap 66.

53

ALCOHOL AND OTHER DRUG ABUSE

Substance abuse, defined as the harmful or hazardous use of alcohol, tobacco, or other legal and illegal drugs, is a leading cause of death and disability in United States. Alcohol and drug abuse are physically damaging and are associated with other leading causes of death, including accidents, suicide, homicide, and HIV infection.

Alcohol abuse is estimated to cost society approximately $85.8 billion annually—nearly twice as much as the abuse of all other drugs combined. Alcohol abuse alone is associated with a dramatic proportion of traffic fatalities (41%), drownings and murders (67%), deaths in fires (70% to 80%), and suicides (35%). Consumption of alcohol during pregnancy can lead to development of fetal alcohol syndrome (FAS), which can produce a variety of deleterious effects ranging from physical anomalies to mental impairment to more subtle cognitive and behavioral dysfunctions. According to the Centers for Disease Control and Prevention an estimated 1 in 3,000 births are affected by FAS each year (Selected References).

Abuse of drugs other than alcohol is estimated to cost society approximately $47 billion per year. Illicit drug use contributes to both social and medical problems. An estimated 5.5 million Americans are affected by drug abuse or dependence, half of whom are within the criminal justice system. Injection drug use and use of crack are major contributors to the spread of HIV. Drug use is also integrally related to problems such as accidents, homicide, and suicide. Estimates of the extent of prescription drug misuse vary, but there is little doubt that misuse of legal medications is responsible for a significant portion of the morbidity and mortality associated with substance abuse. One authority indicates that a 60% to 70% of patients treated in emergency rooms for drug-related episodes are misusing prescription drugs.

According to the National Institute on Drug Abuse, the overall prevalence of drug use does not differ between Caucasian, African American, and Hispanic populations although patterns of use may differ. Primary care providers often fail to recognize alcohol and drug abuse problems in their patients. Some studies report detection rates as low as 30%. Minimal interventions by primary care clinicians, such as advice to modify current use patterns and warnings about adverse health consequences, can have beneficial effects, especially for patients in the early stages of addiction. More intensive interventions, such as referral to outpatient or inpatient/residential treatment facilities, can be life-saving for patients in more advanced stages of alcohol and other drug dependence.

See chapter 18 for information on counseling children and adolescents on alcohol and other drug abuse. See chapter 24 for information on counseling children and adolescents about tobacco use prevention and chapter 60 for information about counseling adults on smoking cessation.

Recommendations of Major Authorities

American College of Obstetricians and Gynecologists—Women should be asked about their use of alcohol and other drugs.

American College of Physicians—The physician's role in recognizing and treating chemical dependence requires knowledge of the symptoms of chronic and excessive drug use and increased sensitivity to and awareness of behavior associated with such problem use. The physician's role in preventing chemical dependency includes patient education and counseling about the appropriate use of substances upon which dependence is likely. Thoughtful and knowledgeable prescribing practices that minimize the likelihood of producing or maintaining iatrogenic chemical dependence are essential.

American Medical Association—All physicians with clinical responsibility for diagnosis of and referral for alcoholism and drug abuse problems should be able to recognize alcohol or drug-caused dysfunction and should be aware of the medical complications, symptoms, and syndromes with which alcoholism or drug abuse commonly presents. All complete health examinations should include an in-depth history of alcohol and other drug use. The physician should evaluate patient requirements and community resources so that an adequate level of care may be prescribed, with patients' needs matched to appropriate resources and with referrals made to a resource that provides appropriate medical care.

Canadian Task Force on the Periodic Health Examination— Routine active case-finding of problem drinking is highly recommended on the basis of the high prevalence of this problem among patients in medical practices, its association with adverse consequences before the stage of dependency is reached, and its amenability to a counseling intervention by clinicians. Detection of biomarkers is not recommended, although this may be useful to confirm suspicions raised by use of patient administered questionnaires (eg, Alcohol Use Disorders Identification Test [AUDIT], the Michigan Alcoholism Screening Test [MAST] and the Drug Abuse Screening Test [DAST]).

US Preventive Services Task Force—Screening to detect problem drinking is recommended for all adult and adolescent patients. Screening should involve a careful history of alcohol use and/or the use of standardized screening questionnaires. Routine measurement of biochemical markers is not recommended in asymptomatic persons. Pregnant women should be advised to limit or cease drinking during pregnancy. Although there is insufficient evidence to prove or disprove harm from light drinking in pregnancy, recommendations that women abstain from alcohol during pregnancy may be made on other grounds. All persons who use alcohol should be counseled about the dangers of operating a motor vehicle or performing other potentially dangerous activities after drinking alcohol.

There is insufficient evidence to recommend for or against routine screening for drug abuse with standardized questionnaires or biologic assays. Including questions about drug use and drug-related problems when taking a history from all adolescents and adult patients may be recommended on other grounds including the prevalence of drug use and the serious consequences of drug abuse and dependence. All pregnant women should be advised of the potential adverse effects of drug use on the development of the fetus. Clinicians should be alert to the signs and symptoms of drug abuse in patients and refer drug abusing patients to specialized treatment facilities where available.

Basics of Identification for Abuse of Alcohol and Other Drugs

1. Conduct an Alcohol/Drug History

Identifying patients with substance abuse problems is critical. Begin history-taking with questions about relatively nonthreatening subjects—such as the number of cups of caffeinated beverages the patient drinks per day—before moving on to questions about the types, amounts, duration, and patterns of use of legal and illegal substances. When asking questions about frequency and use, be aware that there may be a tendency among patients to under-report use. However, such questions may be helpful in identifying individuals who drink large quantities (eg, binge drinkers). Questions about the negative consequences of abuse can also be helpful in assessing the magnitude of the problem. Areas that may be addressed include: driving history, employment history, educational progress, legal problems, family life, social activities, and enrollment in treatment programs. Asking about family history of substance abuse will help assess the patient's genetic vulnerability. If the patient has made previous attempts to stop or moderate use of alcohol or drugs, ask about the methods, barriers encountered, and degree of success. Table 53.1 and Figure 53.1 outline the screening algorithm recommended by the National Institute on Alcohol Abuse and Alcoholism. Table 53.2 provides sample questions for taking clinical histories about drug use.

Figure 53.1. Steps for Alcohol Screening and Brief Intervention

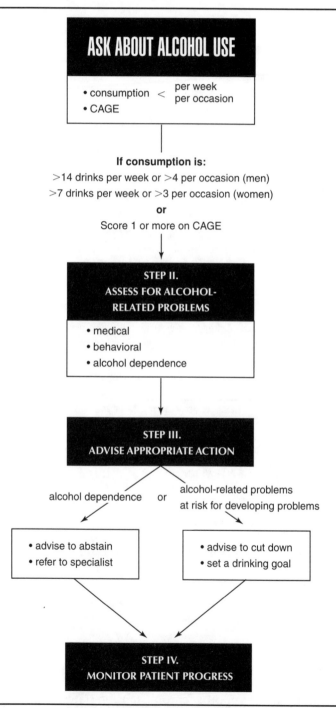

From: National Institute on Alcohol Abuse and Alcoholism. *The Physician's Guide to Helping Patients With Alcohol Problems.* Bethesda, Md. Department of Health and Human Services; 1995. NIH Publication No. 95-3769.

Table 53.1. Screening Procedures for Alcohol-Related Problems

---

Ask all patients:
- Do you drink alcohol, including beer, wine or distilled spirits?

Ask current drinkers about alcohol consumption:
- On average how many days per week do you drink alcohol?
- On a typical day when you drink, how many drinks do you have?
- What is the maximum number of drinks you had on any given occasion during the last month?

Ask current drinkers the **CAGE** questions:*
- Have you ever felt you ought to **C**ut down on drinking?
- Have people **A**nnoyed you by critizing your drinking?
- Have you ever felt bad or **G**uilty about your drinking?
- Have you ever had a drink first thing in the morning to steady your nerves or get rid of a hangover (**E**ye-opener)?

If there is a positive response to any of these questions, ASK:
- Has this occurred during the past year?

A patient may be at risk for alcohol-related problems IF:
- Alcohol consumption is >14 drinks per week or >4 drinks per occasion (MEN)
- Alcohol consumption is >7 drinks per week or >3 drinks per occasion (WOMEN)

OR
- One or more positive responses to the **CAGE** questions refer to the past year

---

* One "yes" response should raise suspicions of alcohol abuse. More than one "yes" response should be considered a strong indication that alcohol abuse exists.

Adapted from: Ewing JA. Detecting alcoholism: the CAGE questionnaire. *JAMA*. 1984;252:1905–1907. Reproduced by permission of the American Medical Association; copyright 1984 and from: National Institute on Alcohol Abuse and Alcoholism. *The Physician's Guide to Helping Patients With Alcohol Problems*. Bethesda, Md: US Department of Health and Human Services; 1995. NIH Publication No. 95-3769.

2. Use Brief Screening Questionnaires

Brief, self-administered screening questionnaires can help identify patients in need of more detailed evaluation. Examples of such tools include: the Alcohol Use Disorders Identification Test (AUDIT), the Michigan Alcoholism Screening Test (MAST), and the Drug Abuse Screening Test (DAST). See Provider Resources.

3. Ask about physical symptoms

Ask the patient about physical symptoms of substance abuse. Examples include frequent headaches or other chronic tension states, absence from work based on vague physical complaints, insomnia, unexplained mood changes,

---

Table 53.2. Examples of Questions for Taking Clinical Histories About Drug Use

---

What type of prescription drugs are you taking?
Have you ever taken prescription medications that were not prescribed for you?
When did you last drink wine, beer, or any alcoholic drink?
Have you ever used marijuana, cocaine, "crack," or any other drug?
Have you ever injected (shot) drugs?
   Which drugs did you inject?
   When did you last inject (shoot) drugs?
   Do you ever use needles, syringes, or "works" that have been or might have been used already
     by another person? How often do you share?
   Do you ever clean needles, syringes, or "works"? How do you clean?
   Do you clean needles, syringes, or "works" with bleach?
   Do you know where and how to obtain sterile syringes?
   Do you know how to inject in a sterile manner?

Adapted from: Gerber AR, Valdiserri RO, Holtgrave DR, et al. Preventive services guidelines for primary care clinicians caring for HIV-infected adults and adolescents. *Arch Fam Med.* 1993;2:969–979. Used with permission of the American Medical Association; copyright 1993.

gastrointestinal disorders, uncontrolled hypertension, impotence and other sexual disorders, and neuropathies.

4. Physical Examination

The physical examination is a relatively insensitive and nonspecific method of detecting alcohol or drug abuse. Some signs of alcohol abuse include weight gain or loss, labile or refractory hypertension, abnormal skin vascularization, conjunctival injection, tongue or hand tremor, epigastric tenderness, and hepatomegaly. Cocaine users may have damaged nasal mucosa and weight loss. Injection drug users may have hypodermic marks. Signs of previous or current trauma are other clues to substance abuse problems.

5. Laboratory Tests

Laboratory tests, such as measurement of liver enzymes and erythrocyte mean corpuscular volume, are helpful in evaluating physiological damage but are not good screening tools for detecting alcohol abuse. Determination of the gamma-glutamyl transferase (GGT) level is the most sensitive biochemical test for alcohol abuse, but this test has a sensitivity of only 25% to 36%. Screening of urine for drugs can help confirm drug use, but such screening provides no information about the quantity or frequency of use. An estimated 5% to 30% of positive drug screens are false positives, depending on the drug, the method of analysis, and the population being tested. In general, these tests should not be used as screening tools in the primary care setting, and certainly they should not be used without patient consent.

Basics of Counseling for Abuse of Alcohol and Other Drugs

1. Establish a Therapeutic Relationship

Express genuine concern and maintain an honest, nonjudgmental approach with substance-abuse patients. Avoid arguing with, confronting, or labeling the patient. Attempt to maintain a partnership with the patient, functioning as an expert consultant. Trust is essential; assure the patient that any information disclosed will be kept confidential to the maximum extent possible.

2. Make the Medical Office or Clinic Off-Limits for Substance Abuse

This policy should apply to use of tobacco, alcohol, and other drugs. Counseling a patient who is under the influence of alcohol or other drugs is not productive and may be counterproductive because of the indirect encouragement of abuse that it gives to the patient. Schedule return appointments for such patients to occur when they are not under the influence.

3. Present Information About Negative Health Consequences

Present such information in a straightforward, nonjudgmental manner. For example, "Your trouble sleeping, the difficulty in controlling your blood pressure, and the recent problems at home with your family make me concerned that alcohol may be the main problem. I would like to discuss this possibility with you more." Warn injection drug users about the risk of HIV infection, hepatitis B infection, and other disorders associated with using contaminated or shared needles. Counseling for injection drug users should also involve proper screening for conditions including infectious hepatitis and HIV (chapters 48 and 59).

4. Emphasize Personal Responsibility and Self-Efficacy

Convey to the patient a sense of optimism and confidence that he or she can control his or her substance use.

5. Convey a Clear Message and Set Goals

Communicate clearly and firmly to the patient a recommendation to stop substance abuse. Assist the patient in setting a date for abstinence or goals for step-wise moderation of substance use. Help the patient to anticipate physiologic and psychologic withdrawal symptoms and to plan for potential relapses or "slips."

6. Involve Family and Other Supports

The assistance and patience of family members can be critical for the success of the patient's efforts at abstinence or moderation. Involve others only with the patient's consent.

7. Establish a Working Relationship with Community Treatment Resources

Many patients may benefit from the structure provided by peer counseling, support groups, in-patient treatment, and other modalities. Become familiar with support and treatment resources available in the community so that appropriate referrals, if needed, can be made.

8. Provide Follow-Up

Monitoring and supporting patient success is essential and desirable, even for patients referred for treatment. Schedule return appointments at regular intervals, particularly during the first weeks of each patient's efforts to stop or moderate use.

Patient Resources

Alcohol: What to Do If It's a Problem for You. American Academy of Family Physicians, 8880 Ward Pkwy, Kansas City, MO 64114-2797; (800)944-0000. Internet address: http://www.aafp.org

Alcohol and Women. American College of Obstetricians and Gynecologists, 409 12th St, SW, Washington, DC 20024; (800)762-2264. Internet address: http://www.acog.com

Drugs and Pregnancy: Often the Two Don't Mix. FDA Office of Consumer Affairs. HFE 88 Room 1675, 5600 Fishers Ln, Rockville, MD 20857; (800)532-4440.

Let's Talk Facts about Substance Abuse. American Psychiatric Association, 1400 K St, NW, Washington, DC 20005; (800)368-5777. Internet address: http://www.psych.org

National Clearinghouse for Alcohol and Drug Information. For information about the numerous publications that are available in both English and Spanish, call: (800)729-6686.

Provider Resources:

Drug Abuse Screening Test. Internet address:
http://www.nida.nih.gov/Diagnosis-Treatment/DAST10.html

Michigan Alcohol Screening Test. Internet address:
http://www.silcom.com/~sbadp/Treatment/MAST.html

The Physician's Guide to Helping Patients With Alcohol Problems. National Institute on Alcohol Abuse and Alcoholism. NIH Publication No. 95-3769. 1995. Internet address:
http://www.niaaa.nih.gov/publications/publications.html

Selected References

American Academy of Family Physicians. *Summary of Policy Recommendations for Periodic Health Examination.* Kansas City, MO: American Academy of Family Physicians; 1997.

American College of Obstetricians and Gynecologists. *Guidelines for Women's Health Care.* Washington, DC: American College of Obstetricians and Gynecologists; 1996.

American College of Physicians. *Chemical Dependence.* Philadelphia, Pa: American College of Physicians; 1984.

American Medical Association, Council on Scientific Affairs. *Guidelines for Alcoholism Diagnosis, Treatment and Referral.* Chicago, Ill: American Medical Association; 1979.

American Medical Association. *Prescribing Controlled Drugs: Source Book.* Chicago, Ill: American Medical Association; 1986.

Babor TF. Alcohol and substance abuse in primary care settings. In: Mayfield J, Grady M, eds. *Primary Care Research: An Agenda for the 90s.* Washington, DC: US Department of Health and Human Services; 1990:113-124.

Babor TF, Ritson EB, Hodgson RJ. Alcohol-related problems in the primary health care setting: a review of early intervention strategies. *Br J Addict.* 1986;81:23-46.

Baird MA. Early detection of alcoholism. *Drug Therapy.* October 1990:29-39.

Barnes HN. Presenting the diagnosis: working with denial. In: Barnes HN, Aronson MD, Delbanco TL, eds. *Alcoholism: A Guide for the Primary Care Physician.* New York, NY: Springer-Verlag; 1987: chap 6.

Batki SL. Drug abuse, psychiatric disorders, and AIDS: dual and triple diagnosis. *West J Med.* 1990;152:547-552.

Bien TH, Miller WR, Tonigan JS. Brief interventions for alcohol problems. *Addiction.* 1993;88:315-336.

Bigby JA. Negotiating treatment and monitoring recovery. In: Barnes HN, Aronson MD, Delbanco TL, eds. *Alcoholism: A Guide for the Primary Care Physician.* New York, NY: Springer-Verlag; 1987: chap 7.

Brown RL. Identification and office management of alcohol and drug disorders. In: Fleming MF, Barry KL, eds. *Addictive Disorders.* St Louis, Mo: Mosby Year Book; 1992.

Bush B, Shaw S, Cleary P, Delbanco TL, Aronson MD. Screening for alcohol abuse using the CAGE questionnaire. *Am J Med.* 1987;82:231-235.

Canadian Task Force on the Periodic Health Examination. Early detection and counseling of problem drinking. In: *The Canadian Guide to Clinical Preventive Health Care*. Ottawa, Canada: Minister of Supply and Services; 1994: chap 42.

Centers for Disease Control and Prevention. Fetal alcohol syndrome—United States, 1979-1992. *MMWR*. 1993;42:339-341.

Colvin R. *Prescription Drug Abuse: The Hidden Epidemic*. Omaha, Neb: Addicts Books; 1995.

Cyr MG, Wartman SA. The effectiveness of routine screening questions in the detection of alcoholism. *JAMA*. 1988;259:51-54.

Delbanco TL. Patients who drink too much: where are their doctors? *JAMA*. 1992;267:702-703.

Ewing JA. Detecting alcoholism: the CAGE questionnaire. *JAMA*. 1984;252:1905-1907.

Gerstein DR, Lewin LS. Treating drug problems. *N Engl J Med*. 1990;323:844-848.

Inciardi JA. *Legal and Illicit Drug Use: Acute Reactions of Emergency Room Populations*. New York: Praeger Publishers; 1978.

Kamerow DB, Pincus HA, Macdonald DI. Alcohol abuse, other drug abuse, and mental disorders in medical practice. *JAMA*. 1986;255:2054-2057.

Magruder-Habib K, Durand M, Frey K. Alcohol abuse and alcoholism in primary health care setting. *J Fam Pract*. 1991;32:406-413.

Moore RD, Bone LR, Geller G, Marmon JA, Stokes EJ, Levine DM. Prevalence, detection, and treatment of alcoholism in hospitalized patients. *JAMA*. 1989;261:403-407.

National Institute on Alcohol Abuse and Alcoholism. *The Physician's Guide to Helping Patients With Alcohol Problems*. Bethesda, Md: US Department of Health and Human Services; 1995. NIH Publication No. 95-3769.

National Institute on Alcohol Abuse and Alcoholism. *Motivational Enhancement Therapy Manual: A Clinical Research Guide for Therapists Treating Individuals With Alcohol Abuse and Dependence*. vol 2. Rockville, Md: US Department of Health and Human Services; 1992. US Department of Health and Human Services Publication ADM 92-894.

National Institute on Alcohol Abuse and Alcoholism. *Seventh Special Report to the US Congress on Alcohol and Health*. Rockville, Md: US Department of Health and Human Services; 1990. US Department of Health and Human Services Publication Publication ADM 90-1656.

Pokorny AD, Miller BA & Kaplan HB. The Brief MAST: A shortened version of the Michigan Alcohol Screening Test. *Am J Psychiatry*. 1972: 129: 342-345.

Rush BR. The use of family medical practices by patients with drinking problems. *Can Med Assoc J*. 1989;140:35-39.

Saunders JB, Aasland OG, Babor TF, de la Fuente JR, Grant M. Development of the Alcohol Use Disorders Identification Test (AUDIT): World Health Organization collaborative Project on Early Detection of Persons with Harmful Alcohol Consumption—II. *Addiction*. 1993;88: 791-804.

Selzer ML. The Michigan Alcoholism Screening Test: the quest for a new diagnostic instrument. *Am J Psychiatry*. 1971;127:89-94.

Skinner HA. The Drug Abuse Screening Test. *Addict Behav*. 1982;7:363-371.

US Preventive Services Task Force. Screening for drug abuse. In: *Guide to Clinical Preventive Services*. 2nd ed. Washington, DC: US Department of Health and Human Services; 1996: chap 53.

US Preventive Services Task Force. Screening for problem drinking. In: *Guide to Clinical Preventive Services*. 2nd ed. Washington, DC: US Department of Health and Human Services; 1996: chap 52.

Walsh DC, Hingson RW, Merrigan DM, et al. The impact of a physician's warning on recovery after alcoholism treatment. *JAMA*. 1992;267:663-667.

54

DENTAL AND ORAL HEALTH

Most Americans are affected by dental and oral health problems at some point in their lives. The most common problems are dental caries (tooth decay) and periodontal diseases, both of which are largely preventable. Although dental caries is more commonly thought of as a childhood disease, adults continue to be at risk for dental decay throughout their lives. The Third National Health and Nutrition Examination Survey (NHANES III) found that 94% of persons older than age 18 years had either untreated decay or fillings in the crowns of their teeth. On average, American adults had 22 decayed or filled coronal surfaces. Root-surface decay associated with gingival recession is a particular concern in older adults. Moderate loss of gingival attachment was present in almost 40% of all Americans. This problem increased significantly with age: 82% of persons older than age 65 years had attachment loss. Periodontal diseases and caries are the predominant causes of tooth loss. Oral mucosal lesions of all types are also prevalent (10% to 25%) in adult and elderly populations.

Numerous clinical trials have demonstrated that personal oral hygiene measures can help control plaque and gingivitis in most individuals. Progression of periodontal diseases can be retarded by the combination of excellent personal oral hygiene practices and regular professional care. Routine use of dentifrices with fluoride has been shown to prevent both coronal and root-surface caries in adult populations.

Oral cancer is also a major concern among adults. In the United States, one person dies from cancers of the oral cavity and pharynx every hour (8000 deaths annually). Some 30,000 individuals are diagnosed with these cancers each year—2% of cancers diagnosed in the US. Men are affected twice as often as women, and 90% of these cancers occur in those over 45 years of age. Use of tobacco in all forms and heavy consumption of alcohol are major causal factors.

See chapter 19 for information on counseling children and adolescents on dental and oral health. See chapter 30 for a discussion of the oral cavity examination.

Recommendations of Major Authorities

American Cancer Society—Patients should be counseled about oral health during cancer-related checkups, which should occur every 3 years for those aged 20 to 40 years, and then yearly for those over 40.

American College of Obstetricians and Gynecologists—Dental hygiene should be included in counseling as part of periodic evaluation visits, which should occur yearly or as appropriate.

American Dental Association—Adults should be seen for routine dental care, preventive services, including oral cancer screening, and oral hygiene counseling at least once every year. This recommendation applies to patients with full dentures as well as patients "with teeth."

Canadian Task Force on the Periodic Health Examination— There is good evidence that the following clinical or personal interventions are effective in preventing dental caries: use of dentifrices containing fluoride; fluoride supplements for patients in areas where there is a low level (0.3 ppm or less) of fluoride in the drinking water; professionally applied topical fluoride and the use of fluoride mouth rinses for patients with very active decay or at a high risk of dental caries; and a selective use of professionally applied fissure sealants on permanent molar teeth. There is poor evidence for: fluoride treatments and fluoride mouth rinses for patients with a low risk of caries; toothbrushing (without a dentifrice containing fluoride) and flossing; professional cleaning of teeth before a fluoride treatment or at a dental visit; and dietary counseling for the general population. There is good evidence to recommend against the use of over-the-counter fluoride mouth rinses by the general population.

US Preventive Services Task Force—Counseling patients to visit a dental provider on a regular basis is recommended based on evidence for risk reduction from such visits when combined with regular personal oral hygiene; the effectiveness of advising patients to visit a dental care provider has not been evaluated. There is little evidence regarding the optimal frequency of visits; this recommendation should be made by the patient's dental care provider. Counseling all patients to brush their teeth daily with fluoride-containing toothpaste and to clean thoroughly between their teeth with dental floss each day is recommended based on the proven efficacy of risk reduction from doing so; the effectiveness of clinician counseling to encourage these behaviors has not been adequately evaluated. When examining the mouth, clinicians should be alert for obvious signs of untreated tooth decay or mottling, inflamed or cyanotic gingiva, loose teeth, and severe halitosis and for signs and symptoms of oral cancer and premalignancy in persons who use tobacco or excessive amounts of alcohol.

Basics of Dental and Oral Health Counseling

1. Encourage all patients (including older adults and edentulous persons) to see an oral health care professional regularly for preventive care. Patients who may need frequent dental care include diabetics; tobacco and alcohol users; persons who are immunocompromised; those with decreased salivary flow (xerostomia), which is caused by many commonly prescribed medications (Table 54.1); persons with Sjögren's syndrome; and persons exposed to head and neck irradiation.

2. Encourage all patients to brush their teeth daily with a fluoride-containing toothpaste and to use dental floss each day.

3. Encourage individuals who have a history of frequent caries to reduce their intake of foods containing refined sugars and to avoid sugary between-meal snacks. Such patients may also benefit from use of a fluoride-containing mouth rinse.

4. Counsel patients not to use of tobacco in any form (chapter 60) and to limit alcohol consumption (chapter 53).

Table 54.1. Effects of Selected Drugs

Effect	Medication
Xerostomia	Anticholinergics, antidepressants, antihypertensives, antipsychotics, diuretics, gastrointestinals, systemic antihistamines/decongestants, systemic bronchodilators
Soft tissue reactions	Methyldopa, barbiturates, sulfonamides, penicillamine, gold salts, chloroquine, isoniazid
Altered host resistance	Antibiotics, insulin, oral hypoglycemics, systemic corticosteroids
Gingival overgrowth	Phenytoin, nifedipine, cyclosporine, diltiazem
Interactions with dental drugs	Barbiturates, benzodiazepines, muscle relaxants, sedative-hypnotics, nonsteroidal anti-inflammatory agents, opiate analgesics

Adapted from: Park BZ, Kinney MB, Steffensen JEM. Putting your teeth into your physical exam. 2: adults. *J Fam Pract.* 1992;35:585–587. Used with permission of the authors and Appleton & Lange; copyright 1992.

5. Encourage individuals who are excessively exposed to sunlight to protect their lips and skin from the harmful effects of ultraviolet rays by using sunscreens and lip balms with an SPF of 15 or more, to wear protective clothing such as hats, and to avoid direct sun exposure between the hours of 10:00 am and 3:00 pm.

6. Encourage individuals who engage in sports that have the potential for oral and dental trauma to use appropriate protective equipment, including headgear and mouth guards. Urge all patients to wear safety belts while in motor vehicles and helmets while riding bicycles and motorcycles.

7. Encourage patients, especially those who use tobacco or alcohol, to see a dentist or physician if they notice any irregularities in the oral cavity—such as color changes, cracks, ulcers, bleeding; or swelling or thickening in the lips, cheeks, gums, tongue, or roof of the mouth—that last longer than 2 weeks.

Table 54.2. Cardiac Conditions* for Which Endocarditis Prophylaxis Is and Is Not Recommended

---

Prophylaxis recommended	Prophylaxis NOT recommended
Prosthetic cardiac valves, including bioprosthetic and homograft valves	Isolated secundum atrial septal defect
Previous bacterial endocarditis, even in the absence of heart disease	Surgical repair, without residua, beyond 6 months for: secundum atrial septal defect, ventricular septal defect, patent ductus arteriosus
Surgically constructed systemic-pulmonary shunts	Previous coronary artery bypass surgery
Most congenital cardiac malformations	Mitral valve prolapse without valvular regurgitation†
Rheumatic and other acquired valvular dysfunction, even after valve surgery	Physiologic, functional, or innocent heart murmurs
Hypertrophic cardiomyopathy	Previous Kawasaki disease without valvular dysfunction
Mitral valve prolapse with valvular regurgitation	Previous rheumatic fever without valvular dysfunction
	Cardiac pacemakers and implanted defibrillators

---

*This table lists selected conditions and is not all-inclusive.

†Persons who have mitral valve prolapse associated with thickening and/or redundancy of valve leaflet(s) may be at increased risk for bacterial endocarditis, particularly men 45 years of age or older.

Adapted from: Dajani AS, Bisno AL, Chung KJ, et al. Prevention of bacterial endocarditis: recommendations by the American Heart Association. *JAMA.* 1990;264:2919–2922. Used with permission from the American Medical Association; copyright 1990.

Table 54.3. Standard Antibiotic Prophylaxis Regimens for Dental or Operative Procedures in the Oral Cavity of Patients Subject to Bacterial Endocarditis*

For patients able to take amoxicillin/penicillin†
Amoxicillin, 3 g orally 1 hr before procedure, then 1.5 g 6 hrs after initial dose

For amoxicillin/pencillin-allergic patients†
Erythromycin ethylsuccinate, 800 mg, or erythromycin stearate, 1 g, orally 2 hrs before procedure, then half the dose 6 hrs after initial dose
OR
Clindamycin, 300 mg orally 1 hr before procedure and 150 mg 6 hrs after initial dose

*Includes those with prosthetic heart valve and other high-risk patients

†Initial pediatric doses are as follows: amoxicillin, 50 mg/kg; erythromycin ethylsuccinate or stearate, 20 mg/kg; clindamycin, 10 mg/kg. Follow-up dose 6 hrs later should be half the initial dose. Total pediatric dose should not exceed total adult dose.

From: Dajani AS, Bisno AL, Chung KJ, et al. Prevention of bacterial endocarditis: recommendations by the American Heart Association. *JAMA.* 1990;264:2919–2922. Used with permission from the American Medical Association; copyright 1990.

8. Counsel patients about the oral effects and complications of medications (Table 54.1).

9. Transient bacteremia is common during dental procedures, including cleaning. Provide antibiotic prophylaxis to patients with certain cardiac conditions before they undergo dental cleaning or other procedures known to induce gingival or mucosal bleeding (Tables 54.2 and 54.3).

Patient Resources

Dental Emergency Procedures; Seal Out Decay; Smokeless Tobacco: Think Before You Chew. American Dental Association, Department of Salable Materials, 211 E Chicago Ave, Chicago, IL 60611; (800)947-4746.

Diet and Dental Health; Smoking Can Really Do a Number on Your Health; Oral Health Care Guidelines for Special Patients (11 different guideline booklets). To order these and other materials, contact the American Dental Association, Department of Salable Materials, 211 E Chicago Ave, Chicago, IL 60611; (800)947-4746.

For a Lifetime of Smiles.... To order this and other material, contact the American Dental Hygienists' Association, 444 N Michigan Ave, Suite 3400, Chicago, IL 60611; (312) 440-8900. Internet address: http://www.adha.org

Dental Tips for Diabetics (English and Spanish); *Dry Mouth (Xerostomia); Fever Blisters and Canker Sores; Fluorides Aren't Just for Kids* (poster); *Periodontal Dis-*

ease and Diabetes: A Guide for Patients; Fluoride to Protect the Teeth of Adults. National Institute of Dental Research, Bldg 31 Room 2C35, 31 Center Dr, MSC 2290, Bethesda, MD 20890-2290; (301) 496-4261. Internet address: http://www.nidr.nih.gov

What You Need to Know About Oral Cancer. Office of Cancer Communications, National Cancer Institute, Bldg 31, Room 10A16, Bethesda MD 20892; (800)4-CANCER.

Provider Resources

Detection and Prevention of Periodontal Disease: A Guide for Health Care Providers. National Institute of Dental Research, Bldg 31, Room 2C35, 31 Center Dr, MSC 2290, Bethesda MD, 20890-2290; (301) 496-4261. Internet address: http://www.nidr.nih.gov

Getting the Picture on Dental X Rays. To order this and other publications, contact the FDA Office of Consumer Affairs. HFE 88 Room 1675, 5600 Fishers Ln, Rockville, MD 20857; (800)532-4440.

Selected References

American Cancer Society. *Cancer Facts and Figures-1996*. Atlanta, Ga: American Cancer Society; 1996.

American Dental Association. *Statement on Diet and Dental Caries*. Chicago, Ill: American Dental Association; 1982.

American Dental Association. Current preventive concepts. In: *Accepted Dental Therapeutics*. 40th ed. Chicago, Ill: American Dental Association; 1984.

American Dental Association. *Importance of Professional Teeth Cleaning*. Chicago, Ill: American Dental Association; 1985.

Brown LJ, Brunelle JA, Kingman A. Periodontal status in the United States, 1988-91: prevalence, extent and demographic variation. *J Dent Res*. 1996;75:672-683.

Canadian Task Force on the Periodic Health Examination. Prevention of periodontal disease. In: *The Canadian Guide to Clinical Preventive Health Care*. Ottawa, Canada: Minister of Supply and Services; 1994: chap 37.

Centers for Disease Control. Deaths from oral cavity and pharyngeal cancer—United States, 1987. *MMWR*. 1991;39:457-472.

Dajani AS, Bisno AL, Chung KJ, et al. Prevention of bacterial endocarditis: recommendations by the American Heart Association. *JAMA*. 1990;264:2919-2922.

Greene JC, Louie R, Wycoff SJ. US Preventive Services Task Force: preventive dentistry: I. dental caries. *JAMA*. 1989;262:3459-3563.

Greene JC, Louie R, Wycoff SJ. US Preventive Services Task Force: preventive dentistry: II. periodontal diseases, malocclusion, trauma, and oral cancer. *JAMA*. 1990;263;421-423.

Kaste LM, Gift HC, Bhat M, Swango PA. Prevalence of Incisor trauma in persons 6 to 50 years of age: United States, 1988-1991. *J Dent Res*. 1996; 75:696-705.

Lewis DW, Ismail AI. Canadian Task Force on the Periodic Health Examination. Periodic health examination, 1995 update: 2. Prevention of dental caries. *Can Med Assn J*. 1995: 152(6):836-846.

Mandel ID. Preventive dental services for the elderly. *Dent Clin North Am*. 1989;33:81-90.

Niessen LC, George CW. Oral health. *Md Med J*. 1989;38:126-128.

Park BZ, Kinney MB, Steffensen JEM. Putting teeth into your physical exam. 2: adults. *J Fam Pract*. 1992;35:585-587.

Thomas JE, Faecher RS. A physician's guide to early detection of oral cancer. *Geriatrics*. 1992; 47:58-63.

US Preventive Services Task Force. Counseling to prevent dental and periodontal disease. In: *Guide to Clinical Preventive Services*. 2nd ed. Washington, DC: US Department of Health and Human Services; 1996: chap 61.

White BA, Albertini TF, Brown LJ, et al. Selected restoration and tooth conditions: United States, 1988-1991. *J Dent Res*. 1996;75:661-671.

Winn DM, Brunelle JA, Selwitz RH, et al. Coronal and root caries in the dentition of adults in the United States, 1988-1991. *J Dent Res*. 1996;75:642-651.

55

INJURY AND DOMESTIC VIOLENCE PREVENTION

Unintentional injuries are the fifth leading cause of death in the United States and the leading cause of death among persons ages 1 to 44 years. Motor vehicle crashes account for half of all unintentional injury deaths. Alcohol is a contributing factor in 20% of non-fatal and 40% of fatal motor vehicle crashes. Nationwide, seat belt use is estimated to be 68%; however, in fatal crashes, seat belt use is lower than 50%. Other major causes of unintentional injury deaths are falls, poisoning, drowning, and residential fires.

Unintentional injury is also a major cause of morbidity and mortality for older adults. Falls are the second leading cause of injury death for adults ages 65-84 years and the leading cause of injury death for those 85 years and older. The number of deaths attributable to falls in the group aged 65 to 74 years is twice that in the general population; among persons older than age 85 years, the fall-related death rate is 15 times that in the general population. Hip fracture is the most common fall-related injury leading to hospitalization in older adults. Roughly half of all persons sustaining hip fractures never regain full function. According to Lindsay, annual expenditures in the United States related to hip fractures are estimated to be between $10 and $20 billion.

Domestic violence is an important health risk for many women. Injury to women as a result of partner abuse is of special concern to primary care clinicians since high rates of violent assault have been detected in patients seen in general medical practices, prenatal clinics, urgent care centers and emergency departments. Although the majority of adults abused by their partners are females, men are also affected by partner violence. Estimates of the magnitude of partner violence vary depending on the data source. Bachman and Saltzman found that over 1 million women and nearly 150,000 men are victims of partner violence each year. Other investigators report that between 2 and 4 million American women each year are victims of partner abuse and that more than 1 million women seek assistance for injuries caused by battering. Abuse of women knows no socioeconomic, racial, ethnic, religious, or age barriers. The risk for domestic violence increases during pregnancy and after separation or divorce. The consequences of partner abuse are serious and alarming ranging from injury to aggravated battery to death. In approximately 30% of all female homicides in the US, the killer is an intimate.

Although primary care clinicians treat a wide range of injuries, studies indicate that they deliver little counseling to adults about injury prevention and do not detect and treat domestic violence in an optimal manner. Considering the amount of death and disability caused by preventable injuries and violence, these topics should be discussed with all patients.

See chapter 26 for information on counseling children and adolescents on violent behavior and firearms; chapter 22 for related information on counseling children and adolescents on safety; chapter 5 for information about screening children and adolescents for depression and suicide; and chapter 33 for information about screening adults for depression.

Recommendations of Major Authorities

Unintentional Injuries

> Most major authorities, including **American College of Physicians, Canadian Task Force on the Periodic Health Examination, National Transportation Safety Board,** and **US Preventive Services Task Force**—Health-care professionals should counsel patients on automobile safety restraint use.
>
> **American Academy of Family Physicians**—Counsel about unintentional injury prevention, including, as appropriate, child safety seats, lap and shoulder belt use, bicycle safety, motorcycle helmet use, smoke detectors, poison control center numbers, and driving while intoxicated.
>
> **American College of Obstetricians and Gynecologists**—Injury prevention should be part of the evaluation and counseling portions of the periodic examination of women of all ages, with particular attention to safety belts and safety helmets, firearms, recreational and occupational hazards, and sports involvement.
>
> **Canadian Task Force on the Periodic Health Examination**—Expert opinion suggests that many patients seen by clinicians could potentially benefit from counseling to modify their injury prone behaviors. In actual practice, however, it is not known how effectively clinicians can alter these behaviors. Since unintentional injuries represent a leading cause of death and nonfatal injury, even modest successes through clinical interventions could have major public health value. Counseling is most relevant for those at increased risk of injury, such as adolescents and young adults, persons who use alcohol and other drugs, and persons with medical conditions that may impair motor vehicle safety. The optimal frequency for counseling patients about unintentional injury has not been determined and is left to clinical discretion. There is insufficient evidence to support including assessment and counseling of elderly patients for the risk of falling in the routine health examination of the elderly. It

may be included, however, on other grounds. There is good evidence for referring elderly patients to multidisciplinary post-fall assessment teams where such a service is available.

US Preventive Services Task Force—Counseling to prevent household and environmental injuries is recommended for adolescents and adults based on the proven efficacy of risk reduction, although the effectiveness of counseling these patients to prevent injuries has not been adequately evaluated. Persons with alcohol or drug problems should be identified and counseled and their progress monitored. Those who use alcohol or illicit drugs should be warned against engaging in potentially dangerous activities while intoxicated. Counseling elderly patients on specific measures to reduce the risk of falling is recommended based on fair evidence that these measures reduce the risk of falls, although the effectiveness of counseling elders to prevent falls has not been adequately evaluated. There is insufficient evidence to recommend for or against the use of external hip protectors to prevent fall injuries, but recommendations for their use in institutionalized elderly may be made on other grounds. More intensive individualized multifactorial intervention is recommended for high-risk elderly patients in settings where adequate resources to deliver such services are available.

Violence/Abuse

American College of Obstetricians and Gynecologists—Women ages 19 to 64 should be counseled on domestic violence as part of periodic evaluation visits, which should occur yearly or as appropriate. Women ages 13 to 18 and over 65 should be counseled on abuse and neglect as part of periodic evaluation visits, which should occur yearly or as appropriate.

American Medical Association—All female patients in emergency, surgical, primary care, pediatric, prenatal, and mental health settings should be screened for domestic violence. Every clinical setting should have a protocol for detection and assessment of elder mistreatment. The physician should assure that a comprehensive medical examination is conducted with elderly patients and the results documented. Physicians can play a critical role in identifying, treating, and preventing elder abuse and neglect in institutional settings. Physicians must be aware of the requirements for reporting elder abuse to adult protective services in the state(s) in which they practice.

American Nurses Association—All women should receive routine assessment and documentation for physical abuse in any health care institution or community setting. Women at increased risk of abuse, such as pregnant women and women presenting in emergency rooms, should receive targeted assessment.

US Preventive Services Task Force—There is insufficient evidence to recommend for or against the use of specific screening instruments for family violence, but including a few direct questions about abuse (physical violence or forced sexual activity) as part of the routine history in adult patients may be recommended on other grounds. These other grounds include the substantial prevalence of undetected abuse among adult female patients, the potential value of this information in the care of the patient, and the low cost and low risk of harm from such screening. All clinicians should be alert to physical and behavioral signs and symptoms associated with abuse and neglect. All individuals who present with multiple injuries and an implausible explanation should be evaluated with attention to possible abuse or neglect. Injured pregnant women and elderly patients should receive special consideration for this problem. Suspected cases of abuse should receive proper documentation of the incident and physical findings (eg, photographs, body maps); treatment of physical injuries; arrangements for counseling by a skilled mental health professional; and the telephone numbers of local crisis centers, shelters, and protective service agencies.

Basics of Injury Prevention Counseling

Adults

1. Make safety counseling an integral part of the primary care practice. Include questions about safety issues on intake questionnaires. Enter significant safety issues on the patient problem list. Keep a record of any counseling interventions that are delivered to patients. Tailor interventions to address concerns and motivations that are important to the patient. Take care to avoid sounding moralistic.

2. Advise all patients to use safety belts when operating or riding in a motor vehicle. Table 55.1 provides guidelines on proper safety belt use.

Table 55.1. Proper Safety Belt Use

The belt should be worn over the shoulder, across the chest, and low on the lap, avoiding excess slack—not behind the back, under the arm, or over the abdomen.

Safety belts should be worn even for short trips. Three out of four motor vehicle crashes occur within 25 miles of home. Unbelted motorists have been killed in crashes when going as slowly as 12 miles per hour.

Safety belts should be worn even when the automobile has airbags.

Adapted from: National Committee for Injury Prevention and Control. Injury prevention: meeting the challenge. *Am J Prev Med.* 1989;5(suppl):1–303. Used with permission of Oxford University Press Journals; copyright 1989.

3. Counsel all patients on the importance of not consuming alcohol when driving, boating, swimming, and using motorized tools and firearms. Encourage use of a nondrinking "designated driver" for return trips from parties and other events at which alcohol will be available.

4. Counsel all patients to wear safety helmets while operating or riding motorcycles or bicycles and to wear mouth guards when playing contact sports.

5. Counsel all patients to install and maintain smoke detectors in their residences and to change the batteries yearly or, if needed, every 6 months. A good way to remember this is to do it when resetting clocks in the spring and fall. Encourage testing of smoke detectors monthly to make sure they are operating correctly.

6. Advise patients about the dangers of keeping guns in the home. Many more children, friends, and family members than intruders are killed every year by guns in the home. If guns are kept in the home, they should be unloaded and locked in a secure location separate from ammunition.

7. Counsel patients to be aware of the hazards and safety rules at the work site. Counsel patients who are at increased risk of back injuries because of occupation or personal history to learn safe lifting techniques and to perform appropriate back-strengthening exercises.

Older Adults

1. Counsel older adults or their caretakers to periodically:

   - Inspect the home for adequate lighting
   - Remove or repair floor structures that predispose to tripping, such as loose rugs, electrical cords, and toys
   - Install handrails and traction strips in stairways and bathtubs
   - Keep hot water set at 49°C (120°F) or lower.

   Safety counseling can be facilitated by advising the patient or caretaker to use a home-safety checklist (Table 55-2). Home visits are also an excellent opportunity to assess home safety for older adults.

2. Periodically check the visual acuity (chapter 45) and assess the physical mobility of patients.

3. Avoid prescribing drugs that increase the risk of falls (ie, long-acting benzodiazepines, tricyclic antidepressants, major tranquilizers, and other sedatives); if such drugs are prescribed, closely monitor the patient. Many falls in older adults are attributable to side effects from polypharmacy (chapter 58).

Table 55.2. Home Safety Checklist for Older Adults

Place a check mark next to each question if the answer is yes. Discuss unmarked items with patient.

Housekeeping
____ Do you clean up spills as soon as they occur?
____ Do you keep floors and stairways clean and free of clutter?
____ Do you put away books, magazines, sewing supplies, and other objects as soon as you are through with them and never leave them on floors or stairways?
____ Do you store frequently used items on shelves that are within easy reach?

Floors
____ Do you keep everyone from walking on freshly washed floors before they are dry?
____ If you wax floors, do you apply two thin coats and buff each thoroughly or use self-polishing wax?
____ Do all area rugs have nonslip backings?
____ Have you eliminated small rugs at the tops and bottoms of stairways?
____ Are all carpet edges tacked down?
____ Are rugs and carpets free of curled edges, worn sports, and rips?
____ Have you chosen rugs and carpets with short, dense pile?
____ Are rugs and carpets installed over good quality, medium thick pads?

Lighting
____ Do you have light switches near every doorway?
____ Do you have enough good lighting to eliminate shadowy areas?
____ Do you have a lamp or light switch within easy reach of every bed?
____ Do you have night lights in your bathrooms and in hallways leading from bedrooms to bathrooms?
____ Are all stairways well lighted with light switches at both top and bottom?

Bathrooms
____ Do you use a rubber mat or nonslip decals in tubs and showers?
____ Do you have a grab bar securely anchored over each tub and shower?
____ Do you have a nonslip rug on all bathroom floors?
____ Do you keep soap in easy-to-reach receptacles?

Traffic Lanes
____ Can you walk across every room in your home, and from one room to another, without detouring around furniture?
____ Is the traffic lane from your bedroom to the bathroom free of obstacles?
____ Are telephone and appliance cords kept away from areas where people walk?

Stairways
____ Do securely fastened handrails extend the full length of the stairs on each side of the stairways?
____ Do the handrails stand out from the walls so you can get a good grip?
____ Are handrails distinctly shaped so you are alerted when you reach the end of a stairway?
____ Are all stairways in good condition with no broken, sagging, or sloping steps?
____ Are all stairway carpeting and metal edges securely fastened and in good condition?
____ Have you replaced any single-level steps with gradually rising ramps or made sure such steps are well lighted?

continued

Table 55.2. Home Safety Checklist for Older Adults—*Continued*

Ladders and Step Stools
____ Do you always use a step stool or ladder that is tall enough for the job?
____ Do you always set up your ladder or step stool on a firm, level base that is free of clutter?
____ Before you climb a ladder or step stool, do you always make sure it is fully open and that the stepladder spreaders are locked?
____ When you use a ladder or step stool, do you face the steps and keep your body between the side rails?
____ Do you avoid standing on the top step of a step stool or climbing beyond the second step from the top on a stepladder?

Outdoor Areas
____ Are walks and driveways in your yard and other areas free of breaks?
____ Are lawns and garden free of holes?
____ Do you put away garden tools and hoses when they are not in use?
____ Are outdoor areas kept free of rocks, loose boards, and other tripping hazards?
____ Do you keep outdoor walkways, steps, and porches free of wet leaves and snow?
____ Do you sprinkle icy outdoor areas with de-icers as soon as possible after a snowfall or freeze?
____ Do you have mats at doorways for people to wipe their feet on?
____ Do you know the safest way of walking when you can't avoid walking on a slippery surface?

Footwear
____ Do your shoes have soles and heels that provide good traction?
____ Do you avoid walking in stocking feet and wear house slippers that fit well and don't fall off?
____ Do you wear low-heeled oxfords, loafers, or good quality sneakers when you work in your house or yard?
____ Do you replace boots or galoshes when their soles or heels are worn too smooth to keep you from slipping on wet or icy surfaces?

Personal Precautions
____ Are you always alert for unexpected hazards, such as out-of-place furniture?
____ If young children visit or live in your home, are you alert for children playing on the floor and toys left in your path?
____ If you have pets, are you alert for sudden movements across your path and pets getting underfoot?
____ When you carry packages, do you divide them into smaller loads and make sure they do not obstruct your vision?
____ When you reach or bend, do you hold onto a firm support and avoid throwing your head back or turning it too far?
____ Do you always move deliberately and avoid rushing to answer the phone or doorbell?
____ Do you take time to get your balance when you change position from lying down to sitting and from sitting to standing?
____ Do you keep yourself in good condition with moderate exercise, good diet, adequate rest, and regular medical checkups?
____ If you wear glasses, is your prescription up to date?
____ Do you know how to reduce injury in a fall?
____ If you live alone, do you have daily contact with a friend or neighbor?

Adapted from: National Safety Council. *Falling—The Unexpected Trip: A Safety Program for Older Adults* (Program Leader's Guide). Chicago, Ill: National Safety Council; 1982. Used with permission of the National Safety Council; copyright 1982.

4. Encourage older adults without medical contraindications to engage in an exercise program to maintain muscle and bone strength, mobility, and flexibility.

5. Assess the need for estrogen replacement therapy to help prevent fractures from osteoporosis in postmenopausal women (chapter 47). Also assess the need for counseling about weight-bearing exercises, calcium supplementation, and other nutritional issues in these women.

Basics of Detecting and Counseling Women Who are Victims of Partner Violence

1. Violence toward women can sometimes be detected on physical examination. The areas most commonly injured in women are the head, neck, chest, abdomen, breasts, and upper extremities. Burns, bruises in patterns resembling hands, belts, cords, or other weapons, and multiple traumatic injuries may be seen.

2. Particular attention should be paid to patients who present repeatedly with somatic complaints such as headaches, insomnia, choking sensation, hyperventilation, gastrointestinal symptoms, and pain in the chest, back, and pelvis.

3. Ask women directly and in a caring and nonjudgmental manner whether they have been physically abused (you may have to ask their partner to leave the exam room). Posing questions such as "did someone you care about do this to you?" or "I am so concerned about the amount of violence in families that I am asking all my patients about it... do you ever feel threatened at home?" are appropriate ways to introduce the subject. Additional questions are listed in Table 55.3.

4. If a woman discloses battering, acknowledge the problem, affirm that it is unacceptable, and advise that she is at risk for future episodes. Let her know that battering is a common problem; she may believe that she is the only one experiencing violence perpetuated by a loved one. She needs to know that she is not alone and that help is available. The patient also needs to know that she does not deserve to be beaten; violence is not an acceptable way to communicate discontent.

5. Have a plan for providing information to abused women. Be sure to include information about community, social, and legal resources; legal rights; and a plan for dealing with the abusive partner. Local referral numbers for such resources can be obtained from the National Council on Child Abuse and Family Violence, (800)222-2000.

Table 55.3. Recommended Questions for Clinicians to Ask Potential Victims of Abuse

Have you been hit, kicked, punched, or otherwise hurt by someone in the past year? If so, by whom?

Are you currently in a relationship in which you have been physically hurt or threatened by your partner?

Have you ever been in such a relationship?

Are you in a relationship in which you are treated badly? In what way?

Has your partner ever destroyed things that you cared about?

Has your partner ever threatened or abused your children?

Has your partner ever forced you to have sex when you didn't want to? Have you been forced to engage in sex that makes you uncomfortable?

We all fight at home. What happens when you and your partner fight or disagree?

Do you ever feel afraid of your partner?

Has your partner ever prevented you from leaving the house, seeking friends, getting a job, or continuing your education?

How does your partner act when drinking or on drugs? Is your partner ever verbally or physically abusive?

Do you have guns in your home? Has your partner ever threatened to use them when angry?

Have police been called to your home because of a partner dispute?

Adapted from: American Medical Association. *Diagnostic and Treatment Guidelines on Domestic Violence.* Chicago, Ill: American Medical Association, 1992. Used with permission of the American Medical Association, copyright 1993.

Patient Resources

Auto Safety Hot Line. National Highway Traffic Safety Administration: (800)424-9393

National Highway Traffic Safety Administration, Office of Occupant Protection, NTS-13, 400 7th St, SW, Washington, DC 20590; (202) 366-2727.

Age Page—Accident Prevention and the Elderly; Age Page—Preventing Falls and Fractures. National Institute on Aging, Bldg 31, Room 5C27, 31 Center Dr,

MSC 2922, Bethesda, MD 20892-2922; (310)496-1752. Internet address: http://www.nih.gov/nia/health/pubpub/pubpub.htm

The Abused Woman. American College of Obstetricians and Gynecologists, 409 12th St, SW, Washington, DC 20024-2188; (202)638-5577. Internet address: http:www.agog.com

Your Home Safety Checklist; Preventing Falls: A Safety Program for Older Adults; Facts About Backs; Playing it Safe: A Pocket Guide to Fitness. To order these and other materials, contact the National Safety Council, 444 N Michigan Ave, Chicago, IL 60601; (800)621-7619, ext 1300.

US Consumer Product Safety Commission, Publication Requests, Washington, DC 20207. Pamphlets on preventing injuries from toys, household goods, and other common items. (800)638-2772 (English and Spanish).

US Consumer Product Safety Commission, Washington, DC 20207. Recorded messages in both English and Spanish. (800)638-2772.

Provider Resources

Domestic Violence. ACOG Technical Bulletin # 209. American College of Obstetricians and Gynecologists, 409 12th St SW, Washington, DC 20024-2188; (202) 638-5577. Internet address: http://www.acog.com

Diagnostic and Treatment Guidelines on Domestic Violence. American Medical Association, Department of Mental Health, 515 N State St, Chicago, IL 60610; (312) 464-5066. Internet address: http://www.ama-assn.org

What Can You Do About Family Violence? (#NC110992) American Medical Association, 515 N State St, Chicago, IL 60610; (800)621-8335. Internet address: http://www.ama-assn.org

Injury Control News. Association for the Advancement of Injury Control, Attn: Harry Teter, 888 17th St NW Suite 1000, Washington, DC 20006; (202) 296-6161.

Auto Safety Hot Line. National Highway Traffic Safety Administration: (800)424-9393.

National Highway Traffic Safety Administration, Office of Occupant Protection, NTS-13, 400 7th St SW, Washington, DC 20590; (202) 366-2727.

Understanding Violence Against Women (Crowell and Burgess, eds.). National Academy Press, 2101 Constitution Ave., NW, Washington DC 20418. (800)624-6242.

US Consumer Product Safety Commission, Washington, DC 20207. For recorded messages in both English and Spanish, call: (800)638-2772.

US Consumer Product Safety Commission, Publication Requests, Washington, DC 20207. Pamphlets on preventing injuries from toys, household goods, and other common items. (800)638-2772 (English and Spanish).

Selected References

American College of Physicians. *Health Promotion/Disease Prevention: Seat Belt Use*. Philadelphia, Pa: American College of Physicians; 1984.

American Academy of Family Physicians. *Summary of Policy Recommendations for Periodic Health Examination*. Kansas City, Mo: American Academy of Family Physicians; 1997.

American College of Obstetricians and Gynecologists. *Guidelines for Women's Health Care*. Washington, DC: American College of Obstetricians and Gynecologists; 1996.

American Medical Association. *Diagnostic and Treatment Guidelines on Domestic Violence*. Chicago, Ill: American Medical Association; 1992.

American Medical Association. *Diagnostic and Treatment Guidelines on Elder Abuse and Neglect*. Chicago, Ill: American Medical Association; 1992.

American Medical Association, Council on Scientific Affairs. Violence against women: relevance for medical practitioners. *JAMA*. 1992;267:3184-3189.

American Nurses Association. *Position Statement on Physical Violence Against Women*. Washington, DC: American Nurses Association; 1991.

Baker SP, O'Neill B, Ginsberg, Li G. *The Injury Fact Book*. New York, NY: Oxford University Press; 1995.

Bachman R, Saltzman LE. *Violence Against Women: Estimates from the Redesigned Survey: Bureau of Justice Statistics Special Report*. Washington DC: US Department of Justice; 1995 Publication NCJ-154348.

Blincoe, LJ. *The Economic Cost of Motor Vehicle Crashes*, 1994. NHTSA Technical Report. July, 1996. Washington DC: National Highway Traffic Safety Administration

Canadian Task Force on the Periodic Health Examination. Prevention of household and recreational injuries in adults. In: *The Canadian Guide to Clinical Preventive Health Care*. Ottawa, Canada: Minister of Supply and Services; 1994: chap 45.

Canadian Task Force on the Periodic Health Examination. Prevention of household and recreational injuries in the elderly. In: *The Canadian Guide to Clinical Preventive Health Care*. Ottawa, Canada: Minister of Supply and Services; 1994: chap 76.

Canadian Task Force on the Periodic Health Examination. Prevention of motor vehicle accident injuries. In: *The Canadian Guide to Clinical Preventive Health Care*. Ottawa, Canada: Minister of Supply and Services; 1994: chap 44.

Canadian Task Force on the Periodic Health Examination. Secondary prevention of elder abuse. In: *The Canadian Guide to Clinical Preventive Health Care*. Ottawa, Canada: Minister of Supply and Services; 1994: chap 77.

Carnaveli D, Patrick M. *Nursing Management of the Elderly*. Philadelphia, Pa: JB Lippincott; 1986.

Hindmarsh JJ, Estes EH. Falls and older persons: causes and interventions. *Arch Intern Med*. 1989;149:2217-2222.

Johnson K, Ford D, Smith G. The current practices of internists in prevention of residential fire injury. *Am J Prev Med.* 1993;9:39-44.

Kellerman AL, Reay DT. Protection or Peril? An Analysis of Firearm-Related Deaths in the Home. *N Engl J Med.* 1986; 31 14(24):1557-60.

Linsday R. The burden of osteoporosis: cost. *Am J Med.* 1995; 98: 9S-11S.

McFarlane J, Parker B, Soeken K, Bullock L. Assessing for abuse during pregnancy. Severity and frequency of injuries and associated entry into prenatal care. *JAMA.* 1992;267:3176-3178.

National Committee for Injury Prevention and Control. Injury prevention: meeting the challenge. *Am J Prev Med.* 1989;5(suppl):1-303.

National Safety Council. *Falling—The Unexpected Trip: A Safety Program for Older Adults* . Chicago, Ill: National Safety Council; 1982. Program Leader's Guide.

Polen MR, Friedman GD. Automobile injury: selected risk factors and prevention in the health care setting. *JAMA.* 1988;259:76-80.

US Department of Health and Human Services. *Surgeon General's Workshop on Violence and Public Health: Report.* US Department of Health and Human Services Publication HRS-D-MC 86-1. Washington, DC: US Public Health Service; 1986.

US Preventive Services Task Force. Counseling to prevent household and environmental injuries. In: *Guide to Clinical Preventive Services.* 2nd ed. Washington, DC: US Department of Health and Human Services; 1996: chap 58.

US Preventive Services Task Force. Screening for family violence. In: *Guide to Clinical Preventive Services*. 2nd ed. Washington, DC: US Department of Health and Human Services; 1996: chap 51.

56

NUTRITION

Four of the 10 leading causes of death in the United States—heart disease, stroke, diabetes mellitus, and certain cancers—are linked to diet. Together these diseases account for nearly two-thirds of the two million annual deaths in this country. Diet-related health conditions in the United States cost an estimated $250 billion annually in medical costs and lost productivity.

Over-consumption of calories, particularly from fat, and declining levels of physical activity have made overweight a major public health problem in the United States. Obesity[1] is a risk factor for several chronic diseases, and the proportion of overweight Americans, presently over one-third, continues to increase. High sodium intake is associated with hypertension. High alcohol intake increases risk for hypertension, stroke, heart disease, and certain cancers. Under-consumption of nutrients such as calcium, iron, and folate causes health problems for some individuals, particularly women.

Good nutrition is essential to maintain good health throughout life, and dietary intervention is an important component of both the prevention and treatment of many chronic conditions. Patients often look to their primary care providers for nutritional guidance; simple, focused interventions by clinicians can be beneficial to patients.

See chapter 20 for information on nutrition counseling for children and chapter 29 for information on body measurement and obesity.

Recommendations of Major Authorities

Most major authorities, including **American Academy of Family Physicians, American College of Obstetricians and Gynecologists, American College of Physicians, American Dietetic Association, American Heart Association, Canadian Task Force on the Periodic Health Examination (CTFPHE),** and **US Preventive Services Task Force (USPSTF)**—Clinicians should routinely provide nutritional assessment and counseling to their patients. The **USPSTF** has

---

[1]Obesity is an excess of body fat. Overweight refers to an excess of body weight relative to height. Because it is more readily quantified than obesity, overweight is often used as a proxy for obesity.

stated that there is insufficient evidence that nutritional counseling by physicians has an advantage over dietitian counseling or community interventions in changing the dietary habits of patients. The **AAFP** targets obesity (for all patients over 2 years) and calcium intake (for females 11 years and over). **AAFP** recommends directing obese patients to replace calories from fat with increased dietary fiber and counseling age-appropriate females with regard to adequate calcium intake. The **CTFPHE** has stated that it is reasonable for physicians to provide general dietary advice, while for patients at increased risk, such as alcoholics and the elderly living alone, it is prudent to consider referral to a clinical nutritionist or other professional with specialized nutritional expertise.

The American Academy of Family Physicians (AAFP), American College of Obstetricians and Gynecologists (ACOG),US Preventive Services Task Force (USPSTF) and the Canadian Task Force on the Periodic Health Examination (CTFPHE) recommend that women of childbearing age who are capable of becoming pregnant consume 0.4 mg of folic acid per day.

Basics of Nutrition Counseling

1. Weigh and measure every patient on a regular basis. Chapter 29 contains information on performing and assessing body measurement. Advise patients of their healthy weight range based on such factors as age, gender, and distribution of body fat.

2. Talk with all patients about their dietary habits. Ask them if they are taking any dietary supplements. Short patient questionnaires can be useful in identifying patients in need of more in-depth evaluation. See Table 56.1 for a brief questionnaire developed for screening older adults. Questionnaires for more general use have also been developed (see Block, et al, in Selected References).

3. Provide patients with basic information about managing a healthy diet. The US Department of Agriculture and the US Department of Health and Human Services recommend the following in their publication, *Dietary Guidelines for Americans:*

   ■ Eat a variety of foods.

   ■ Balance the food you eat with physical activity; maintain or improve your weight.

   ■ Choose a diet with plenty of grain products, vegetables, and fruits.

   ■ Choose a diet low in fat (less than 30% of calories), saturated fat (less than 10% of calories), and cholesterol (300 mg or less per day).

   ■ Choose a diet moderate in sugars.

Table 56.1. Determining Your Nutritional Health: Checklist for Older Adults*

	Yes
I have an illness or condition that made me change the kind and/or amount of food I eat.	2
I eat fewer than two meals per day.	3
I eat few fruits and vegetables or milk products.	2
I have three or more drinks of beer, liquor, or wine almost every day.	2
I have tooth or mouth problems that make it hard for me to eat.	2
I don't always have enough money to buy the food I need.	4
I eat alone most of the time.	1
I take three or more different prescribed or over-the-counter drugs a day.	1
Without wanting to, I have lost or gained 10 pounds in the last 6 months.	2
I am not always physically able to shop, cook, or feed myself.	2
	TOTAL

*Instructions: Read the statements above. Circle the number in the "yes" column for those that apply. For each "yes" answer, score the circled number. Total your nutrition score. If it is:

- 0–2   Good! Recheck your nutritional score in 6 months.
- 3–5   You are at moderate risk. See what can be done to improve your eating habits and lifestyle. Your office on aging, senior nutrition program, senior citizens center, or health department can help. Recheck your nutritional score in 3 months.
- ≥6   You are at high nutritional risk. Talk with your clinician, dietitian, or other qualified health or social service professional about this checklist. Ask for help to improve your nutritional health.

Adapted from: *The Nutrition Screening Initiative.* (Educational material and office aids for screening elderly patients for nutritional deficiencies). Washington, DC: Nutrition Screening Initiative. Reprinted with permission of the Nutrition Screening Initiative; copyright 1993.

- ■ Choose a diet moderate in salt and sodium (less than 2400 mg per day).

- ■ If you drink alcoholic beverages, do so only in moderation (no more than one drink daily for women or 2 drinks daily for men). One drink is 12 oz of regular beer, 5 oz of wine, or 1.5 oz of 80-proof distilled spirits.

4. Use the Food Guide Pyramid (Figure 56.1) and the Nutrition Facts label (Figure 56.2) as educational tools for helping patients plan healthful diets.

Figure 56.1. Food Guide Pyramid: A Guide to Daily Food Choices

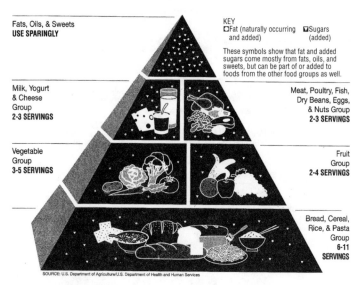

Fats, Oils, & Sweets
USE SPARINGLY

KEY
□Fat (naturally occurring   ▼Sugars
and added)   (added)

These symbols show that fat and added sugars come mostly from fats, oils, and sweets, but can be part of or added to foods from the other food groups as well.

Milk, Yogurt
& Cheese
Group
2-3 SERVINGS

Meat, Poultry, Fish,
Dry Beans, Eggs,
& Nuts Group
2-3 SERVINGS

Vegetable
Group
3-5 SERVINGS

Fruit
Group
2-4 SERVINGS

Bread, Cereal,
Rice, & Pasta
Group
**6-11
SERVINGS**

SOURCE: U.S. Department of Agriculture/U.S. Department of Health and Human Services

What Counts as One Serving?

Grain Products Group (bread, cereal, rice, and pasta)
1 slice of bread
1 ounce of ready-to-eat cereal
½ cup of cooked cereal, rice, or pasta

Vegetable Group
1 cup of raw leafy vegetables
½ cup of other vegetables, cooked or chopped raw
¾ cup of vegetable juice

Fruit Group
1 medium apple, banana, or orange
½ cup of chopped, cooked, or canned fruit
¾ cup of fruit juice

Milk Group (milk, yogurt, and cheese)
1 cup of milk or yogurt
1½ ounces of natural cheese
2 ounces of processed cheese

Meat and Beans Group (meat, poultry, fish, dry beans, eggs, and nuts)
2 to 3 ounces of cooked lean meat, poultry, or fish
½ cup of cooked dry beans or 1 egg counts as 1 ounce of lean meat
2 tablespoons of peanut butter or ⅓ cup of nuts count as 1 ounce of meat

Fats, Oils, and Sweets
Limit calories from these, especially if weight loss is needed

Note: The amount eaten may be more than one serving. For example, a dinner portion of spaghetti would count as two or three servings of pasta.

How Many Servings Are Needed?
Teenaged boys and active men need the highest number of servings shown. Women and some older adults need the lowest number of servings shown. Children, teenaged girls, active women, and most men need a number of servings somewhere in the middle of those shown.

From: Human Nutrition Information Service. *Food Guide Pyramid: A Guide to Daily Food Choices.* Washington, DC: US Department of Agriculture; 1992. (Leaflet No 572) and US Department of Agriculture, US Department of Health and Human Services. *Nutrition and Your Health: Dietary Guidelines for Americans.* 4th ed. Washington, DC: US Government Printing Office; 1995.

Figure 56.2. Guide To Using the New Food Label

Serving sizes are now more consistent across product lines, stated in both household and metric measures, and reflect the amounts people actually eat.

Nutrition Facts

Serving Size ½ cup (114g)
Servings Per Container 4

Amount Per Serving

Calories 90   Calories from Fat 30

% Daily Value*

Total Fat 3g	**5%**
Saturated Fat 0g	**0%**
Cholesterol 0mg	**0%**
Sodium 300mg	**13%**
Total Carbohydrate 13g	**4%**
Dietary Fiber 3g	**12%**
Sugars 3g	
Protein 3g	

Vitamin A	80%	•	Vitamin C	60%
Calcium	4%	•	Iron	4%

* Percent Daily Values are based on a 2,000 calorie diet. Your daily values may be higher or lower depending on your calorie needs:

		Calories	2,000	2,500
Total Fat	Less than		65g	80g
Sat Fat	Less than		20g	25g
Cholesterol	Less than		300mg	300mg
Sodium	Less than		2,400mg	2,400mg
Total Carbohydrate			300g	375g
Fiber			25g	30g

Calories per gram:
Fat 9   •   Carbohydrate 4   •   Protein 4

* This label is only a sample. Exact specifications are in the final rules.

New title signals that the label contains the newly required information.

Calories from fat are now shown on the label to help consumers meet dietary guidelines that recommend people get no more than 30 percent of their calories from fat.

% Daily Value shows how a food fits into the overall daily diet.

The **list of nutrients** covers those most important to the health of today's consumers, most of whom need to worry about getting <u>too much</u> of certain items (fat, for example), rather than too few vitamins or minerals, as in the past.

The label of larger packages must now tell the number of calories per gram of fat, carbohydrate, and protein.

Daily Values are also something new. Some are maximums, as with fat (65 grams <u>or less</u>); others are minimums, as with carbohydrate (300 grams <u>or more</u>). The daily values for a 2,000- and 2,500-calorie diet must be listed on the label of larger packages. Individuals should adjust the values to fit their own calorie intake.

From: US Food and Drug Administration. The new food label. *FDA Backgrounder*. Dec 10, 1992:1–9.

5. Women have special dietary needs, particularly for calcium and folic acid. Counsel women of all ages to consume adequate calcium, which helps build optimal bone mass during the teen years and early adulthood and, after menopause, helps control bone loss and delay development of osteoporosis. Dairy products are major sources of calcium. Other sources of calcium are canned fish with soft bones, vegetables such as broccoli and spinach, and fortified cereals and grains. See Table 56.2 for calcium re-

Table 56.2. Optimal Calcium Requirements Recommended by the National Institutes of Health Consensus Panel

Group	Optimal daily intake of calcium (mg)
Birth to 6 months	400
6 months to 1 year	600
1 to 5 years	800
6 to 10 years	800–1200
11 to 24 years	1200–1500
Men aged 25 to 65 years	1000
Women aged 25 to 50 years	1000
Men over age 65 years	1500
Women who are pregnant or nursing	1200–1500
Postmenopausal women (aged 50 to 65 years)	1500 (1000 if receiving estrogen)
Women over age 65 years	1500

From: National Institutes of Health. *Optimal Calcium Intake: National Institute of Health Consensus Statement.* Bethesda MD: National Institutes of Health; 1994.

quirements. The National Academy of Science is expected to publish reference intakes for calcium in late 1997.

6. Advise women of the following options for consuming adequate amounts of folic acid:

■ Consumption of a diet consistent with the *Dietary Guidelines for Americans* and the Food Guide Pyramid (Figure 56.1) is likely to provide the proper amount of folic acid. Some good sources are dry beans, leafy green vegetables, and citrus fruits.

■ Consumption of fortified foods, such as breakfast cereals, may help patients consume enough folic acid.

■ Folic acid-supplement pills and multivitamin preparations containing 0.4 mg folic acid are available.

Caution patients against consuming more than 1 mg of folic acid daily, because the effects of excess folic acid are not well known. Such effects may include a delay in the detection of vitamin B_{12} deficiency, thus allowing neurologic damage to progress. However, advise women who have had a previous neural tube defect-affected pregnancy to consult with their clinicians several months before planning to become pregnant about consuming a higher dose of folic acid. Public health measures to fortify the US food supply with folic acid are currently being implemented.

7. For patients who are overweight, recommend a diet with fewer total calories from fat and a modest increase in physical activity. See chapter 57 for information on physical activity counseling. In general, the goal should be a weight loss of $1/2$ to 1 pound per week. Although more rapid weight loss may be achieved with a very-low-calorie (800 kcal/day or less) diet, weight loss from these diets usually is not well maintained, and such diets may lead to health problems. Selected patients who have failed at conservative methods of weight loss and who are severely obese or have obesity-related medical problems may benefit from the short-term weight loss associated with very-low-calorie diets or from prescription weight loss medications, under medical supervision. Behavior therapy and physical activity have been shown to help maintain weight loss.

8. The National Cholesterol Education Program (NCEP) recommends that primary care providers instruct patients with borderline or elevated cholesterol levels in the use of a cholesterol-lowering diet. The Step I diet recommended by the NCEP has less than 300 mg per day of cholesterol and derives only 8% to 10% of total calories from saturated fatty acids. The Step II diet is recommended for patients whose cholesterol levels are not adequately reduced by the Step I diet. The Step II diet has less than 200 mg of cholesterol per day and derives less than 7% of total calories from saturated fatty acids. Referral to a dietitian is recommended for patients in need of the Step II diet. See Table 56.3 for examples of foods to choose for the Step I or Step II diet.

9. Provide ongoing support and reinforcement to patients undertaking significant dietary changes. This support can take several forms, including follow-up visits, telephone calls, and postcards. Recommend making changes gradually, in small, achievable steps over time. Encourage patients through the plateaus and regressions that occur as a normal part of efforts at long-term change.

10. Patients with multiple or severe nutritional problems should be referred, if possible, for counseling from a nutrition professional. Information on consulting registered nutrition professionals in the community can be obtained from the American Dietetic Association: (800)366-1655.

Table 56.3. Examples of Foods To Choose or Decrease for the NCEP Step I and Step II Diets*

Food Group	Choose	Decrease
Lean meat, poultry, and fish ≤ 5-6 oz per day	Beef, pork, lamb—lean cuts well trimmed before cooking	Beef, pork, lamb—regular ground beef, fatty cuts, spare ribs, organ meats
	Poultry without skin	Poultry with skin, fried chicken
	Fish, shellfish	Fried fish, fried shellfish
	Processed meat—prepared from lean meat, eg, lean ham, lean frankfurters, lean meat with soy protein or carrageen	Regular luncheon meat, eg, bologna, salami, sausage, frankfurters
Eggs ≤4 yolks per week, Step I ≤2 yolks per week Step II	Egg whites (whites can be substituted for 1 whole egg in recipes), cholesterol-free egg substitute	Egg yolks (if more than 4 per week on Step I or if more than 2 per week on Step II); includes eggs used in cooking and baking
Low-fat Dairy Products 2–3 servings per day	Milk—skim, ½%, or 1% fat (fluid, powdered, evaporated), buttermilk	Whole milk (fluid, evaporated, condensed), 2% fat milk (lowfat milk), imitation milk
	Yogurt—nonfat or low-fat yogurt or yogurt beverages	Whole milk yogurt, whole milk yogurt beverages
Dairy products	Cheese—low-fat natural or processed cheese	Regular cheeses (American, blue, Brie, cheddar, Colby, Edam, Monterey Jack, whole-milk mozzarella, Parmesan, Swiss), cream cheese, Neufchatel cheese
	Low-fat or non-fat varieties, eg, cottage cheese—low-fat, nonfat, or dry curd (0% to 2%)	Cottage cheese (4% fat)
	Frozen dairy dessert—ice milk, frozen yogurt (low-fat or nonfat)	Ice cream
	Low-fat coffee creamer	Cream, half & half, whipping cream
	Low-fat or nonfat sour cream	Nondairy creamer, whipped topping, sour cream

continued

Table 56.3. Examples of Foods To Choose or Decrease for the NCEP Step I and Step II Diets* —*Continued*

Food Group	Choose	Decrease
Fats and oils ≤6–8 teaspoons per day	Unsaturated oils—safflower, sunflower, corn, soybean, cottonseed, canola, olive, peanut	Coconut oil, palm kernel oil, palm oil
	Margarine—made from unsaturated oils listed above, light or diet margarine, especially soft or liquid forms	Butter, lard, shortening, bacon fat, hard margarine
	Salad dressings—made with unsaturated oils listed above, low-fat or fat-free	Dressing—made with egg yolk, cheese, sour cream, whole milk
	Seeds and nuts—peanut butter, other nut butters	Coconut
	Cocoa powder	Milk chocolate
Breads and Cereals 6 or more servings per day	Breads—whole-grain bread, English muffins, bagels, buns, corn or flour tortilla	Bread in which eggs, fat, and/or butter are a major ingredient; croissants
	Cereals—oat, wheat, corn, multigrain	Most granolas
	Pasta	
	Rice	
	Dry beans and peas	
	Crackers, low-fat—animal-type, graham, soda crackers, breadsticks, melba toast	High-fat crackers
	Homemade baked goods using unsaturated oil, skim or 1% milk, and egg substitute—quick breads, biscuits, cornbread muffins, bran muffins, pancakes, waffles	Commercial baked pastries, muffins, biscuits

continued

Table 56.3. Examples of Foods To Choose or Decrease for the NCEP Step I and Step II Diets* —*Continued*

Food Group	Choose	Decrease
Soups	Reduced- or low-fat and reduced-sodium varieties, eg, chicken or beef noodle, minestrone, tomato, vegetable, potato, reduced-fat soups made with skim milk	Soup containing whole milk, cream, meat fat, poultry fat, or poultry skin
Vegetables 3–5 servings per day	Fresh, frozen, or canned, without added fat or sauce	Vegetables fried or prepared with butter, cheese, or cream sauce
Fruits 2–4 servings per day	Fruit—fresh, frozen, canned, or dried Fruit juice—fresh, frozen, or canned	Fried fruit or fruit served with butter or cream sauce
Sweets and modified-fat desserts	Beverages—fruit-flavored drinks, lemonade, fruit punch	
	Sweets—sugar, syrup, honey, jam, preserves, candy made without fat (candy corn, gumdrops, hard candy), fruit-flavored gelatin	Candy made with milk chocolate, coconut oil, palm kernel oil, palm oil
	Frozen dessert—low-fat and nonfat yogurt, ice milk, sherbert, sorbert, fruit ice, popsicles	Ice cream and frozen treats made with ice cream
	Cookies, cake, pie, pudding—prepared with egg whites, egg substitutes, skim milk or 1% milk, and unsaturated oil or margarine; ginger snaps, fig and other fruit bar cookies, fat-free cookies, angel food cake	Commercial baked pies, cakes, doughnuts, high-fat cookies, cream pies

*Careful selection of processed foods is necessary to stay within the sodium guideline (<2400 mg).

From: National Cholesterol Education Program. *Second Report of the National Cholesterol Education Program Expert Panel on Detection, Evaluation, and Treatment of High Blood Cholesterol in Adults (Adult Treatment Panel II).* Bethesda, Md: National Institutes of Health, National Heart, Lung, and Blood Institute; 1993. NIH Publication 93-3095.

Patient Resources

CHATS: A Guide to Sensible Eating (scripted slide show); *Osteoporosis in Women: Keeping Your Bones Healthy and Strong.* American Academy of Family Physicians, 8880 Ward Parkway, Kansas City, MO 64114-2797; (800)944-0000. Internet address: http://www.aafp.org

Diet, Nutrition and Cancer Prevention: The Good News. Office of Cancer Communications, National Cancer Institute, Bldg 31, Room 10A24, Bethesda, MD 20892; (800)4-CANCER.

Eating Right To Lower Your Blood Cholesterol; Eating Right to Lower Your High Blood Pressure. National Heart, Lung, and Blood Institute Information Center, PO Box 30105, Bethesda, MD 20824-0105; (301) 251-1222.

The Food Guide Pyramid; Nutrition and Your Health: Dietary Guidelines for Americans. 4th ed; *Nutritive Value of Foods.* Superintendent of Documents, US Government Printing Office, Washington, DC 20402; (202) 783-3238.

Choosing a Safe and Successful Weight-Loss Program;/ Physical Activity and Weight Control; Prescription Medications for the Treatment of Obesity; Very Low Calorie Diets. The National Institute of Diabetes and Digestive and Kidney Disease, 1 WIN Way, Bethesda, MD 20892-3665; (800)946-8098; http://www.niddk.nih.gov/NutritionDocs.html

Provider Resources

Physician's Guide to Outpatient Nutrition. American Academy of Family Physicians, 8880 Ward Parkway, Kansas City, MO 64114-2797; (800)944-0000. Internet address: http:www.aafp.org.

Diet, Nutrition and Cancer Prevention: A Guide to Food Choices. Office of Cancer Communications, National Cancer Institute, Bldg 31, Room 10A24, Bethesda, Maryland 20892; (800)4-CANCER.

Nutrition Screening Initiative. Educational material and office aids for screening elderly patients for nutritional deficiencies. Nutrition Screening Initiative, 1010 Wisconsin Ave NW, Suite 800, Washington, DC 20007; (202)625-1662.

Selected References

American Academy of Family Physicians. *Summary of Policy Recommendations for Periodic Health Examination.* Kansas City, Mo: American Academy of Family Physicians; 1997.

American College of Obstetricians and Gynecologists. *Guidelines for Women's Health Care.* Washington, DC: American College of Obstetricians and Gynecologists; 1996.

American College of Physicians. *Nutrition.* Washington, DC: American College of Physicians; 1985.

American Heart Association. Dietary guidelines for healthy American adults: a statement for physicians and health professionals by the Nutrition Committee. *Circulation.* 1988;77:721A-724A.

American Medical Association, Counsel on Scientific Affairs. *Medical Evaluation of Healthy Persons.* Chicago, Ill: American Medical Association; 1983.

American Societies for Experimental Biology, Life Sciences Research Office. *Third Report on Nutrition Monitoring in the United States.* Washington, DC: US Government Printing Office; 1995.

Ammerman AS, DeVellis RF, Carey TS, et al. Physician-based diet counseling for cholesterol reduction: current practices, determinants, and strategies for improvement. *Prev Med.* 1993; 22:96-109.

Block G, Clifford C, Naughton MD, Henderson M, McAdams M. A brief dietary screen for high fat intake. *J Nutr Educ.* 1989;21:199-207.

Canadian Task Force on the Periodic Health Examination. Nutritional counseling for undesirable dietary patterns and screening for protein/calorie malnutrition disorders in adults. In: *The Canadian Guide to Clinical Preventive Medicine.* Ottawa, Canada: Minister of Supply and Services; 1994: chap 49.

Canadian Task Force on the Periodic Health Examination. Primary and secondary prevention of neural tube defects. In: *The Canadian Guide to Clinical Preventive Medicine.* Ottawa, Canada: Minister of Supply and Services; 1994: chap 7.

Expert Panel on Detection, Evaluation, and Treatment of High Blood Cholesterol in Adults. Summary of the second report of the National Cholesterol Education Program (NCEP) Expert Panel on Detection, Evaluation, and Treatment of High Blood Cholesterol in Adults (Adult Treatment Panel II). *JAMA.* 1993;269:3015-3023.

Human Nutrition Information Service. *Food Guide Pyramid: A Guide to Daily Food Choices.* Washington, DC: US Department of Agriculture; 1992. (Leaflet No 572)

Lin-Fu JS, Anthony MA. *Folic Acid and Neural Tube Defects: A Fact Sheet for Health Care Providers.* Rockville, Md: Maternal and Child Health Bureau, Health Resources and Services Administration, Public Health Service; May 1993.

National Cholesterol Education Program. *Report of the Expert Panel on Population Strategies for Blood Cholesterol Reduction.* Bethesda, Md: National Institutes of Health, National Heart, Lung, and Blood Institute; 1990. US Department of Health and Human Services, Public Health Service, publication NIH 90-3046.

National Cholesterol Education Program. *Second Report of the National Cholesterol Education Program Expert Panel on Detection, Evaluation, and Treatment of High Blood Cholesterol in Adults (Adult Treatment Panel II).* Bethesda, Md: National Institutes of Health, National Heart, Lung, and Blood Institute; 1993. NIH Publication 93-3095.

National Institutes of Health. *Optimal Calcium Intake: National Institutes of Health Consensus Statement.* Bethesda MD: National Institutes of Health; 1994.

National Task Force on the Prevention and Treatment of Obesity. Very low-calorie diets. *JAMA.* 1993;270:967-974.

Rosenberg HM, Ventura SJ, Maurer JD, et al. Births and Deaths: United States, 1995. Hyattsville MD: National Center for Health Statistics; 1996: Monthly vital statistics report; vol 45, no 3, supp 2.

US Department of Agriculture and US Department of Health and Human Services. *Nutrition and Your Health: Dietary Guidelines for Americans*. 4th ed. Washington, DC: US Government Printing Office; 1995: Home and Garden Bulletin No 232.

US Department of Health and Human Services. *Surgeon General's Report on Nutrition and Health*. Washington, DC: Department of Health and Human Services; 1988. DHHS Publication PHS 88-50210.

US Food and Drug Administration. The new food label. *FDA Backgrounder*. Dec 10, 1992:1-9.

US Preventive Services Task Force. Counseling to promote a healthy diet. In: *Guide to Clinical Preventive Services*. 2nd ed. Washington, DC: US Department of Health and Human Services; 1996: chap 56.

US Preventive Services Task Force. Screening for neural tube defects (and folate prophylaxis). In: *Guide to Clinical Preventive Services*. 2nd ed. Washington, DC: US Department of Health and Human Services; 1996: chap 42.

57

PHYSICAL ACTIVITY

In the last 25 years, the United States has seen a steady decline in age-adjusted deaths from cardiovascular disease (CVD). Despite this trend, cardiovascular disease continues to be the leading cause of death for Americans. Growing evidence indicates that physical inactivity is a major risk factor for CVD. In addition, physical inactivity is associated with other leading causes of disease and disability such as type 2 diabetes mellitus, colon cancer, obesity, osteoporosis, and falls.

Regular exercise reduces cardiovascular disease risk, promotes weight loss and control, improves musculoskeletal functioning, helps prevent diabetes, helps to control stress, and may help prevent bone loss associated with aging. Despite these advantages, physical activity levels among Americans are low. According to the 1996 Surgeon General's Report on Physical Activity and Health, more than 60% of Americans are not regularly physically active and 25% report no physical activity at all. The prevalence of physical inactivity is higher among women than men, among African Americans and Hispanics than Caucasians, among older than younger adults, and among the less affluent than the more affluent.

The relationship of physical activity to chronic health problems and the high prevalence of physical inactivity in the American population makes physical activity counseling an important role for clinicians. Surveys of primary care clinicians indicate that only about 30% routinely provide counseling on physical activity to their sedentary patients. Clinicians may consider referring patients to an exercise physiologist or a rehabilitation specialist for evaluation and in-depth counseling.

See chapter 21 for information on physical activity counseling for children and adolescents.

Recommendations of Major Authorities

American Academy of Family Physicians, American College of Obstetricians and Gynecologists, and the **US Preventive Services Task Force (USPSTF)**—Providers should routinely assess patients' physical activity practices and counsel them in engaging in a program of regular physical activity that is tailored to their health status and lifestyle. **USPSTF** recommends that women receive counseling regarding the use of weight-bearing exercise to help prevent postmenopausal osteoporosis. Both the **USPSTF** and **Canadian Task Force on the Periodic Health Examination** state that the effectiveness of clinician counseling to promote increased patient physical activity is not established.

The National Institutes of Health Consensus Panel on Physical Activity and Cardiovascular Health—All Americans should engage in regular physical activity at a level appropriate to their capacity, needs, and interest. Children and adults should set a goal of accumulating at least 30 minutes of moderate-intensity physical activity on most, and preferably all, days of the week.

Basics of Physical Activity Counseling

1. Ask all patients about their physical activity habits. Include organized activities, general activities, and occupational activities.

2. Determine if the patient's level of activity is sufficient. Experts agree that physical activity that is at least of moderate intensity, for 30 minutes or longer, and performed on most days of the week is sufficient to confer health benefits. The Surgeon General's Report defines moderate-intensity physical activity as 50% to 69% of maximal heart rate. (Table 57.1).

3. Assist patients who lack activity sufficient for health benefits and those wishing to improve physical activity habits in planning a program of physical activity. Such a program should be:

   ■ *Medically Safe:* Existing heart disease presents the biggest risk.

   □ Medical Evaluation: The NIH consensus Panel recommends a medical evaluation prior to embarking on a vigorous exercise program for the following individuals: persons with cardiovascular disease; men over 40 years and women over 50 years of age with multiple CVD risk factors (such as hypertension, diabetes, elevated cholesterol, current smoker, or obesity).

   □ Exercise testing: The use of exercise testing is controversial. The American College of Cardiology and the American Heart Association do not recommend routine screening by exercise testing in asymptomatic patients. They indicate that screening by exercise testing may be reasonable in patients with two or more cardiac risk factors prior to starting a vigorous exercise program.

   Additional advice to promote medically safe physical activity includes:

   □ Increase the level of exercise gradually rather than abruptly.

   □ Decrease the risk of musculoskeletal injuries by performing alternate-day exercises and using stretching exercises in the warm-up and cool-

Table 57.1. Heart Rates (Beats/Minute) According to Age*†

Age (Years)	55% of Maximum[a]	60% of Maximum[b]	90% of Maximum[c]	Maximum[d]
20	110	120	180	200
25	107	117	177	195
30	104	114	173	190
35	102	111	168	185
40	99	108	163	180
45	96	105	159	175
50	93	102	153	170
55	91	99	149	165
60	88	96	143	160
65	85	93	140	155
70	82	90	135	150
75	80	87	132	145
80	77	84	129	140

*This table should not be used for individuals with coronary artery disease.

†This formula is only an approximation of any individual's response and will not apply when certain rate-altering medications are being taken, such as beta blockers and some calcium antagonists.

a. Minimum exercise heart rate for health benefit designated by ACSM

b. Minimum exercise heart rate for fitness designated by ACSM

c. Maximum exercise heart rate designated by ACSM

d. Maximum average heart rate adjusted for age (according to formula: maximum = 220-age)

Adapted from: American College of Sports Medicine, Preventive and Rehabilitative Exercise Committee. *Guidelines for Exercise Testing and Prescription.* 4th ed. Philadelphia, Pa: Lea & Febiger; 1991. Used with permission of Lea & Febiger; copyright 1991.

down phases of exercise sessions. (This is particularly important for older adults and those who have not been physically active recently.)

- *Enjoyable:* Patients will not continue activities that they do not enjoy. Counsel patients to choose activities they find inherently pleasurable, to vary activities, and to share activities with friends or family. Encourage patients to identify barriers to enjoyment and to find ways to overcome these barriers. For most people, the hardest aspect of starting a regular exercise program is the "regular," not the "exercise." Help patients focus on making the time to exercise, starting with ordinary walking before they concern themselves with choosing a sport or sports. See Table 57.2 for examples of methods for overcoming barriers.

- *Convenient*: Encourage participation in activities that can be enjoyed with a minimum of special preparation, ideally those that fit into daily activities. The patient's effort should go into the exercise, not the preparation.

Table 57.2. Overcoming Barriers to Exercise

Barrier	Suggested Response
Exercise is hard work.	Start with ordinary walking, or an exercise that is not work for most people. See where it might lead.
I do not have the time.	That may be true, but you will never know for sure unless you try to make it.
I am usually too tired for exercise.	Tell yourself, "This activity will give me more energy." See if it doesn't happen.
I hate to fail, so I will not start.	Physical activity is not a test. You will not fail if you choose an activity you like and start off slowly. Setting reasonable, realistic goals reduces the chances for failure.
I do not have anyone to work out with.	Maybe you have not asked. A neighbor or a coworker may be a willing partner. Or you can choose an activity that you enjoy doing by yourself.
There is not a convenient place.	Pick an activity you can do at a convenient place. Walk around your neighborhood or a nearby mall, or do exercises with a TV show or a videotape at home.
I am afraid of being injured.	Walking is very safe and is excellent exercise. Choose a safe, well-lighted area.
The weather is too bad.	There are many activities that you can do in your own home or at a shopping mall in any weather.
Exercise is boring.	Some ways to make exercise more fun are: listening to music, exercising with a companion, varying the exercise with the season, setting a non-exercise related goal such as getting an errand or two done in the course of it, or giving yourself a reward periodically.
I am too overweight.	You can benefit regardless of your weight. Pick an activity that you are comfortable with, like walking.
I am too old.	It is never too late to start. People of any age, including older people, can benefit from physical exercise.

Adapted from: Jonas S. The Exercise Recommendations in Clinical Practice. Presented at the 16th Annual Medical Seminar, ISC Division of Wellness Role of Exercise and Nutrition in Preventive Medicine, 1997. Originally adapted from: Project PACE. *Physician-based Assessment and Counseling for Exercise*. San Diego, Calif: San Diego State University; 1991. Used with the permission of the publisher; copyright 1991.

- *Realistic:* A program that is too difficult in terms of goals and integration with other daily activities will lead to disappointment. Gradual change leads to permanent change; therefore, stress the importance of gradually increasing the intensity, frequency, and duration of exercise. Use of an exercise log may help patients keep track of gradual progress toward attainable goals.

- *Structured:* Having defined activities, goals for performance, and a set schedule and location may help improve some patients' compliance. Signing a physical activity "contract" may be helpful. However, too much structure may cause some patients to lose interest. The definition of activities should be individualized for each patient.

4. Encourage patients who are unwilling or unable to participate in a regular exercise program to increase the amount of physical activity in their daily lives. Ways in which to implement such increases include taking the stairs rather than the elevator when possible, leaving the subway or bus one or two stops early and walking the rest of the way, doing household chores and yard work on a regular basis, and substituting walking or bicycling for driving whenever convenient.

5. Involve nursing and office staff in monitoring patient progress and providing information and support to patients. Some form of routine follow-up with patients about their progress is very helpful.

6. Use posters, displays, videotapes, and other resources to create an office or clinic environment that conveys positive messages about exercise and physical activity.

7. Providers should try to engage in adequate physical activity themselves. Studies show that providers who exercise regularly are significantly better at providing exercise counseling to their patients than those who do not.

Patient Resources

Weight Control: Losing Weight and Keeping It Off. American Academy of Family Physicians, 8880 Ward Pkwy, Kansas City, MO 64114-2797; (800)944-0000. Internet address: http://www.aafp.org

Women and Exercise (educational bulletin 173); *Exercise and Fitness: A Guide for Women.* American College of Obstetricians and Gynecologists, 409 12th St, SW, Washington, DC 20024; (800)762-2264. Internet address: http://www.acog.com

Weight Control: Eating Right and Keeping Fit (AP064; 50/pack). American College of Obstetricians and Gynecologists. (800)762-2264. Internet address: http://www.acog.com

Check Your Healthy Heart IQ; Check Your Physical Activity and Heart Disease IQ; Exercise and Your Heart; Aprenda a Reconocer un Corazon Sano. National Heart, Lung, and Blood Institute Smoking Education Program, PO Box 30105, Bethesda, Md 20824-0105; (301) 251-1222 (English and Spanish). Internet address: http://www.nhlbi.nih.gov/nhlbi/nhlbi.html

Provider Resources

Anabolic Steroids and Athletes. American College of Sports Medicine, PO Box 1440, Indianapolis, IN 46206-1440; (317) 637-9200. Internet address: http://www.acsm.org/sportsmed

The Physician's Rx: Exercise. President's Council on Physical Fitness and Sports, 701 Pennsylvania Ave, NW, Suite 250, Washington, DC 20004; (202) 272-3421.

Physician-based Assessment and Counseling for Exercise. Project PACE, San Diego State University, San Diego, CA 92182-0567; (619) 594-5949.

Selected References

American Academy of Family Physicians. *Summary of Policy Recommendations for Periodic Health Examination.* Kansas City, MO: American Academy of Family Physicians; 1997.

American College of Obstetricians and Gynecologists. *Guidelines for Women's Health Care.* Washington, DC: American College of Obstetricians and Gynecologists; 1996.

American College of Obstetricians and Gynecologists. *Women and Exercise.* Washington, DC: American College of Obstetricians and Gynecologists; 1992. Technical bulletin 173.

American College of Sports Medicine, Preventive and Rehabilitative Exercise Committee. *Guidelines for Exercise Testing and Prescription.* 4th ed. Philadelphia, Pa: Lea & Febiger; 1991.

American College of Sports Medicine. The recommended quantity and quality of exercise for developing and maintaining cardiorespiratory and muscular fitness in healthy adults. *Med Sci Sports Exerc.* 1990;22:265-274.

American College of Sports Medicine. *American College of Sports Medicine's Guidelines for Exercise Testing and Prescription,* 5th ed. Philadelphia, Pa: Williams and Wilkins; 1995.

Canadian Task Force on the Periodic Health Examination. Physical activity counseling. In: *The Canadian Guide to Clinical Preventive Medicine.* Ottawa, Canada: Minister of Supply and Services; 1994: chap 47.

Centers for Disease Control. Prevalence of sedentary lifestyle—Behavioral Risk Factor Surveillance System, United States, 1991. *MMWR.* 1993;42:576-579.

Fletcher GF, Balady G, Froelicher VF, Hartley H, Haskell WL & Pollock ML. Exercise standards: a statement for healthcare professionals from the American Heart Association. *Circulation.* 1995; 91:580-615.

Fletcher GF, Blair SN, Blumenthal J, et al. Statement on exercise: benefits and recommendations for physical activity programs for all Americans. *Circulation.* 1992;86(1) 340-344.

Gibbons RJ, Ballady GJ, Beesley JW, et al. American College of Cardiology/American Heart Association guidelines for exercise testing. *J Am Coll Cardiology.* 1997;30:260-315.

Harris SS, Caspersen CJ, DeFriese GH, Estes EH. Physical activity counseling for healthy adults as a primary preventive intervention in the clinical setting. *JAMA.* 1989;261:3590-3598.

Jonas S. *Regular Exercise: A Handbook for Clinical Practice.* New York, NY: Springer Publishing Co; 1995.

Jonas S. *A Guidebook for the Regular Exerciser.* New York, NY: Springer Publishing Co; 1995.

King AC, Blair SN, Bild DE, et al. Determinants of physical activity and interventions in adults. *Med Sci Sports Exerc.* 1992;24(suppl):S221-S236.

Haskell WL, Leon AS, Caspersen CJ, et al. Cardiovascular benefits and assessment of physical activity and physical fitness in adults. *Med Sci Sports Exerc.* 1992;24(suppl):S201-S215.

Lewis BS, Lynch WD. The effect of physician advice on exercise behavior. *Prev Med.* 1993;22: 110-121.

Pate RR, Pratt M, Blair SN, et al. Physical activity and health: a recommendation from the Centers for Disease Control and Prevention and the American College of Sports Medicine. *JAMA.* 1995;273:402-407.

National Institutes of Health. *Physical Activity and Cardiovascular Health.* NIH Consensus Statement. Bethesda, Md: 1995; Dec 18-20; 13(3):1-33.

US Department of Health and Human Services. Physical activity and fitness. In: *Healthy People 2000: National Health Promotion and Disease Prevention Objectives.* Washington DC: US Department of Health and Human Services, Public Health Service; 1991: part II, chap 1. USDHHS publication PHS 91-50212.

US Department of Health and Human Services. *Physical Activity and Health: A Report of the Surgeon General.* Atlanta, Ga: US Department of Health and Human Services, Centers for Disease Control and Prevention, National Center for Chronic Disease Prevention and Health Promotion; 1996.

US Preventive Services Task Force. Counseling to promote physical activity. In: *Guide to Clinical Preventive Services.* 2nd ed. Washington, DC: US Department of Health and Human Services; 1996: chap 55.

US Preventive Services Task Force. Screening for postmenopausal osteoporosis. In: *Guide to Clinical Preventive Services.* 2nd ed. Washington, DC: US Department of Health and Human Services; 1996: chap 46.

58

POLYPHARMACY

Polypharmacy, the prescribing of multiple drugs for an individual patient, is most common in older adults, who tend to have more illnesses for which medications are prescribed. Adults aged 65 years and older represent 12% of the population but consume 30% of all prescription medications. Among persons older than age 65 years, the rate of nonprescription (over-the-counter) drug use is seven times that of the general population. The incidence of adverse drug reactions increases with advancing age and the number of drugs taken. Deteriorating vision and cognitive function cause older adults to make many mistakes when taking medications, often with serious consequences. Up to 10% of all hospital admissions for patients over 65 years of age involve medication toxicity.

Clinicians contribute significantly to the problem if they prescribe medications without considering changes in drug metabolism that occur with aging. Renal and hepatic function decrease with advancing age, slowing the clearance of medications. Increases in the proportion of body fat and decreases in the proportion of body water that occur with aging lead to an accumulation of fat-soluble medications in adipose tissue and increases in the concentration of hydrophilic medications in the blood.

Polypharmacy can occur in younger patients as well. As the number of symptoms and diseases increases in an individual, so does the risk of polypharmacy and the attendant risk of overmedication and adverse effects.

Recommendations of Major Authorities

American College of Obstetricians and Gynecologists—Clinicians should assess the use of prescription and nonprescription medications by women 65 years of age and older at each periodic health evaluation (annually or as appropriate).

American Nurses Association—Clinicians should maintain a drug profile on older adults to evaluate/monitor for unnecessary and excessive drug use.

Basics of Polypharmacy Counseling

1. Use flow sheets or summary lists in patient charts to document prescription and nonprescription medication dosages, frequencies, dates of use, and adverse reactions. A computerized medication list, if available, is helpful for this purpose.

2. Encourage patients to keep an up-to-date list of medications with dosage and usage schedules. Ask older adults to bring all their medications to each health care visit for inspection. Inspection of the patient's medication is especially important if the patient is visually or cognitively impaired.

3. Ask patients about their use of alcohol or other drugs and recreational substances that may interact with medications.

4. Inform all patients and caretakers of the possible side effects and symptoms of toxicity caused by medications. Printed information sheets are helpful for this purpose.

5. Evaluate potential medication interactions each time a new medication is prescribed or dosages of existing medications are changed. Several good printed references and software programs are available for this purpose. Computerized medication monitoring systems are very helpful.

6. Consider discontinuing any medications that have not shown clear benefit in well-designed studies or for the individual patient. Avoid prescribing medications for minor or self-limiting symptoms that may be treated safely with counseling and reassurance. Simplify medication regimens whenever possible. Table 58.1 provides guidelines for simplifying the medication regimen.

7. For older adults, consider using lower initial doses of medication unless an initial high plasma concentration is needed, as with antibiotics and certain cardiac medications.

8. Use particular caution when prescribing medications with the following characteristics to older adults:

   - Central nervous system effects
   - Anticholinergic side effects
   - Long half-lives.

Table 58.1. How To Simplify the Medication Regimen

Eliminate pharmacologic duplication and complications
Avoid combinations that augment side effects
Avoid combinations that duplicate therapy
Use monotherapy to manage multiple diseases when possible
Avoid drugs that can exacerbate the patient's other medical conditions

---

Decrease dosing frequency
Choose the best medication for the patient with the least frequent dosing interval
Consider sustained-release formulations (beware of cost)

Review drug regimens regularly
Include *all* medications—over-the-counter medications as well as *all* those prescribed by other health care providers
Ask the following questions:
■ Is the patient taking the medication as prescribed?
■ Are all agents still needed?
■ Can the regimen be simplified?

Adapted from: Colley CA, Lucas LM. Polypharmacy: the cure becomes the disease. *J Gen Intern Med.* 1993;8:278–283. Used with permission from Hanley & Belfus, Inc; copyright 1993.

Patient Resources

Age Page—Medicines—Use Them Safely; Age Page—Safe Use of Tranquilizers by Older People. National Institute on Aging, Bldg 31, Room 5C27, 31 Center Dr MSC 2922, Bethesda, MD 20892-2922; (301)496-1752. Internet address: http://www.nih.gov/nia/health/pubpub/pubpub.htm

Provider Resources

Patient Counseling Handbook. American Pharmaceutical Association, 2215 Constitution Ave NW, Washington, DC 20037, (202)628-4410, (800)878-0729.

FDA Ensures Equivalence of Generic Drugs; FDA Guide to Non Prescription Pain Relievers; FDA Guide to Choosing Medical Treatments; FDA's Tips for Taking Medicines. FDA Office of Consumer Affairs. HFE 88 Room 1675, 5600 Fishers Ln, Rockville, MD 20857; (800)532-4440.

National Council on Patient Education has forms available for providers to distribute to patients to assist with management of prescription medications. Phone: (202)347-6711; fax: (202)638-0773.

Selected References

American College of Obstetricians and Gynecologists. *Guidelines for Women's Health Care.* Washington, DC: American College of Obstetricians and Gynecologists; 1996.

Beers MH, Ouslander JG. Risk factors in geriatric drug prescribing: a practical guide to avoiding problems. *Drugs.* 1989;37:105.

Colley CA, Lucas LM. Polypharmacy: the cure becomes the disease. *J Gen Intern Med.* 1993; 8:278-283.

Everitt DE, Avorn J. Drug prescribing for the elderly. *Arch Intern Med.* 1986;146:2393-2396.

Porter J, Jick H. Drug-related deaths among inpatients. *JAMA.* 1977;237:879-881.

Royal College of General Physicians. Medication for the elderly. *J Roy Coll Physicians London.* 1984;18:7-17.

Williamson J, Chopin JM. Adverse reactions to prescribed drugs in the elderly: a multicenter investigation. *Age Aging.* 1980;9:73.

World Health Organization. Health care in the elderly: report of the technical group on use of medicaments by the elderly. *Drugs.* 1981;22:279.

US Department of Health and Human Services. Food and drug safety. In: *Healthy People 2000: National Health Promotion and Disease Prevention Objectives.* Washington, DC: US Department of Health and Human Services, Public Health Service; 1991: part II, chap 12. USDHHS publication PHS 91-50212.

59

SEXUALLY TRANSMITTED DISEASES AND HIV INFECTION

Almost 12 million cases of sexually transmitted diseases (STDs) occur annually in the United States. Eighty-six percent of such cases occur in persons aged 15 through 29 years. In addition to syphilis and gonorrhea, the list of STDs now includes human immunodeficiency virus (HIV) infection, *Chlamydia trachomatis* infection, genital herpes virus infection, human papilloma virus (HPV) infection, chancroid, genital mycoplasmas, cytomegalovirus infection, hepatitis B infection, vaginitis, enteric infections, and ectoparasitic diseases. Chlamydial infection is the most common STD, causing an estimated 4 million acute cases annually. Although the incidence of gonorrhea and syphilis decreased in the early 1990s, these diseases remain a persistent public health problem.

Acquired immunodeficiency syndrome (AIDS) is the eighth leading cause of death in the United States. It is now the leading cause of death among men aged 25 to 44 years and the third leading cause of death among women of the same age group. AIDS is the sixth leading cause of years of potential life lost in the United States. The Centers for Disease Control and Prevention estimate that 650,000 to 900,000 people in the United States are infected with HIV. No cure for AIDS currently exists, although treatment can delay onset of symptoms.

The consequences of STDs are particularly troublesome for women and children. Apart from AIDS, the most serious complications of STDs for women are pelvic inflammatory disease (PID), an increased risk of cervical cancer, ectopic pregnancy, congenital infection and malformations, delivery of premature and low-birth-weight infants, and fetal death. Persons who are poor or medically underserved and racial and ethnic minorities also contract a disproportionate number of STDs and the disabilities associated with them.

Individuals who are at increased risk for STDs and HIV infection include: (1) those who are or were recently sexually active, especially persons with multiple sexual partners; (2) those who use alcohol or illicit drugs; (3) gay or bisexual men who have sex with other men; (4) persons with a previous history of a documented STD/HIV infection and their close contacts; (5) persons involved in the exchange of sex for drugs or money; and (6) persons living in areas where the prevalence of HIV infection and STDs is high.

Many sexually transmitted diseases (AIDS, chancroid; *Chlamydia trachomatis* [genital infections only]; gonorrhea; hepatitis B; hepatitis C/non-A, non-B; HIV infection [pediatric cases only]; and syphilis) are currently designated as infectious diseases notifiable at the national level. Refer to Appendix C for further information on nationally notifiable diseases.

See chapter 40 for information on screening for STDs and HIV infection, chapter 23 for information on counseling children and adolescents about STDs and HIV infection, and chapters 25 and 61 for information about counseling to prevent unintended pregnancy among adolescents and adults, respectively.

Recommendations of Major Authorities

American Academy of Family Physicians—Adolescents and adults should be counseled about the risks for sexually transmitted diseases and how to prevent them.

American College of Obstetricians and Gynecologists (ACOG) and **American College of Physicians**—Patients should be counseled on measures to prevent STDs and HIV infection. **ACOG** recommends offering HIV counseling and testing to all pregnant women and strongly encourages it for high-risk women. HIV and STD counseling should be included for all women as a part of their routine preventive services whether pregnant or not.

The Canadian Task Force on the Periodic Health Examination—There is insufficient evidence to recommend for or against the inclusion or exclusion of the following from the periodic health examination of asymptomatic individuals: obtaining a history of sexual practices and injection drug use or counseling on high-risk sexual practices and condom use. There is fair evidence to include counseling to prevent the spread of gonorrhea.

Centers for Disease Control and Prevention—Latex condoms should be made more widely available by health care providers in STD, family planning, and drug treatment clinics. HIV seronegative pregnant women and women of childbearing age who are at increased risk of becoming infected with HIV should receive additional counseling regarding the maternal and fetal risks associated with pregnancy should they become infected. STD and HIV screening should be offered to high-risk individuals; counselors should take advantage of all available opportunities to provide patients with HIV-prevention messages. HIV pretest counseling must include a personalized patient-risk assessment and should result in a personalized plan for the patient to reduce the risk of HIV infection.

US Preventive Services Task Force (USPSTF)—All adolescent and adult patients should be advised about risk factors for sexually transmitted diseases and HIV infection and counseled appropriately about effective measures to reduce risk of infection. This recommendation is based on the proven efficacy of risk reduction, although the effectiveness of clinician counseling in the primary care setting is uncertain. Counseling should be tailored to the individual risk factors, needs, and abilities of each patient. Assessment of risk should be based on a careful sexual and drug use history and consideration of the local epidemiology of STDs and HIV infection. Patients at risk of STDs and HIV infection should receive information on their risk and be advised about measures to reduce their risk. Effective measures include abstaining from sex, maintaining a mutually faithful monogamous sexual relationship with a partner known to be uninfected, regular use of latex condoms, and avoiding sexual contact with high-risk individuals (eg, injection drug users, commercial sex workers, and persons with numerous sex partners). Women at risk of STDs should be advised of options to reduce their risk in situations when their male partner does not use a condom, including the female condom. Warnings should be provided that using alcohol and drugs can increase high-risk sexual behavior. Persons who inject drugs should be referred to available drug treatment facilities, warned against sharing drug equipment and, where possible, referred to sources for uncontaminated injection equipment and condoms. All patients at risk for STDs should be offered testing in accordance with **USPSTF** recommendations for screening for syphilis, gonorrhea, chlamydia, genital herpes, hepatitis B, and HIV infection (chapter 40).

Basics of STD/HIV Counseling

1. Determine every patient's risk for STDs (Table 59.1), including HIV infection. Tailor counseling to the behaviors, circumstances, and special needs of the person being served. Risk-reduction messages must be personalized and realistic. Counseling should be culturally appropriate, sensitive to issues of sexual identity, developmentally appropriate, and linguistically specific. HIV counseling is not a lecture; an important aspect of HIV counseling is the clinician's ability to listen to the patient.

2. Provide patients with materials about HIV transmission and prevention that are appropriate for their culture and educational level.

3. Advise all patients that any unprotected sexual behavior poses a risk for STDs and HIV infection. A person who is infected can infect others during sexual intercourse, even if no symptoms are present. Caution patients to avoid sexual intercourse with persons who may be infected with HIV,

Table 59.1. Examples of Questions for Taking Clinical Histories About Sexual Behavior

Are you currently or were you recently in a sexual relationship?

Do you have sex with men, women, or both?

How many men or women did you have sex with in the last week, last month, last year?

How often do you have sex with each man or woman?

Is each partner new, casual, or regular?

Do you know if your partners have other sex partners?

Have any of your partners been men who have had sex with other men?

Have any of your partners injected (shot) drugs?

Have you had sex with someone that you know or suspect has HIV?

Has anyone ever given you money, drugs, or other things of value in exchange for sex?

Adapted from: Gerber AR, Valdiserri RO, Holtgrave DR, et al. Preventive services guidelines for primary care clinicians caring for HIV-infectd adults and adolescents. *Arch Fam Med.* 1993;2:969–979. Used with permission of the American Medical Association, copyright 1993.

such as those who have injected drugs, individuals with multiple or anonymous sex partners, or those who have had any STD within the past 10 years, even if they have no symptoms. Advise patients not to make decisions about sexual intercourse while they are under the influence of alcohol or other drugs that cloud judgment and permit risk-taking behavior.

4. Provide patients with educational materials and information that explain that STDs and HIV infection are best prevented by the following measures:

   ■ Abstinence

   ■ Limiting sexual relationships to those between mutually monogamous partners known to be HIV-negative

   ■ Avoiding sex with high-risk partners

   ■ Avoiding anal intercourse

   ■ Using latex condoms if having sex with anyone other than a single, mutually monogamous partner known to be HIV-negative.

5. Provide patients with educational materials and information indicating that partners can transmit infection even if males withdraw before ejaculating. Infection can be transmitted during all forms of sexual intercourse, including oral sex.

6. Provide educational information indicating that the risk of HIV infection is increased through co-infection with other STDs, such as syphilis, genital herpes, and gonorrhea.

7. Instruct all sexually active patients about the effective use and limitations of condoms, stressing that they are not foolproof, must be used properly, and may break during intercourse. The best preventive measure against transmission of HIV and other STDs, after abstinence, is use of latex condoms (not "lambskin" or natural-membrane condoms). Scientific research has demonstrated that latex condoms, when used consistently and correctly, are highly effective in stopping HIV transmission. Condom failure (slip, break, or leak) usually is caused by user error. See Table 23.1 for guidelines regarding condom use.

8. Dispel myths about HIV transmission by informing patients that they cannot become infected from mosquito bites; contact with toilet seats or other everyday objects, such as doorknobs, telephones, or drinking fountains; or casual contact with someone who is infected with HIV or has AIDS, such as shaking hands, hugging, or a kiss on the cheek.

9. Use patient-centered counseling to assess, inform, and advise about STDs and HIV prevention. In patient-centered counseling, the provider asks the patient what they know about HIV transmission and provides the correct information in response to any misconceptions the patient expresses.

   ■ Establish a trusting, caring relationship with the patient to enhance the efficacy of counseling on safe sex practices and risks for STD and HIV infection.

   ■ Listen carefully to the patient to identify any specific barriers to preventing STD and HIV infection that the patient has and to assist the patient in identifying a personal, workable preventive plan without lecturing the patient.

   ■ Provide counseling that is culturally appropriate. Present information and services in a manner that is sensitive to the culture, values, and traditions of the patient.

   ■ Counseling should be sensitive to issues of sexual orientation.

   ■ Provide information and services at a level of comprehension that is consistent with the age and learning skills of the patient, using a dialect and terminology consistent with the patient's language and communication style.

10. Advise all patients of the adverse health consequences of injection drug use. Refer patients with evidence of drug dependence to appropriate drug-treatment providers and community programs specializing in treatment of drug dependencies. Providers should actively assist the patient in obtaining assessment for drug treatment.

11. Persons who continue to inject drugs should have periodic screening for HIV and hepatitis B. Hepatitis B vaccination should be considered for individuals lacking immunity who are negative for hepatitis B surface antigen (chapter 48). Measures to reduce the risk of infection caused by drug

use should also be discussed: use a new, sterile syringe for each injection; never share or reuse injection equipment; use clean (if possible, sterile) water to prepare drugs; clean the injection site with alcohol before injection; and safely dispose of syringes after use. Patients should also be informed of available resources for obtaining sterile supplies.

12. Contact the state or local health agency responsible for communicable disease reporting to determine the local prevalence of HIV infection and other STDs. This agency also can provide information regarding state and local laws regulating patient testing and confidentiality. Requirements regarding which infections to report, when, and to whom may vary from state to state (Appendix C). Chapter 40 discusses the types of HIV tests available.

Patient Resources

How to Prevent Sexually Transmitted Diseases, Genital Herpes, Gonorrhea and Chlamydia, Pelvic Inflammatory Disease. American College of Obstetricians and Gynecologists, 409 12th St, SW, Washington, DC 20024; (800)762-2264. Internet address: http://www.acog.com

HIV Infection and Women. ACOG Patient Education Pamphlet AP082. American College of Obstetricians and Gynecologists, 409 12th St, SW, Washington, DC 20024; (800)762-2264. Internet address: http://www.acog.com

Giving and Receiving Blood (#329 546); Testing for HIV Infection (#329 547); Women, Sex, and HIV (#329 537); HIV Infections and AIDS (#329 560). Available through your local chapter of the American Red Cross.

Surgeon General's Report to the American Public on HIV Infection and AIDS; Condoms and Sexually Transmitted Diseases ... Especially AIDS. To order these and many other materials, contact the CDC National AIDS Information Hot Line: (800)342-AIDS (English speaking); (800)344-SIDA (Spanish speaking); (800)AIDS-TTY (hearing impaired). All phone calls are confidential.

HIV in America: A Profile of the Challenges Facing Americans Living With HIV. National Association of People Living with AIDS, 1413 K St, NW, Washington, DC 20005; (202)898-0435.

National STD Hot Line: (800)227-8922; (809)765-1010 (Spanish; call collect).

Information on hemophilia and HIV: Hemophilia and AIDS Network for the Dissemination of Information, 110 Green St, New York, NY 10012; (800)424-2634.

Women, AIDS, and Drug Use Annotated Client Education Directory. NOVA Research Co, 4600 East-West Hwy, Suite 700, Bethesda, MD 20814; (301)986-1891.

National AIDS Information Hotline, Centers for Disease Control and Prevention, (800)342-AIDS.

Provider Resources

HIV Infection and AIDS (monograph); *HIV Infection in the Family Physician's Office* (brochure); *Clinical and Psychosocial Aspects of Caring for HIV Patients* (audiotape); *HIV Infection and Physician Emotions* (videotape and discussion guide). American Academy of Family Physicians, 8880 Ward Pkwy, Kansas City, MO 64114-2797; (800)944-0000. Internet address: http://www.aafp.org

Gynecologic Herpes Simplex Virus Infection (technical bulletin 119). American College of Obstetricians and Gynecologists, 409 12th St SW, Washington, DC 20024; (800)762-2264. Internet address: http://www.acog.com

National AIDS Information Clearinghouse. PO Box 6003, Rockville, MD 20850; (800)458-5231. General information (in both English and Spanish) on STDS, HIV, AIDS and AIDS-related diseases (seven brochures) and fact sheet packet (10 brochures).

National HIV Telephone Consultation Service is a clinical consultation service of health care providers: (800)933-3413.

National AIDS Information Hotline, Centers for Disease Control and Prevention, (800)342-AIDS.

Selected References

American Academy of Family Physicians. *Summary of Policy Recommendations for Periodic Health Examination.* Kansas City, Mo: American Academy of Family Physicians; 1997.

American College of Obstetricians and Gynecologists. *Guidelines for Women's Health Care.* Washington, DC: American College of Obstetricians and Gynecologists; 1996.

American College of Obstetricians and Gynecologists and American Academy of Pediatrics. *Guidelines for Perinatal Care.* 4th ed. Washington, DC and Elk Grove Village, Ill: American College of Obstetricians and Gynecologists and American Academy of Pediatrics; 1997.

American College of Physicians. Acquired immunodeficiency syndrome. *Ann Intern Med.* 1986;104:575-581.

American Medical Association. Prevention and control of acquired immunodeficiency syndrome: an interim report. *JAMA.* 1987;258:2097-2103.

Canadian Task Force on the Periodic Health Examination. Prevention of gonorrhea. In: *The Canadian Guide to Clinical Preventive Health Care.* Ottawa, Canada: Minister of Supply and Services; 1994: chap 59.

Canadian Task Force on the Periodic Health Examination. Screening for HIV antibody. In: *The Canadian Guide to Clinical Preventive Health Care.* Ottawa, Canada: Minister of Supply and Services; 1994: chap 58.

Centers for Disease Control and Prevention. Technical guidance on HIV counseling. *MMWR.* 1993;42(RR-2):8-17.

Centers for Disease Control. Sexually transmitted diseases treatment guidelines. *MMWR.* 1989;38(S-8):1-43.

Centers for Disease Control. CDC estimates of HIV prevalence and projected AIDS cases: summary of a workshop, October 31-November 1, 1989. *MMWR.* 1990;39:110-112, 117-119.

Gerber AR, Valdiserri RO, Holtgrave DR, et al. Preventive services guidelines for primary care clinicians caring for HIV-infected adults and adolescents. *Arch Fam Med.* 1993;2:969-979.

Higgins DL, Galavotti C, O'Reilly KR, et al. Evidence for the effects of HIV antibody counseling and testing on risk behaviors. *JAMA.* 1991;266:2419-2429.

Janssen RS, Sattan GA, Critchley SE. HIV infection among patients in US acute care hospitals: strategies for the counseling and testing of hospital patients. *N Engl J Med.* 1992;327: 445-452.

US Department of Health and Human Services. Sexually transmitted diseases. In: *Healthy People 2000: National Health Promotion and Disease Prevention Objectives.* Washington, DC: US Department of Health and Human Services, Public Health Service; 1991: chap 19. USDHHS publication PHS 91-50212.

US Preventive Services Task Force. Counseling to prevent human immunodeficiency virus infection and other sexually transmitted diseases. In: *Guide to Clinical Preventive Services.* 2nd ed. Washington, DC: US Department of Health and Human Services; 1996: chap 62.

US Preventive Services Task Force. Screening for drug abuse. In: *Guide to Clinical Preventive Services.* 2nd ed. Washington, DC: US Department of Health and Human Services; 1996: chap 53.

60

SMOKING CESSATION

More than 400,000 people die of tobacco-related causes annually. Cigarette smoking is the leading cause of preventable death in the United States, and smoking cessation is a critically important topic for patient counseling because of its potential benefit. Figure 60.1 shows the benefits of smoking cessation for different parts of the smoker's body. Evidence also suggests that nonsmokers who are exposed to environmental tobacco smoke are susceptible to lung cancer and possibly coronary heart disease. Rates of chronic middle ear effusions, pneumonia, and asthma are increased among children who are exposed to environmental tobacco smoke.

Primary care clinicians can play a key role in helping patients quit smoking. Even very simple interventions by clinicians can lead to long-term quit rates of 5% to 10%. More extensive interventions, including use of nicotine gum and patches, can lead to quit rates that are significantly higher. If all primary care providers used simple interventions such as asking about smoking status and suggesting that patients quit smoking, the national smoking cessation rate could double. Recent studies indicate, however, that fewer than half of patients who smoke receive any assistance in quitting from their health care providers.

See chapter 24 for information on counseling children and adolescents on prevention of tobacco use. See chapters 19 and 54 for information about counseling on dental and oral health for children and adolescents and for adults, respectively. See chapters 18 and 53 for information about counseling on alcohol and other drug abuse for children and adolescents and for adults, respectively.

Recommendations of Major Authorities

All major authorities, including the **American Academy of Family Physicians (AAFP), American Cancer Society, American College of Obstetricians and Gynecologists, American College of Physicians, American Medical Association, Canadian Task Force on the Periodic Health Examination, National Heart, Lung, and Blood Institute, National Institute of Dental Research,** and **US Preventive Services Task Force, and the Smoking Cessation Guideline Panel convened by the Agency for Health Care Pol-**

Figure 60.1. Benefits of Smoking Cessation

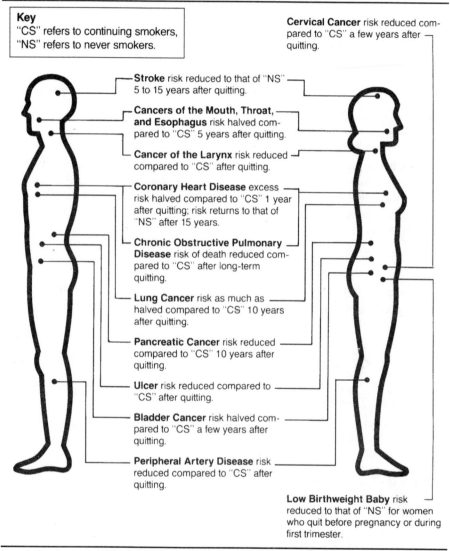

Key
"CS" refers to continuing smokers, "NS" refers to never smokers.

Cervical Cancer risk reduced compared to "CS" a few years after quitting.

Stroke risk reduced to that of "NS" 5 to 15 years after quitting.

Cancers of the Mouth, Throat, and Esophagus risk halved compared to "CS" 5 years after quitting.

Cancer of the Larynx risk reduced compared to "CS" after quitting.

Coronary Heart Disease excess risk halved compared to "CS" 1 year after quitting; risk returns to that of "NS" after 15 years.

Chronic Obstructive Pulmonary Disease risk of death reduced compared to "CS" after long-term quitting.

Lung Cancer risk as much as halved compared to "CS" 10 years after quitting.

Pancreatic Cancer risk reduced compared to "CS" 10 years after quitting.

Ulcer risk reduced compared to "CS" after quitting.

Bladder Cancer risk halved compared to "CS" a few years after quitting.

Peripheral Artery Disease risk reduced compared to "CS" after quitting.

Low Birthweight Baby risk reduced to that of "NS" for women who quit before pregnancy or during first trimester.

From: Centers for Disease Control, Office on Smoking and Health. *The Health Benefits of Smoking Cessation: A Report of the Surgeon General, At a Glance, 1990.* Rockville, Md: Centers for Disease Control; 1990. USDHHS publication CDC 90-8419.

icy and Research and the Centers for Disease Control and Prevention—For patients who smoke, clinicians should provide smoking cessation counseling, consider drug therapy with nicotine products, and referral as appropriate to smoking cessation programs. The **AAFP** recommends counseling be done on a regular basis to smokers, as multiple messages are often needed, and the harmful effect of smoking on children's health be emphasized to smoking parents.

Several major authorities, including **Joint Commission on Accreditation of Health Care Organizations**—Smoking should be prohibited in health-care facilities.

Basics of Smoking Cessation Counseling[1]

1. Consider designating an office smoking cessation coordinator who will be responsible for the administration of the smoking cessation program.

2. Systematically identify smokers:

   ■ Treat smoking status as a vital sign.

   ■ Place a sticker or other visual cue on the charts of patients who smoke as a reminder of the need to address the issue of smoking at every visit. (Similar stickers may be placed on the charts of children of smokers to serve as cues to talk to parents about the ways in which smoking endangers their children).

   ■ Use a flow chart in patient records to keep track of smoking cessation interventions.

   ■ Use of a brief, self-administered questionnaire (Table 60.1) may facilitate assessment of smoking status.

3. Strongly advise all smokers to stop smoking:

   Advice should be:

   ■ *Clear:* "I think it is important for you to quit smoking now and I will help you. Cutting down when you are ill is not enough."

   ■ *Strong*: "As your clinician I need you to know that quitting smoking is the most important thing you can do to protect your current and future health."

   ■ *Personalized*: Tie smoking to current health or illness; the social and economic costs of tobacco use; motivation level/readiness to quit; and /or the impact of smoking on children and others in the household.

4. Ask every smoker if he/she is ready to make a quit attempt.

5. Assist patients who are ready to quit:

   ■ Set a quit date: ideally, within 2 weeks

   ■ Counsel patients who are preparing to quit to:

      □ Inform their families, friends, and co-workers of their intention to quit smoking and request their understanding and support.

[1]Adapted from: Fiore MC, Bailey WC, Cohen S.J., et al. Smoking Cessation. Clinical Practice Guideline No 18. Rockville, Md: US Department of Health and Human Services, Public Health Service, Agency for Health Care Policy and Research, 1996. AHCPR publication 96-0692.

Table 60.1. Smoking Assessment Form

Name: _____   Date: _____
1. Do you now smoke cigarettes?   ____Yes   ____No
2. Does the person closest to you smoke cigarettes?   ____Yes   ____No
3. How many cigarettes do you smoke a day?   _____Cigarettes
4. How soon after you wake up do you smoke your first cigarette?
   ____Within 30 minutes   ____More than 30 minutes
5. How interested are you in stopping smoking?
   ____Not at all   ____A little   ____Some   ____A lot   ____Very
6. If you decided to quite smoking completely during the next 2 weeks, how confident are you that
   you would succeed?
   ____ Not at all   ____A little   ____Some   ____A lot   ____Very

From: Glynn TJ, Manley MW. *How To Help Your Patients Stop Smoking: A National Cancer Institute Manual for Physicians.* Bethesda, Md: National Institutes of Health; 1995. NIH publication NIH 95-3064.

□ Remove cigarettes from their environment. Before attempting to quit, they should consider avoiding smoking in places where they spend a lot of time (eg, home, car).

□ Review previous quit attempts. What helped? What led to relapse?

□ Anticipate challenges to the planned quit attempt, particularly during the critical first few weeks. These challenges include nicotine withdrawal symptoms.

■ Encourage Nicotine Replacement Therapy (NRT): Tables 60.2 through 60.7 present information related to pharmacologic aids to smoking cessation.

■ Provide key advice on successful quitting:

□ Abstinence—Total abstinence is essential. "Not even a single puff after the quit date."

□ Alcohol—Drinking alcohol is highly associated with relapse. Persons who stop smoking should review their alcohol use and consider limiting/abstaining from alcohol during the quit process.

□ Other smokers in the household—The presence of other smokers in the household, particularly a spouse, is associated with lower success rates. Patients should consider quitting with their significant others and/or developing specific plans to stay abstinent in a household where others still smoke.

■ Referral: Consider referring patients to a group clinic or intensive smoking cessation program. Information on reputable programs can be obtained by calling the National Cancer Institute Information Service: (800)4-CANCER.

■ Provide self-help materials (see Patient Resources).

Table 60.2. Availability of Pharmacologic Agents for Smoking Cessation

	Patch	Gum	Other
Over-the-counter	Nicoderm® CQ Patch Nicotrol® Patch	Nicorette® gum	
Prescription	Pro-Step® Patch* Habitrol® Patch*		Nicotrol® Inhaler† Nicotrol®Nasal Spray† Zyban™ Tablets†

*May be available as over-the-counter in late 1997
†Not available at time of AHCPR guideline panel (1996)

6. Schedule follow up contact:

   ■ A member of the office staff should call or write patients within 7 days after the quit date. A second follow up contact is recommended within the first month. Schedule further follow up contacts as indicated.

   ■ Actions during follow-up:

      □ Congratulate success

      □ If smoking occurred, review circumstances and elicit recommitment of total abstinence. Remind patient that a lapse can be a learning experience. Identify problem areas already encountered and anticipate challenges in the immediate future. Assess NRT use and problems. Consider referral to more intense or specialized program.

Creating a Smoke Free Office:[2]

■ Select a date for the office to become smoke-free. Advise all staff and patients of this plan.

■ Post no-smoking signs in all office areas.

■ Remove ashtrays.

■ Display nonsmoking materials and cessation information prominently.

■ Do not use waiting room magazines that contain tobacco advertising. A list of such magazines is available (Glynn and Manley, 1995; Goldsmith, 1991).

---

[2]Adapted from: Glynn TJ, Manley MW. How To Help Your Patients Stop Smoking: A National Cancer Institute Manual for Physicians. Bethesda, Md: National Institutes of Health; 1995. NIH publication 95-3064,

Table 60.3. Information About Nicotine Patch Use

Preparation	■ Patient should stop smoking before using the patch. ■ Apply the patch immediately upon awakening on the quit day.
Dosage	■ Dose varies according to product. ■ Most manufacturers advise starting with the highest-dose patch available, except small patients (less than 100 lb) and those with a history of cardiovascular disease.
Administration	■ Apply the patch only once a day to a clean, dry, and non-hairy site on the trunk or upper arm. ■ Apply the patch immediately after removing it from its protective pouch to prevent evaporative loss of nicotine from the system. ■ To prevent skin irritation, do not reuse an application site for at least a week.
Duration of therapy	■ Ranges from 6 to 10 weeks depending on the type of patch and the smoker.
Adverse reactions	■ Local skin reactions are the most common side effect of the nicotine patch. This reaction is usually a mild, transient (15 to 60 minutes) itching or burning at the site. Erythema, sometimes accompanied by edema, also occurs frequently at the patch site. ■ Other side effects—headache, vertigo, insomnia, somnolence, abnormal dreams, myalgia, arthralgia, abdominal pain, nausea, dyspepsia, diarrhea, and nervousness. Anxiety, irritability, and depression may also occur but are more often symptoms of nicotine withdrawal than patch toxicity.
Contraindications and Precautions	**Contraindications:** ■ Serious cardiac arrhythmias, severe or worsening angina, recent myocardial infarction, and hypersensitivity or allergy to nicotine. **Precautions:** ■ Use the patch with caution in patients with psoriasis, dermatitis (atopic or eczematous), active peptic ulcers, severe renal impairment, accelerated hypertension, hyperthyroidism, pheochromocytoma, or insulin-dependent diabetes mellitus. ■ As with the nicotine gum, the nicotine patch, should be used in pregnancy only if the increased likelihood of smoking cessation, with its potential benefits, outweighs the risks of nicotine replacement and potential concomitant smoking.

Adapted from: Glynn TJ, Manley MW. *How To Help Your Patients Stop Smoking: A National Cancer Institute Manual for Physicians.* Bethesda, Md: National Institutes of Health; 1995. NIH publication 95-3064; and Fiore MC, Bailey WC, Cohen SJ, et al *Smoking Cessation.* Clinical Practice Guideline No 18. Rockville, Md: US Department of Health and Human Services, Public Health Service, Agency for Health Care Policy and Research, 1996. AHCPR publication 96-0692.

Table 60.4. Information About Nicotine Gum Use

Preparation	■ Patients should stop smoking before beginning nicotine gum use.
Dosage	■ Two doses are available: 2 mg and 4 mg ■ Research supports tailoring nicotine gum treatment to the individual smoker. The 4-mg gum can be used with patients who are highly dependent on nicotine (eg, those smoking more than 25 cigarettes daily). Clinicians may also recommend the higher dosage if patients request it or have failed to quit using the 2-mg gum. ■ Patients using the 2-mg strength should use no more than 30 pieces daily; those using the 4-mg strength should not use more than 20 pieces daily.
Administration	■ Instruct patients to chew the gum on a fixed schedule (at least one piece every 1 to 2 hours) for at least 1 to 3 months. ■ Patients should use one piece of gum whenever they have the urge to smoke. Patients commonly use the gum too sparingly in the first few days after quitting and relapse because of lack of nicotine. ■ Each piece of nicotine gum should be chewed slowly and intermittently for about 30 minutes. Chewing quickly can release the nicotine too rapidly and reduce the effect of the gum. ■ Each piece of gum should be chewed enough to soften it or until the "peppery" taste or "tingling" from the nicotine is felt. Then it should be "parked" in contact with the oral mucosa to allow absorption of the nicotine. The gum should be rechewed gently every few minutes to release more nicotine. ■ Acidic beverages (eg, coffee, juices, soft drinks) interfere with the buccal absorption of nicotine, so eating and drinking anything except water should be avoided for 15 minutes before and during chewing. ■ Patients should not smoke while using nicotine gum.
Duration of therapy	■ Taper the dose of nicotine gum after about 3 months. ■ Use of the gum for more than 6 months is not recommended; however, continued use of the gum is preferable to returning to smoking.
Adverse reactions	■ Sore jaw, mouth irritation, heartburn, nausea, sore throat, and palpitations.
Contraindications and Precautions	**Contraindications:** ■ Patients who have had a recent myocardial infarction, severe or worsening angina, or life-threatening arrhythmias. It is also contraindicated for patients who are unable to chew. **Precautions:** ■ As with the nicotine patch, nicotine gum should be used in pregnancy only if the increased likelihood of smoking cessation, with its potential benefits, outweighs the risks of nicotine replacement and potential concomitant smoking.

Adapted from: Glynn TJ, Manley MW. *How To Help Your Patients Stop Smoking: A National Cancer Institute Manual for Physicians*. Bethesda, Md: National Institutes of Health; 1995. NIH publication 95-3064; and Fiore MC, Bailey WC, Cohen SJ, et al *Smoking Cessation*. Clinical Practice Guideline No 18. Rockville, Md: US Department of Health and Human Services, Public Health Service, Agency for Health Care Policy and Research, 1996. AHCPR publication 96-0692.

Table 60.5. Information About Nicotrol® Inhaler Use

Preparation	■ Patient should stop smoking completely when initiating therapy.
Dosage	■ Each cartridge delivers 4 mg nicotine from a porous plug containing 10 mg of nicotine. ■ The dosage is individualized. ■ Patients may self-titrate to the level of nicotine they require. ■ Patients should use at least 6 cartridges per day for the first 3 to 6 weeks of treatment. Maximum recommended initial dose is 16 cartridges per day for up to 12 weeks.
Administration	■ A new cartridge should be attached to the mouthpiece before each use. ■ Frequent continuous puffing is recommended for best effect. (About 80 deep inhalations over 20 minutes.) ■ Nicotine vapor inhaled through the mouthpiece is absorbed buccally.
Duration of Therapy	■ Patients who are successfully abstinent should be treated at their selected dosage for up to 12 weeks. ■ Use of the inhaler should then preferably be gradually reduced over an additional 6 to 12 weeks. However, gradual reduction is not required; some patients may abruptly stop therapy successfully. ■ If the patient is unable to stop smoking by the fourth week of therapy, treatment should probably be discontinued. ■ Continued use for periods longer than 6 months is not recommended.
Adverse Reactions	■ Common local side effects: mouth and throat irritation, cough, rhinitis, pharyngitis, stomatitis, sinusitis, dry mouth. ■ Systemic effects: headache, dyspepsia, and nausea are the most common complaints.

continued

Table 60.5. Information About Nicotrol® Inhaler Use—*Continued*

Contraindications and Precautions	**Contraindications:** ■ Hypersentivity or allergy to nicotine or menthol. **Precautions:** ■ Do not use during the immediate post-myocardial infarction period, in patients with serious arrhythmias, or with severe angina. ■ Use with caution in patients with bronchospastic disease, coronary heart disease, vasospastic diseases, hyperthyroidism, pheochromocytoma, insulin-dependent diabetes, active peptic ulcer disease, or accelerated hypertension. ■ Discontinue if tachycardia or palpitations occur. ■ Pregnancy: Encourage pregnant smokers to attempt cessation without pharmacologic treatment. Use during pregnancy only if the likelihood of smoking cessation justifies the potential risk of using it by the pregnant patient, who might continue to smoke. ■ Nursing mothers: Nicotine passes freely into breast milk. The risk of exposure of the infant to nicotine from Nicotrol Inhaler should be weighed against the risks associated with the infant's exposure to nicotine from continued smoking by the mother and from Nicotrol Inhaler alone, or in combination with continued smoking. ■ Drug interactions: Smoking cessation, with or without nicotine replacement, may alter the pharmacokinetics of certain concomitant medications. ■ Dependence might occur from transference of tobacco-related nicotine dependence to the Nicotrol® Inhaler. ■ Safety note concerning children: This product contains nicotine and should be kept out of the reach of children and pets.

Adpated from: "Nicotrol®Inhaler (nicotine inhalation system) 10 mg/unit Physician Insert". McNEIL Consumer Products Co, Fort Washington, Pa; 1997. Used with permission of the publisher.

Table 60.6. Information About Nicotrol® Nasal Spray (Nicotrol® NS) Use

Preparation	■ Patient should stop smoking completely when initiating therapy.
Dosage	■ Each use of the device delivers a spray containing 0.5 mg of nicotine. One dose is 1 mg of nicotine (2 sprays, one in each nostril). ■ Patients should be started with 1 or 2 doses per hour, which may be increased up to a maximum of 40 doses per day (maximum 5 doses per hour.) ■ No particular tapering strategy is recommended.
Administration	■ Patients should administer the spray with the head titled slightly backward. ■ Patients should be instructed not to sniff, swallow, or inhale through the nose as the spray is being administered. ■ Patient should spray once in each nostril per dose.
Duration of Therapy	■ Maximum recommended duration of therapy is 3 months. ■ Patients who are successfully abstinent on Nicotrol® NS should be treated at the selected individualized dose for up to 8 weeks, following which use of the spray should be discontinued over the next 4 to 6 weeks. Some patients may not require gradual reduction of dosage and may abruptly stop treatment successfully. ■ If the patient is unable to stop smoking by the fourth week of therapy, treatment should probably be discontinued.
Adverse Reactions	■ The most common type of adverse reaction involves irritant effects of the nasophrayngeal and ocular tissues. During the first 2 days of treatment, nearly all patients report nasal irritation. Although the frequency and severity of nasal irritation declines with continued use, most patients continue to experience this effect to some degree. ■ Other common local side effects: runny nose, throat irritation, watering eyes, sneezing, and cough. ■ Systemic side effects: headaches and dizziness

continued

Table 60.6. Information About Nicotrol® Nasal Spray (Nicotrol® NS) Use—*Continued*

Contraindications and Precautions	**Contraindications:** ■ Hypersensitivity or allergy to nicotine or other product component. **Precautions:** ■ Not recommended in patients with severe reactive airways disease because of potential to exacerbate bronchospasm. ■ Do not use during immediate post-myocardial infarction period, in patients with serious arrhythmias, or with severe or worsening angina. ■ Discontinue if tachycardia occurs. ■ Use with caution in patients with coronary heart disease, vasospastic diseases, hyperthyroidism, pheochromocytoma, insulin-dependent diabetes, active peptic ulcer disease, and accelerated hypertension. ■ Nicotrol® NS has a dependence potential intermediate between other nicotine-based therapies and cigarettes. ■ Pregnancy: Encourage pregnant smokers to attempt cessation without pharmocologic treatment. Use during pregnancy only if the likelihood of smoking cessation justifies the potential risk of using it by the pregnant patient, who might continue to smoke. ■ Nursing mothers: Nicotine passes freely into breast milk. The risk of exposure of the infant to nicotine from Nicotrol® NS should be weighed against the risks associated with the infant's exposure to nicotine from continued smoking by the mother and from Nicotrol® NS alone, or in combination with continued smoking. ■ Drug interaction: Smoking cessation, with or without nicotine replacement, may alter the pharmacokinetics of certain concomitant medications. ■ Safety note concerning children: Keep both used and unused containers of Nicotrol® NS out of reach of children and pets.

Adapted from: "Nicotrol® NS (nicotine nasal spray) 10 mg/ml Physician Insert" McNEIL Consumer Products Co, Fort Washington, Pa, 1996. Used with permission of the publisher.

Table 60.7. Information About Use of Zyban™ (Bupropion Hydrochloride) Sustained-Release Tablets

Preparation	■ Treatment should be initiated while the patient is still smoking. ■ Patients should set a "target quit date" within the first two weeks of treatment, generally in the second week.
Dosage	■ Usual dosage: 150 mg twice daily. ■ Start dosing at 150 mg once daily. Increase on day 4 to 150 mg twice daily and maintain for duration of therapy. ■ Maximum dosage: 300 mg/day. ■ Dose tapering on discontinuation is not required.
Administration	■ Oral tablet swallowed whole. Patient should not chew, divide, or crush tablets. ■ Combination treatment with Zyban™ and a nicotine transdermal system (NTS) may be used. Add NTS after patient reaches target quit date. Refer to table 60-3 for more information about NTS.
Duration of Therapy	■ 7 to 12 weeks. If a patient has not made significant progress towards smoking abstinence by the seventh week of therapy, the manufacturer recommends discontinuation of therapy.
Adverse Reactions	■ Most common reactions: Insomnia and dry mouth. ■ Most common reactions leading to discontinuation of therapy: nervous system disturbances, primarily tremor, and skin disorders, primarily rashes. ■ Other side effects: arthralgia, dizziness, constipation, rash, nausea, pruritus, taste perversion.

continued

Table 60.7. Information About Use of Zyban™ (Bupropion Hydrochloride) Sustained-Release Tablets—*Continued*

Warnings, Contraindications and Precautions	**Warnings:** ■ Because the use of bupropion is associated with a dose-dependent risk of seizures, clinicians should not prescribe doses over 300 mg/day for smoking cessation. The risk of seizures is also related to patient factors, clinical situation, and concurrent medications, which must be considered in selection of patients for therapy with bupropion. **Contraindications:** ■ Patients with a seizure disorder. ■ Patients taking other medications containing bupropion. ■ Current or prior diagnosis of bulimia or anorexia nervosa. ■ Concurrent administration of a monoamine oxidase (MAO) inhibitor or administration of an MAO inhibitor less than 14 days prior to initiation of Zyban™. **Precautions:** ■ Pregnancy: not recommended ■ Nursing mothers: not recommended. ■ Use caution with concurrent administration of Zyban™ and agents that lower seizure threshold (eg antipsychotics, antidepressants, theophylline, systemic steroids, etc.) ■ Be aware that the antidepressant Wellbutrin® contains bupropion, the same active ingredient in Zyban. ■ If combining Zyban™ with NTS use, monitor for treatment-induced hypertension.

Adapted from: "Zyban™ (bupropion hydrocholoride) Sustained-Release Tablets Product Information". Glaxo Wellcome Inc. Research Triangle Park, NC. 1997. Reproduced with permission of Glaxo Wellcome Inc.

Patient Resources

Smoking: Steps To Help You Break the Habit. American Academy of Family Physicians, 8880 Ward Pkwy, Kansas City, MO 64114-2797; (800)944-0000; Internet address: http://www.aafp.org

How to Quit Cigarettes; The Fifty Most Often Asked Questions about Smoking and Health and the Answers. To order these and other materials, contact your local office of the American Cancer Society or call (800)ACS-2345.

Smoking in Women. American College of Obstetricians and Gynecologists, 409 12th St SW, Washington, DC 20024; (800)762-2264. Internet address: http://www.acog.com

Smoking Can Really Do a Number on Your Health. To order this and other material, contact the American Dental Association, Department of Salable Materials, 211 E Chicago Ave, Chicago, IL 60611; (800)947-4746.

Chew or Snuff Is Real Bad Stuff; Why Do You Smoke? National Cancer Institute. Superintendent of Documents, Consumer Information Center—3C, PO Box 100, Pueblo, CO 81002.

Check Your Smoking I.Q.: An Important Quiz for Older Smokers. To order this and other material, contact the National Heart, Lung, and Blood Institute Smoking Education Program, PO Box 30105, Bethesda, MD 20824-0105; (301)251-1222 (English and Spanish); Internet address: http://www.nhlbi.nih.gov/nhlbi/nhlbi.html

You Can Quit Smoking: Smoking Cessation Consumer Guide, Clinical Practice Guideline Number 18. Publication number 96-0695. Call or write: Agency for Health Care Policy and Research, Publications Clearinghouse, P.O. Box 8547, Silver Spring MD 20907; 1-800-358-9295, Also available through InstantFAX at (301)594-2800 (push 1 and start, wait for directions); Internet address: http://www.ahcpr.gov

Provider Resources

Stop Smoking Kit. American Academy of Family Physicians, 8880 Ward Pkwy, Kansas City, MO 64114-2797; (800)944-0000; Internet address: http://www.aafp.org

Smoking and Reproductive Health. American College of Obstetricians and Gynecologists, 409 12th St SW, Washington, DC 20024; (800)762-2264. Technical Bulletin AT180.

Doctors Helping Smokers. To order this office-based tobacco cessation program and video by the same name, contact Doctors Helping Smokers at Blue Plus, PO Box 64179 R 3-11, St. Paul, MN 55164; (800)382-2000, ext 1975.

How To Help Your Patients Stop Smoking: A National Cancer Institute Manual for Physicians; How To Help Your Patients Stop Using Tobacco: A National Cancer Institute Manual for the Oral Health Team. To order these and other materials, contact the Office of Cancer Communications, National Cancer Institute, Bldg 31, Room 10A16, Bethesda, MD 20892; (800)4-CANCER; Internet address: http://wwwicic.nci.nih.gov

Helping Smokers Quit: A Guide for Primary Care Clinicians, Clinical Practice Guideline No. 18, AHCPR Publication No. 96-0693. Call or write: Agency for Health Care Policy and Research, Publications Clearinghouse, P.O. Box 8547, Silver Spring, MD 20907; (800)-358-9295, Also available through InstantFAX at (301)594-2800 (push 1 and start, wait for directions); Internet address: http://www.ahcpr.gov

Nurses: Help Your Patients Stop Smoking. National Heart, Lung, and Blood Institute Smoking Education Program, PO Box 30105, Bethesda, MD 20824-0105; (301)251-1222 (English and Spanish); Internet access: http://www.nhlbi.nih.gov/nhlbi/nhlbi.html

Selected References

American Academy of Family Physicians. *Summary of Policy Recommendations for Periodic Health Examination.* Kansas City, Mo: American Academy of Family Physicians; 1997.

American College of Obstetricians and Gynecologists. *Guidelines for Women's Health Care.* Washington, DC: American College of Obstetricians and Gynecologists; 1996.

American College of Obstetricians and Gynecologists. *Smoking and Reproductive Health: ACOG Technical Bulletin.* 1993;180:1-5.

American College of Physicians, Health and Public Policy Committee. Methods for stopping cigarette smoking. *Ann Intern Med.* 1986;105:281-291.

American Medical Association. *How to help patients stop smoking: guidelines for diagnosis and treatment of nicotine dependence.* Chicago, Ill: American Medical Association, 1994.

Canadian Task Force on the Periodic Health Examination. Prevention of tobacco-caused disease. In: *The Canadian Guide to Clinical Preventive Health Care.* Ottawa, Canada: Minister of Supply and Services; 1994: chap 43.

Centers for Disease Control. *The Health Benefits of Smoking Cessation.* Washington, DC: US Department of Health and Human Services; 1990. USDHHS publication CDC 90-8416.

Centers for Disease Control, Office on Smoking and Health. *The Health Benefits of Smoking Cessation: A Report of the Surgeon General, 1990 at a Glance.* Rockville, Md: Centers for Disease Control; 1990. USDHHS publication CDC 90-8419.

Fiore MC. The new vital sign: assessing and documenting smoking status. *JAMA.* 1991;266: 3183-3184.

Fiore MC, Bailey WC, Cohen SJ, et al. *Smoking Cessation. Clinical Practice Guideline No. 18.* Rockville, MD: US Department of Health and Human Services, Public Health Service, Agency for Health Care Policy and Research; 1996. AHCPR Publication No. 96-0692.

Fiore MC, Jorenby DE, Baker TB, Kenfor SL. Tobacco dependence and the nicotine patch: clinical guidelines for effective use. *JAMA.* 1992;268:2687-2694.

Frank E, Winkleby MA, Altman DG, Rockhill B, Fortmann SP. Predictors of physicians' smoking cessation advice. *JAMA.* 1991;266:3139-3144.

Glynn TJ, Manley MW. *How To Help Your Patients Stop Smoking: A National Cancer Institute Manual for Physicians.* Bethesda, Md: National Institutes of Health; 1995. NIH publication 95-3064.

Goldsmith MS. Magazines without tobacco advertising (Medical News and Perspectives). *JAMA.* 1991;266:3099-3102.

Kottke TE, Battista RN, DeFriese GH, Brekke ML. Smoking cessation: attributes of successful interventions. *JAMA.* 1988;259;2883-2889.

Solberg LI, Maxwell PL, Kottke TE, Gepner GJ, Brekke ML. A systematic primary care office-based smoking cessation program. *J Fam Pract.* 1990;30:647-654.

Steenland K. Passive smoking and the risk of heart disease. *JAMA.* 1992;267:94-99.

US Preventive Services Task Force. Counseling to prevent tobacco use. In: *Guide to Clinical Preventive Services.* 2nd ed. Washington, DC: US Department of Health and Human Services; 1996: chap 54.

61

UNINTENDED PREGNANCY

Modern contraceptives have enabled women to increase control over their reproductive lives. However, in the United States 60% of all pregnancies are unintended. Unplanned pregnancies affect women of all ages and circumstances; however, their number is higher in certain population groups, such as teenagers (82% of pregnancies unintended) and never-married women (88% of pregnancies unintended). The consequences of these pregnancies in the United States include approximately 1.5 million abortions annually, children who are at increased risk of health and behavior problems in childhood and later in life, and pregnancies that have not benefitted from preconception risk identification and management.

Screening, counseling, and preventive services are particularly needed for older women of childbearing age. For women aged 35 to 39, 56% of pregnancies are unintended. For women aged 40 to 44, the number is 77%, and 59% of these end in abortion, the highest percentage for any age group from age 15 to 44. Pregnancies of women aged 40 to 44 and beyond, while small in absolute numbers, are disproportionately unintended, likely to end in abortion, and likely to entail other adverse outcomes. The large percentage of unintended pregnancies for women approaching age 44 suggests that both women and their care givers underestimate the potential for, and fall short of, adequate protection against pregnancy during these years when fertility is expected to decline.

Modern contraceptives marketed in the United States have been shown to be safe and effective (Table 61.1). Although most are relatively inexpensive, their costs vary.

See chapter 25 for information on counseling to prevent unintended pregnancy in adolescents. See chapters 23 and 59 for information on counseling to prevent sexually transmitted diseases and HIV infection among adolescents and adults, respectively.

Table 61.1. Percentage of women experiencing an unintended pregnancy during the first year of typical use and the first year of perfect use of contraception and the percentage continuing use at the end of the first year, United States.

Method	% of Women Experience an Unintended Pregnancy within the First Year of Use		% of Women Continuing Use at One Year[3]
	Typical Use[1]	Perfect Use[2]	
Chance[4]	85	85	
Spermicides[5]	26	6	40
Periodic abstinence	25		63
Calendar		9	
Ovulation method		3	
Sympto-thermal[6]		2	
Post-ovulation		1	
Withdrawal	19	4	
Cap[7]			
Parous women	40	26	42
Nulliparous women	20	9	56
Sponge			
Parous women	40	20	42
Nulliparous women	20	9	56
Diaphragm[7]	20	6	56
Condom[8]			
Female (Reality®)	21	5	56
Male	14	3	61
Pill	5		71
Progestin only		0.5	
Combined		0.1	
IUD			
Progesterone T	2.0	1.5	81
Copper T 380A	0.8	0.6	78
LNg 20	0.1	0.1	81
Depo-Provera	0.3	0.3	70
Norplant® (6 capsules)	0.05	0.05	88
Female sterilization	0.5	0.5	100
Male sterilization	0.15	0.10	100

[1] Among *typical* couples who initiate use of a method (not necessarily for the first time), the percentage who experience an accidental pregnancy during the first year if they do not stop use for any other reason.

[2] Among couples who initiate use of a method (not necessarily for the first time) and who use it *perfectly* (both consistently and correctly), the percentage who experience an accidental pregnancy during the first year if they do not stop use for any other reason.

[3] Among couples attempting to avoid pregnancy, the percentage who continue to use a method for 1 year.

[4] The percents becoming pregnant in columns (2) and (3) are based on data from populations where contraception is not used and from women who cease using contraception in order to become pregnant. Among such populations, about 89% become pregnant within 1 year. This estimate was lowered slightly (to 85%) to represent the percent who would become pregnant within 1 year among women now relying on reversible methods of contraception if they abandoned contraception altogether.

[5] Foams, creams, gels, vaginal suppositories, and vaginal film.

[6] Cervical mucus (ovulation) method supplemented by calendar in the pre-ovulatory and basal body temperature in the post-ovulatory phases.

[7] With spermicidal cream or jelly.

[8] Without spermicides.

Adapted from: Hatcher RH, Stewart F, Trussel J, et al. *Contraceptive Technology*. 17th Rev Ed. New York, NY: Irvington Publishing; 1998 (in press). Used with permission of the publisher. Copyright 1997.

Recommendations of Major Authorities

American College of Obstetricians and Gynecologists and US Preventive Services Task Force—Primary care providers should obtain a history of sexual practices and provide counseling on the prevention of unintended pregnancy and contraceptive options to all sexually active women who do not want to become pregnant and men who do not want to have a child. Counseling should also be provided regarding high-risk sexual behavior and the prevention of STDs and HIV infection.

Basics of Counseling to Prevent Unintended Pregnancy

1. The main goal is to make sure family planning is a part of primary care for all sexually active patients. Assess sexual practices and the need for contraceptive counseling for every patient, including women in their forties and men. This can be done as a part of periodic health examinations or during acute care visits for issues of a related nature, such as STDs, postpartum care, or family stress. As with all counseling of patients regarding sensitive topics, address this issue with openness and a nonjudgmental attitude.

2. Determine each patient's level of knowledge about contraceptive options. What methods have they tried in the past? Have these methods been acceptable and effective for the patient and partner or partners? What medical and life-style factors could influence the patient's choice of an appropriate contraceptive?

3. Educate patients about the important characteristics of different contraceptive methods (Table 61.2). Present the patient with a range of contraceptive options. Assist patients in carefully choosing a contraceptive method that is appropriate for their abilities, motivation, and life-style, thereby increasing the likelihood that it will be used correctly and consistently. Encourage patients who are already using a method correctly and successfully to continue to do so.

4. Discuss the ability of different contraceptive methods to protect against sexually transmitted diseases (STDs) and human immunodeficiency virus (HIV) infection. Latex condoms, used consistently and correctly, are effective for both birth control and reducing the risk of disease. Other forms of birth control, such as IUDs, diaphragms, cervical caps, and oral contraceptives, do not give the same protection. Stress to patients that even if they use another form of birth control, if they are not involved in a mutually monogamous relationship with a person known to be free of infection, they also need to use condoms to reduce the risk of STDs.

5. Contraception is a responsibility of both partners. If possible, involve both partners in counseling and discussion of contraceptive options. See Table 61.1 for an evaluation of the effectiveness of various contraceptive methods. Also discuss ways in which males can participate in family planning.

Table 61.2. Complications, Side Effects, and Benefits of Major Methods of Contraception

Methods	Potential Complications	Potential Side Effects	Noncontraceptive Benefits
Pill	Cardiovascular complications (stroke, heart attack, blood clots, high blood pressure, hepatic adenomas)	Nausea, heachaches, dizziness, spotting, weight gain, breast tenderness, chloasma	Protects against pelvic inflammatory disease (PID), some cancers (ovarian, endometrial) and some benign tumors (leiomyomata, benign breast masses) and ovarian cysts; decreases menstrual blood loss and pain
IUD	Pelvic inflammatory disease, uterine perforation, anemia	Menstrual cramping, spotting, increased bleeding	None known except for progestin-releasing IUDs, which may decrease menstrual blood loss and pain
Male condom	None known	Decreased sensation, allergy to latex, loss of spontaneity	Protects against transmission of sexually transmitted diseases, including AIDS; delays premature ejaculation
Female condom	None known	Aesthetically unappealing and awkward to use for some	Protects against sexually transmitted diseases
Implant	Infection at implant site	Tenderness at site, menstrual changes	May protect against PID; lactation not disturbed; may decrease menstrual cramps, pains and blood loss
Injectable	None definitely proven	Menstrual changes, weight gain, headaches	May protect against PID; lactation not disturbed; may have protective effects against ovarian and endometrial cancers
Sterilization	Infection	Pain at surgical site, psychological reactions, subsequent regret that the procedure was performed	None known; may protect against PID
Abstinence	None known	Psychological reactions	Prevents infections including AIDS

continued

Table 61.2. Complications, Side Effects, and Benefits of Major Methods of Contraception—*Continued*

Methods	Potential Complications	Potential Side Effects	Noncontraceptive Benefits
Abortion	Infection pain, perforation, psychologic trauma	Cramping	None known
Barriers: diaphragm, cap, sponge	Vaginal and urinary tract infections, toxic shock syndrome	Pelvic pressure, vaginal discharge if left in too long, allergy	Provides modest protection against some sexually transmitted infections
Spermicides	Urinary tract infections	Tissue irritation, allergy	Provides modest protection against some sexually transmitted infections
Lactational amenorrhea method (LAM)	None known	Mastitis from staphylococcal infection	Provides excellent nutrition for infants under 6 months old

Adapted from: Trussel J. Contraceptive efficacy. In Hatcher RA, Trussel J, Stewart F et al. *Contraceptve Technology.* 17th rev ed. New York, NY: Irvington Publishers; 1998, in press. Used with permission of the publisher; copyright 1997.

6. After patients choose a method, conduct an in-depth discussion of:

   ■ How it works

   ■ Theoretical and actual effectiveness

   ■ Advantages/benefits

   ■ Disadvantages/risks

   ■ How to use the method

   ■ Nuisance side effects

   ■ Warning signs

   ■ Back-up methods.

   Provide patients with printed material about the contraceptive method chosen (Patient Resources).

7. Follow-up counseling is particularly important in the first few weeks of contraceptive use to deal with any difficulties associated with use and side effects. Ask patients how they are using the method, correct misinformation, and discuss any impediments to proper use of the method. Continue

counseling during each patient visit, especially until patients are very comfortable with use of the contraceptive method. Many compliance problems can be resolved relatively simply with reassurance and changes in dose or technique of use.

8. Oral contraceptives (OCs) can also be prescribed as a postcoital ("morning after") method to prevent pregnancy (Table 61.3). The Food and Drug Administration announced in February 1997 that certain combined oral contraceptives containing ethinyl estradiol and norgestrel or levonorgestrel were safe and effective for use as postcoital emergency contraception . This approach to emergency contraception has been reported to reduce the risk of pregnancy by 55.3% to 94.2% after unprotected intercourse if treatment is initiated within 72 hours.

Instruct the patient to take the first dose as soon as possible (but no more than 72 hours) after unprotected intercourse; the second dose is taken 12 hours after the first dose. The most common side effects of these regimens are nausea and vomiting.

Table 61.3. Oral Contraceptives for Use as Postcoital Emergency Contraception

Brand Name	Pill Color	Number of pills to swallow within 72 hours after unprotected sex	Number of pills to swallow 12 hours later
Ovral®	white	2	2
Lo/Ovral®	white	4	4
Nordette®	light orange	4	4
Levlen®	light orange	4	4
Triphasil®	yellow	4	4
Tri-Levlen®	yellow	4	4

Adapted from: Food and Drug Administration. Prescription Drug products; certain combined oral contraceptives for use as postcoital emergency contraception. *Federal Register.* 1997:62(37):8610–8612.

Patient Resources

Birth Control: Choosing the Method That's Right for You. American Academy of
Family Physicians, 8880 Ward Pkwy, Kansas City, MO 64114-2797; (800)944-
0000. Internet address: http://www.aafp.org

Barrier Methods of Contraception; Contraception (in English and Spanish); *Family
Planning by Periodic Abstinence; The Intrauterine Device; Oral Contraceptives; Post-
partum Sterilization; Sterilization by Laparoscopy; Sterilization for Women and
Men.* American College of Obstetricians and Gynecologists, 409 12th St SW,
Washington, DC 20024; (800)762-2264. Internet address:
http://www.acog.com

Drugs and Pregnancy: Often the Two Don't Mix; Choosing a Contraceptive. FDA
Office of Consumer Affairs. HFE 88 Room 1675, 5600 Fishers Ln, Rockville,
MD 20857; (800)532-4440.

Emergency Contraception Website. The Office of Population Research at
Princeton University. Internet address:
http://opr.princeton.edu//ec/hotline.html

Emergency Contraception Hotline. The Office of Population Research at
Princeton University. (800)584-9911.

Facts About Birth Control. Planned Parenthood, 810 7th Ave, New York, NY
10019; (212) 541-7800; Internet address: http://www.ppfa.org/ppfa

Provider Resources

Hormonal Contraception. (ACOG Educational Bulletin #198). American College
of Obstetricians and Gynecologists. 409 12th St SW, Washington, DC 20024;
(800)762-2264. Internet address: http://www.acog.com

Emergency Contraception. (ACOG Practice Pattern #3). American College of
Obstetricians and Gynecologists. 409 12th St SW, Washington, DC 20024;
(800)762-2264. Internet address: http://www.acog.com

Food and Drug Administration. Prescription Drug Products; Certain Combined Oral contraceptives for Use as Postcoital Emergency Contraception; Notice. *Federal Register.* 1997; 62(37)8610-8612.

The Intrauterine Device (technical bulletin 164). American College of Obstetricians and Gynecologists, 409 12th St SW, Washington, DC 20024; (800)762-
2264. Internet address: http://www.acog.com

Managing Contraceptive Pill Patients. EMIS Publishers, Dallas, TX; (800)225-0694.

Oral Contraceptive User Guide (Second Edition). EMIS Publishers, Dallas, TX. (800)225-0694.

Planned Parenthood. Planned Parenthood at 810 7th Ave, New York, NY 10019; (212) 541-7800. Internet address: http://www.ppfa.org/ppfa

Selected References

American College of Obstetricians and Gynecologists. *Guidelines for Women's Health Care.* Washington, DC: American College of Obstetricians and Gynecologists; 1996.

Baird D, Glasier AF. Hormonal contraception. *N Engl J Med.* 1993;328:1543-1549.

Canadian Task Force on the Periodic Health Examination. The periodic health examination: 2. 1987 update. *Can Med Assoc J.* 1988;138:618-626.

Hatcher RA, Trussell J, Stewart F, et al. *Contraceptive Technology 1994-1996.* 16th rev ed. New York, NY: Irvington Publishers, 1996.

Hatcher RA, Stewart F, Trussell J, et al. *Contraceptive Technology.* 17th rev ed. New York, NY: Irvington Publishers; 1998, in press.

Trussell J, Stewart F. The effectiveness of postcoital hormonal contraception. *Family Planning Perspectives.* 1992;24:262-264.

Trussell J, Stewart F, Guest F, Hatcher RA. Emergency contraceptive pills: a simple proposal to reduce unintended pregnancies. *Family Planning Perspectives.* 1992;24:269-273.

US Department of Health and Human Services, Public Health Service. *Healthy People 2000 Progress Review: Family Planning.* Washington, DC: US Department of Health and Human Services, Public Health Service; March 26, 1996.

US Preventive Services Task Force. Counseling to prevent unintended pregnancy. In: *Guide to Clinical Preventive Services.* 2nd ed. Washington, DC: US Department of Health and Human Services; 1996: chap 63.

62

OSTEOPOROSIS

According to the National Osteoporosis Foundation, more than 25 million Americans have osteoporosis, and each year more than 1.3 million fractures occur as a result. Osteoporosis is the most common metabolic bone disorder, and the risk for osteoporosis and osteoporosis-related fractures increases with advancing age. As the population of the United States ages, osteoporosis becomes an increasing public health concern.

About 70% of fractures in persons aged 45 or older are related to osteoporosis. The earliest and most predominant fractures involve the lower thoracic and lumbar vertebrae. These are often asymptomatic and may be diagnosed through spinal x-rays obtained for other reasons. These fractures produce loss of height and the development of a "dowager's hump," a distortion of the spine. As these fractures progress, they produce compression of the abdominal cavity, resulting in difficulties eating and digesting. After age 65, fractures of the hip and of the arm produce greater morbidity and are associated with pain, disability, and decreased functional ability. In the first year following a hip fracture, a patient's expected survival decreases 15% to 20%. The economic impact of osteoporosis is also high. In 1995, an estimated $13.8 billion was spent in the United States for osteoporosis-related medical, nursing home, and social costs. These numbers are expected to increase over the next 20 years.

Important risk factors for osteoporosis are female gender, low dietary intakes of calcium during adolescence, age, and early menopause. Women of Caucasian or Asian ancestry and those whose mothers have had osteoporosis are at greatest risk. Dietary intake of calcium during childhood and adolescence is a determinant of adult peak bone mass. Peak bone mass is achieved in the third decade, after which bone loss begins. In women, bone loss is accelerated by menopause, particularly premature menopause induced by oophorectomy. Low body weight, excessive alcohol intake, and sedentary life style have been associated with osteoporosis as well. Parity, lactation history, caffeine intake, and smoking have been suggested in the past as possible risk factors but are poor predictors of bone mass.

The main techniques available for screening for osteoporosis include single photon absorption (SPA), dual photon absorption (DPA), dual energy x-ray absorption (DXA), and quantitative computed tomography (QCT). DXA is currently the favored method because of its ease of use, good precision, relatively low procedure time (5 to 10 minutes), and very low radiation dose. Like the SPA and DPA, however, it cannot discriminate between cortical bone and trabecular bone; QCT must be used to accomplish this. DXA measures bone mineral content (g/cm) or areal density (g/cm^2) and may be used over the total body or for a specific area. Most experts agree that DXA is a safe, accurate, and precise modality for measuring bone density. Ultrasound technology for assessing bone density is under development and may be of use in the future.

DXA can identify at risk persons who can most benefit from interventions; however, because the rate of postmenopausal bone loss varies among women, bone mass at menopause correlates only moderately with bone mass 10 to 20 years later when most fractures occur. Also, no consensus exists regarding what interventions are indicated for patients with any particular level of bone density.

See chapter 47 for information on hormone replacement therapy. See Chapter 56 for information on nutrition counseling and Chapter 57 for information on physical activity counseling.

Recommendations of Major Authorities (Includes Screening)

American Academy of Family Physicians—All patients should be counseled about the importance of adequate calcium intake, regular weight-bearing exercise, smoking cessation, and moderate alcohol use. Patients at risk and those diagnosed with osteoporosis should be advised of treatment options. Bone densitometry cannot be recommended for routine use at this time. Bone mineral densitometry may be useful for high-risk patients, to monitor therapy, and for patients who are unable to come to a decision about hormone replacement therapy.

American College of Obstetricians and Gynecologists—All women should be counseled on diet and exercise as part of routine preventive visits. Women over 40 should be counseled on use of hormone replacement therapy. Women 65 and over should be counseled on fall prevention.

American College of Physicians—Routine screening of all postmenopausal women by bone densitometry for osteoporosis is not recommended. Bone density measurements may be indicated in specific clinical situations where the decision to treat must be based on knowledge of bone mass and related to risk of fracture.

Canadian Task Force on Periodic Health Examination —Does not recommend routine radiologic screening for osteoporosis. Bone density measurements may be useful to guide treatment in selected postmenopausal women considering hormone replacement therapy. The **CTFPHE** recommends counseling all peri-menopausal women regarding the benefits and risks of estrogen replacement therapy; however, there is insufficient evidence to recommend for or against the inclusion or exclusion of counseling premenopausal and postmenopausal women to engage in regular weight-bearing exercise to reduce osteoporosis risk.

National Osteoporosis Foundation—Recommends a comprehensive program to prevent osteoporosis in women and men of all ages that includes adequate calcium and vitamin D intake, weight-bearing exercises, a healthy lifestyle with no smoking and limited alcohol consumption, and medication when appropriate. A bone mineral density (BMD) test is the only way to detect bone loss before a fracture occurs. A BMD test is indicated when risk factors are present and a decision must be made regarding osteoporosis medications to reduce fracture risk.

National Institutes of Health—A 1984 consensus conference on osteoporosis recommended that estrogen therapy after menopause should be considered in high-risk women who have no medical contraindications and who are willing to adhere to a program of careful follow-up.

US Preventive Services Task Force—There is insufficient evidence to recommend for or against routine screening for osteoporosis with bone densitometry in postmenopausal women. Recommendations against routine screening may be made on other grounds. All postmenopausal women should be counseled about hormone prophylaxis and advised of the importance of smoking cessation, regular exercise and adequate calcium intake. For those high-risk women who would consider estrogen only to prevent osteoporosis, screening may be appropriate to assist treatment decisions.

World Health Organization—Bone density measurements may be useful to guide treatment in selected postmenopausal women considering hormone replacement therapy.

Basics of Osteoporosis Counseling

The most effective management for osteoporosis is the prevention of osteoporosis through counseling about dietary and behavioral practices to maximize the peak bone mass achieved by the third decade and to slow the rate of bone loss after that period.

1. Counsel all patients about consuming adequate amounts of calcium and vitamin D (chapter 56). Also advise patients to avoid smoking and excessive alcohol intake.

2. Counsel all patients to exercise (chapter 57). Weight bearing activities such as walking and stair climbing promote achievement of peak bone mass and delay bone loss. Once fractures have occurred, the patient should limit exercise to tolerable walking and avoid lifting and vigorous muscle straining.

3. Advise perimenopausal women of the probable risks and benefits of hormone replacement therapy (HRT) (chapter 47).

4. For all older persons, assess the risk of falls and provide appropriate counseling to implement precautionary measures such as removal of throw rugs and installation of hand rails next to stairs and in the bathroom (chapter 55).

5. Evaluate for the presence of clinical risk factors (Table 62.1) to identify individuals who may profit from more precise evaluation of bone mineral content as a procedure for selection and monitoring of specific therapy.

6. Discuss with patients the drugs currently approved by the FDA for the prevention of osteoporosis (HRT and alendronate [Fosamax]) and for the treatment of osteoporosis (estrogen replacement therapy, alendronate, and calcitonin). The protective effects of all therapies appear to be lost soon after discontinuation of treatment.

   ■ **Hormone Replacement Therapy (HRT):** Recent studies have shown that women who start HRT late after menopause receive the same protective effect against risk of subsequent fractures as those who start treatment during or immediately after menopause. Counsel each patient about the risks and benefits of hormone replacement therapy (chapter 47).

   ■ **Alendronate:** This third-generation amino-bisphosphonate that acts as an osteoclast inhibitor, has been approved for the prevention and treatment of osteoporosis. Initial studies have shown that alendronate not only arrests further loss of bone mineral content, but in many cases leads to an actual increase in bone mineral density. Alendronate treatment is also associated with decreases in fractures in people with low bone mass density who have already had a spine fracture. Other bisphosphonate agents are currently under review, and these agents may increase treatment options for patients.

   ■ **Calcitonin:** Calcitonin, a hormone that helps control bone remodeling, is administered by injection (subcutaneously or intramuscularly) or by nasal spray. Side effects include flushing, rash, nausea, dizziness, and faintness. Calcitonin does not offer the other benefits of estrogen (control of hot flashes, lowering of cholesterol, protection against coronary heart disease), and its efficacy in fracture prevention has not been proven. Its effectiveness has been demonstrated only in women with established osteoporosis who are more than 5 years postmenopausal.

Table 62.1 Risk Factors for Hip Fractures

Age ≥80 years
Maternal history of hip fracture
Any other fracture since age 50 years
Self-reported fair, poor, or very poor health
Previous hyperthyroidism
Anticonvulsant therapy
Current weight less than weight at age 25 years
Height at age 25 ≥168 cm (5 ft, 6 in)
Caffeine intake >2 cups daily
On feet ≤4 hours daily
No walking for exercise
Inability to rise from a chair without using arms
Lowest quartile of visual depth perception
Lowest quartile of contrast sensitivity

Adapted from: Cummings, SR, Nevitt MC, Browner WS, et al. Risk factors for hip fractures in white women. *N Engl J Med.* 1995;332(12):767–773.

Patient Resources

Osteoporosis in Women: Keeping Your Bones Healthy and Strong. American Academy of Family Physicians, 8880 Ward Pkwy, Kansas City MO 64114-2797; (800)944-0000.

Preventing Osteoporosis (ACOG Patient Education Pamphlet AP048). American College of Obstetricians and Gynecologists. 409 12th St, SW, Washington, DC 20024; (800)762-2264. Internet address: http://www.acog.com

National Osteoporosis Foundation, Osteoporosis and Related Bone Disorders National Resource Center, 1150 17th St, NW, Suite 500, Washington, DC 20036; (800)624-BONE.

Provider Resources

National Osteoporosis Foundation, Osteoporosis and Related Bone Disorders National Resource Center, 1150 17th St, NW, Suite 500, Washington, DC 20036; (800)624-BONE.

Selected References

Alexeera L, Burkhardt P, Christiansen C, et al. *Assessment of Fracture Risk and Application of Screening for Postmenopausal Osteoporosis.* World Health Organization. Technical Report Series 843. Geneva: World Health Organization, 1994.

American Academy of Family Physicians. *Diagnosis and Management of Osteoporosis.* Kansas City, Mo: American Academy of Family Physicians; 1996.

American Academy of Family Physicians. *Summary of Policy Recommendations for Periodic Health Examination.* Kansas City, MO: American Academy of Family Physicians; 1997.

American College of Obstetricians and Gynecologists. *Guidelines for Women's Health Care.* Washington, DC: American College of Obstetricians and Gynecologists; 1996.

American College of Obstetricians and Gynecologists. *Osteoporosis.* ACOG Technical Bulletin #167. Washington, DC: American College of Obstetricians and Gynecologists; 1992.

American College of Physicians. Guidelines for counseling postmenopausal women about preventive hormone therapy. *Ann Intern Med.* 1992;117:1038-1041.

Black DM, Cummings SR, Karpf DB et al. Randomized trial of effect of alendronate on risk of fracture in women with existing vertebral fractures. *Lancet.* 1996;348:1535-41.

Cummings SR, Nevitt MC, Browner WS, et al. Risk factors for hip fractures in white women. *N Engl J Med.* 1995;332(12):767-773.

Canadian Task Force on the Periodic Health Examination. *Canadian Guide to Clinical Preventive Health Care.* Ottawa, Canada: Canadian Communication Group; 1994:602-631.

Canadian Task Force on the Periodic Health Examination. Physical Activity Counselling. In: *The Canadian Guide to Clinical Preventive Health Care.* Ottawa, Canada: Minister of Supply and Services; 1994: chap 47.

Canadian Task Force on the Periodic Health Examination. Prevention of Osteoporotic fractures in women by estrogen-replacement therapy. In: *The Canadian Guide to Clinical Preventive Health Care.* Ottawa, Canada: Minister of Supply and Services; 1994: chap 52.

Melton LJ, Eddy DM, Johnston CC. Screening for osteoporosis. *Ann Intern Med.* 1990;112:516-528.

National Institutes of Health. Consensus conference: osteoporosis. *JAMA.* 1984;252:799-802.

Ray NF, Chan JK, Thamer M, Melton LJ. Medical expenditures for the treatment of osteoporotic fractures in the United States in 1995: report from the National Osteoporosis Foundation. *J Bone and Mineral Research.* 12(1)1997;24-35.

US Preventive Services Task Force. *Guide to Clinical Preventive Services.* 2nd ed. Washington, DC: US Department of Health and Human Services; 1996: chap 25.

Appendices

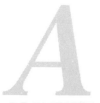

PREVENTIVE CARE TIMELINES AND RISK FACTOR TABLES

A prevention strategy based on risk factors may increase or decrease the priority of specific services, increase or decrease the frequency of particular services, change the ages at which certain services become appropriate, or add or delete some services for individuals or populations. Appendix A contains timelines for preventive care (Figures A.1[a], A.1[b], A.2[a] and A.2[b]) for both children and adults at normal risk as well as tables of clinical preventive services organized by risk factor category and target conditions (Tables A.1 through A.11).

The timeline and risk factor tables may help guide risk-based prevention strategies for populations and individual patients. They may also be used to augment discussions between patients and clinicians when considering preventive services. Ultimately, the decision to perform a particular service is based on the needs and preferences of informed patients in consultation with their health care providers.

Preventive Care Timelines

The preventive care timelines for children are presented in Figures A.1(a) and A.1(b). The preventive care timelines for adults are presented in Figures A.2(a) and A.2(b). Figures A.1(a) and A.2(a) are graphical representations of the clinical preventive services that are recommended by most major authorities cited in the *Clinician's Handbook*. These timelines, applicable to a general practice population, present a core set of clinical preventive services for which a strong consensus exists among authorities. However, differences in recommendations exist regarding the periodicity and age of onset of certain clinical preventive services. Figures A.1(b) and A.2(b) illustrate the range of these recommendations. All four timelines illustrate the core clinical interventions around which clinicians can prioritize preventive services.

The timelines represent the most basic approach to risk assessment, one based on age and gender. A more individualized prevention strategy would be based on further information gathered in a patient history or health risk assessment, as illustrated in the risk factor tables.

Risk Factor Tables

These tables highlight prevention strategies based on risk factors identified through patients' histories or from health risk assessment surveys. Clinicians should consider the need for particular preventive services based on the knowledge of an individual's risk factors. Tables B.1 to B.11 include risk factors mentioned in the *Clinician's Handbook* as well as in the *Guide to Clinical Preventive Services, 2nd edition* of the US Preventive Services Task Force. Detection of the risk factors (primary prevention) or preclinical conditions (secondary prevention) presented in these tables can modify clinical management and health outcomes.

These 11 tables include risk factors cited in the *Clinician's Handbook* and are grouped by risk factor or by target condition. The lists of risk factors, risk factor categories, and target conditions are not exhaustive.

Table A.1—Age and Gender Profile: Children and Adolescents
Table A.2—Age and Gender Profile: Adults
Table A.3—Social Circumstances and Living Conditions: All Ages
Table A.4—Geographic and Ethnic Background: All Ages
Table A.5—Occupational, Recreational, Environmental & Residential
          Exposures: All Ages
Table A.6—Substance Abuse: Adolescents and Adults
Table A.7—Personal Medical History: All Ages
Table A.8—Family Medical History: All Ages
Table A.9—Sexual History: Adolescent and Adult Male
Table A.10—Sexual History: Adolescent and Adult Female
Table A.11—Reproductive History: Female

Each table has five column headings:
- Risk Factor
- Prevention Target Condition
- Preventive Service and/or Referrals
- Reimbursement Strategy
- *Clinician's Handbook* Chapters

Changes from the First Edition

Although much of the basic structure of Appendix A has been maintained from the first edition of the *Clinician's Handbook*, the following changes have been made:

- The 'Preventive Care Timelines', previously in the introductory section, are included in Appendix A to illustrate the complementary nature of the timelines and the risk tables.

■ The categories within the risk factor tables have been modified and expanded. Risk factors may be identified in more than one category to emphasize the overlap among many categories and to acknowledge that different practitioners categorize risk factors differently.

■ Two new column headings have been added to the Risk Factor Tables: "Preventive Service and/or Referrals" and "Reimbursement Strategy." The latter aids clinicians in identifying preventive services covered by Medicare or Medicaid's Early and Periodic Screening, Diagnosis, and Treatment Program (EPSDT). This column may be tailored to particular practice settings by identifying the services covered by local health plans and state Medicaid policies.

Figure A.1(a)

Clinical Preventive Services for Normal-Risk Children

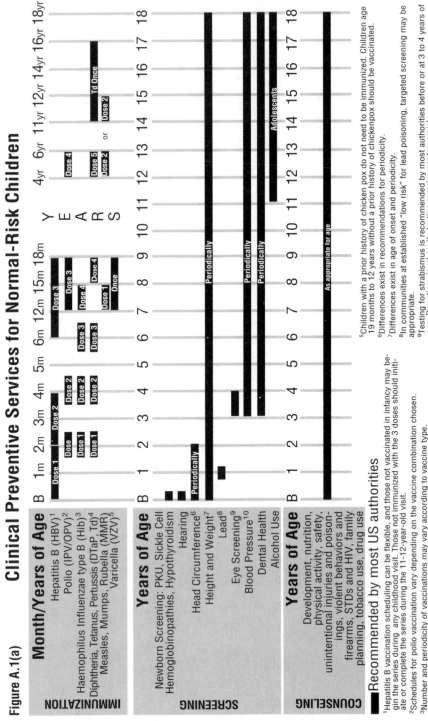

1Hepatitis B vaccination scheduling can be flexible, and those not vaccinated in infancy may begin the series during any childhood visit. Those not immunized with the 3 doses should initiate or complete the series during the 11-12-year-old visit.

2Schedules for polio vaccination vary depending on the vaccine combination chosen.

3Number and periodicity of vaccinations may vary according to vaccine type.

4DTaP (diphtheria and pertussis toxoids and acellular pertussis) is the preferred vaccine for all doses. Whole cell DTP is an acceptable alternative.

5Children with a prior history of chicken pox do not need to be immunized. Children age 19 months to 12 years without a prior history of chickenpox should be vaccinated.

6Differences exist in recommendations for periodicity.

7Differences exist in age of onset and periodicity.

8In communities at established "low risk" for lead poisoning, targeted screening may be appropriate.

9Testing for strabismus is recommended by most authorities before or at 3 to 4 years of age. Routine visual acuity testing remains controversial.

10Differences exist in age of onset and periodicity.

■ **Recommended by most US authorities**

Figure A.1(b)

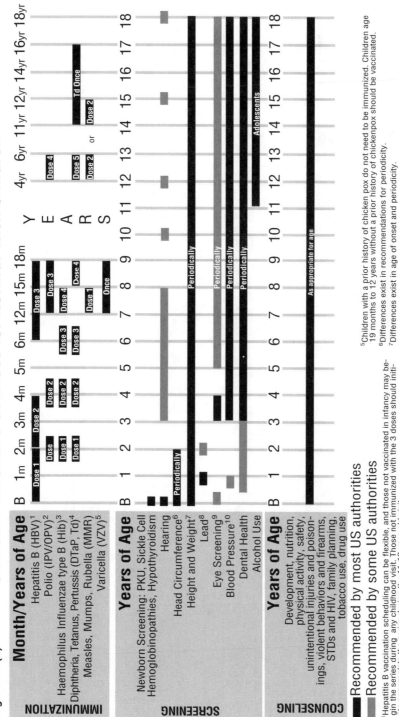

Clinical Preventive Services for Normal-Risk Children

■ Recommended by most US authorities
■ Recommended by some US authorities

[1]Hepatitis B vaccination scheduling can be flexible, and those not vaccinated in infancy may begin the series during any childhood visit. Those not immunized with the 3 doses should initiate or complete the series during the 11-12-year-old visit.

[2]Schedules for polio vaccination vary depending on the vaccine combination chosen.

[3]Number and periodicity of vaccinations may vary according to vaccine type.

[4]DTaP (diphtheria and pertussis toxoids and acellular pertussis) is the preferred vaccine for all doses. Whole cell DTP is an acceptable alternative.

[5]Children with a prior history of chicken pox do not need to be immunized. Children age 19 months to 12 years without a prior history of chickenpox should be vaccinated.

[6]Differences exist in recommendations for periodicity.

[7]Differences exist in age of onset and periodicity.

[8]In communities at established "low risk" for lead poisoning, targeted screening may be appropriate.

[9]Testing for strabismus is recommended by most authorities before or at 3 to 4 years of age. Routine visual acuity testing remains controversial.

[10]Differences exist in age of onset and periodicity.

Figure A.2(a)

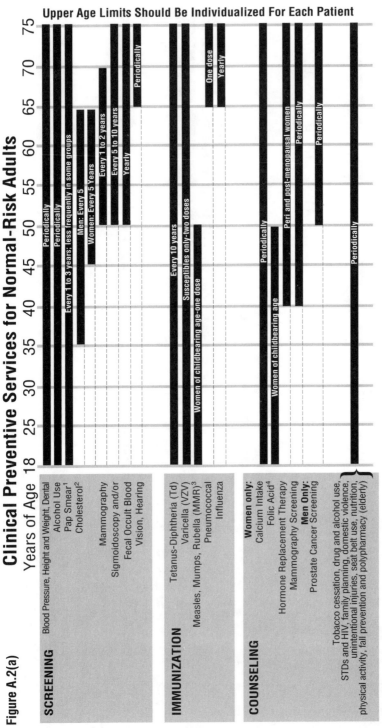

Clinical Preventive Services for Normal-Risk Adults

Upper Age Limits Should Be Individualized For Each Patient

Years of Age: 18, 25, 30, 35, 40, 45, 50, 55, 60, 65, 70, 75

SCREENING

- Blood Pressure, Height and Weight, Dental — Periodically
- Alcohol Use — Periodically
- Pap Smear[1] — Every 1 to 3 years; less frequently in some groups
- Cholesterol[2] — Men: Every 5 / Women: Every 5 Years
- Mammography — Every 1 to 2 years
- Sigmoidoscopy and/or — Every 5 to 10 years
- Fecal Occult Blood — Yearly
- Vision, Hearing — Periodically

IMMUNIZATION

- Tetanus-Diphtheria (Td) — Every 10 years
- Varicella (VZV) — Susceptibles only-two doses
- Measles, Mumps, Rubella (MMR)[3] — Women of childbearing age-one dose
- Pneumococcal — One dose
- Influenza — Yearly

COUNSELING

Women only:
- Calcium Intake — Periodically
- Folic Acid[4] — Women of childbearing age
- Hormone Replacement Therapy — Peri and post-menopausal women
- Mammography Screening — Periodically
Men Only:
- Prostate Cancer Screening — Periodically

Tobacco cessation, drug and alcohol use, STDs and HIV, family planning, domestic violence, unintentional injuries, seat belt use, nutrition, physical activity, fall prevention and polypharmacy (elderly) — Periodically

■ Recommended by most US authorities

[1]There is no upper age limit for pap smears, but regular testing in women over age 65 may be discontinued in those who have had regular screening with consistently normal results. Pap smears are not necessary in women who have undergone a hysterectomy in which the cervix was removed for reasons other than cervical cancer or its precursors.

[2]Some authorities recommend initiating screening at age 19. Screening at less frequent intervals may be reasonable in low risk individuals, including those with previously normal levels.

[3]MMR need only be given to women of childbearing age who lack documented evidence of immunization and are capable of becoming pregnant.

[4]Folic acid 0.4mg per day is recommended for women of childbearing age who are capable of becoming pregnant.

Figure A.2(b)

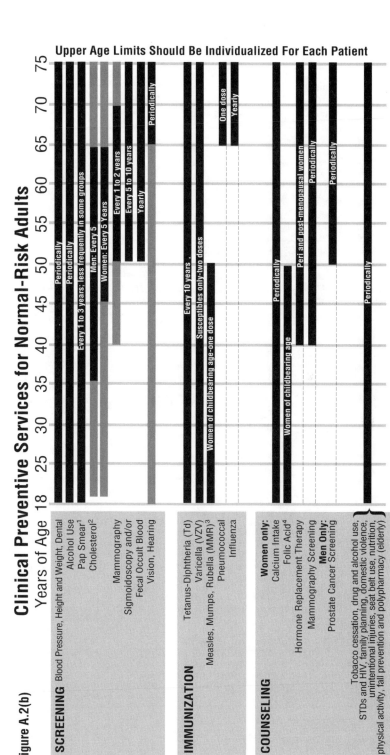

Clinical Preventive Services for Normal-Risk Adults

Upper Age Limits Should Be Individualized For Each Patient

Years of Age: 18 25 30 35 40 45 50 55 60 65 70 75

SCREENING

- Blood Pressure, Height and Weight, Dental — Periodically
- Alcohol Use — Periodically
- Pap Smear[1] — Every 1 to 3 years: less frequently in some groups
- Cholesterol[2] — Men: Every 5 / Women: Every 5 Years
- Mammography — Every 1 to 2 years
- Sigmoidoscopy and/or — Every 5 to 10 years
- Fecal Occult Blood — Yearly
- Vision, Hearing — Periodically

IMMUNIZATION

- Tetanus-Diphtheria (Td) — Every 10 years
- Varicella (VZV) — Susceptibles only-two doses
- Measles, Mumps, Rubella (MMR)[3] — Women of childbearing age-one dose
- Pneumococcal — One dose
- Influenza — Yearly

COUNSELING

Women only:
- Calcium Intake — Periodically
- Folic Acid[4] — Women of childbearing age
- Hormone Replacement Therapy — Peri and post-menopausal women
- Mammography Screening — Periodically

Men Only:
- Prostate Cancer Screening — Periodically

- Tobacco cessation, drug and alcohol use, STDs and HIV, family planning, domestic violence, unintentional injuries, seat belt use, nutrition, physical activity, fall prevention and polypharmacy (elderly) — Periodically

■ Recommended by most US authorities
▨ Recommended by some US authorities

[1] There is no upper age limit for pap smears, but regular testing in women over age 65 may be discontinued in those who have had regular screening with consistently normal results. Pap smears are not necessary in women who have undergone a hysterectomy in which the cervix was removed for reasons other than cervical cancer or its precursors.

[2] Some authorities recommend initiating screening at age 19. Screening at less frequent intervals may be reasonable in low risk individuals, including those with previously normal levels.

[3] MMR need only be given to women of childbearing age who lack documented evidence of immunization and are capable of becoming pregnant.

[4] Folic acid 0.4mg per day is recommended for women of childbearing age who are capable of becoming pregnant.

Table A.1. Risk Factor Category: Age and Gender Profile - Children and Adolescents Ages 0–18 Years

Risk Factor	Prevention Target Condition	Prevention Service and/or Referral	Reimbursement Strategy	*Clinician's Handbook* Chapter
Newborn infants	Ophthalmia neonatorum (gonorrhea)	Ocular antibiotic prophylaxis		
	Congential hypothyroidism	Thyroid function tests	EPSDT	8
	Hemoglobinopathy	Hemoglobin electrophoresis or other comparable test	EPSDT	8
Newborn infants >1 day old	Phenylketonuria	Blood phenylalanine level	EPSDT	8
Infants and toddlers	Iron-deficiency anemia	CBC, serum ferritin	EPSDT	1
		Nutritional counseling		20
		Breast-feeding counseling		
Children ages 3–4 years	Amblyopia and strabismus	Visual acuity screening	EPSDT	11
		Ocular alignment		
Infants, children and adolescents	Infectious diseases	Immunizations		12, 13, 14, 15, 16, 17
Children and adolescents	Hypertension	Blood pressure screening		2
		Nutritional counseling		20
		Exercise counseling		21
	Obesity, malnutrition	Obesity screening		3
		Nutritional counseling		20
		Exercise counseling		21
	Unintentional injury	Counsel regarding: lap belts, car seats, bicycle helmets, poison control phone number, syrup of ipecac, safe storage of drugs, firearms, toxic substances, and matches		22
	Dental hygiene	Counsel regarding regular dental checks		19
	Tobacco-related complications	Tobacco counseling		19, 24
Adolescents	Scoliosis	Visual inspection (state-specific recommendations)		

Table A.2. Risk Factor Category: Age and Gender Profile - Adults Ages >18 years

Risk Factor	Prevention Target Condition	Preventive Service and/or Referral	Reimbursement Strategy	*Clinician's Handbook* Chapter
All adults	Obesity	Obesity screening		29
	Hypertension	Blood pressure screening		28
	Coronary heart disease	Cholesterol screening		31
		Nutritional counseling		56
		Exercise counseling		57
		Smoking cessation counseling		60
		Aspirin therapy (if indicated)		46
	Diabetes mellitus	Plasma glucose		38
	Malnutrition	Nutritional counseling		56
	Dental disease	Dental check-ups		54
	Alcohol-related problems	Assess for problem drinking		53
	Injuries: intentional, unintentional, and related to drugs/alcohol	Counsel about various preventive measures		53, 55
	Measles, mumps (persons born after 1956 only)	Serology for immune status (if no record of vaccination) Measles and mumps vaccines (if non-immune)		15
Women of childbearing age	Neural tube defects	Folate		20, 56
	Congenital rubella syndrome	Screen for rubella immunity (if no record of prior vaccination) Rubella vaccine (if non-immune)		15, 51
Men 35–65 years Women 45–65 years	Elevated cholesterol	Cholesterol screening		31
		Nutritional counseling		56
		Exercise counseling		57
		Aspirin therapy (if indicated)		46
Women ≥40 years of age	Breast cancer	Mammography	Medicare	36
		Clinical breast exam		30

continued

Table A.2. Risk Factor Category: Age and Gender Profile - Adults Ages >18 years—*Continued*

Risk Factor	Prevention Target Condition	Preventive Service and/or Referral	Reimbursement Strategy	*Clinician's Handbook* Chapter
Men ages ≥40 years	Prostate cancer	Digital rectal exam*		30
		Prostate specific antigen*		39
Persons ages ≥50 years	Colorectal cancer	Fecal occult blood test		30, 34
		Sigmoidoscopy		41
All peri- and post-menopausal women	Osteoporosis	Hormone replacement		47, 62
		Nutritional counseling		56
		Exercise counseling		57
	Coronary heart disease	Obesity screening		29
		Blood pressure screening		28
		Cholesterol screening		31
		Nutritional screening		56
		Exercise counseling		57
		Smoking cessation counseling		60
		Aspirin therapy (if indicated)		46
Persons ≥60 years	Thyroid dysfunction	Thyroid function tests		42
Persons age ≥65 years	Influenza	Influenza vaccine	Medicare	49
	Pneumococcal disease	Pneumococcal vaccine	Medicare	50
	Tetanus	Check for last tetanus booster		52
	Visual problems including glaucoma	Snellen acuity test		45
		Referral for glaucoma screening		
	Hearing impairment	Question regarding hearing		35
Persons >70 years with one or more of the following risk factors: psychoactive, antihypertensive or cardiac medication; impaired cognition, balance or strength	Falls	Counsel regarding home safety		55
		Assess vision		45
		Counsel regarding polypharmacy		58
		Assess for cognitive/functional impairment		32

*Whether these procedures diminish the morbidity and mortality associated with prostate cancer is controversial.

Table A.3. Risk Factor Category: Social Circumstances and Living Conditions - All Ages

Risk Factor	Prevention Target Condition	Preventive Service and/or Referral	Reimbursement Strategy	*Clinician's Handbook* Chapter
Low-income household/community	Iron-deficiency anemia (infants)	CBC, serum ferritin Nutritional counseling Breast-feeding counseling	EPSDT	1 20
	Lead poisoning (ages 1–5 years)	Blood lead level		7
	Tuberculosis	PPD		9, 43
Living in large metropolitan areas, or living in any homes built before 1950 with dilapidated paint or recent renovation	Lead poisoning (ages 1–5 years)	Blood lead level Residential lead hazard control (notify department of health)	EPSDT	7
Institutionalized persons (eg, persons living in correctional facilities or chronic-care facilities)	Tuberculosis	PPD		9, 43
	Hepatitis B	Hepatitis B vaccine	Medicare	14, 48
	Influenza	Influenza vaccine	Medicare	49
	Pneumococcal disease	Pneumococcal vaccine	Medicare	50
Homelessness	Tuberculosis	PPD		9, 43
	Hepatitis B	Hepatitis B vaccine	Medicare	14, 48
	Influenza	Influenza vaccine	Medicare	49
	Pneumococcal disease	Pneumococcal vaccine	Medicare	50
Close contact of person(s) with tuberculosis	Tuberculosis	PPD		9, 43
Resident of American Indian reservation or Alaska Native community	Tuberculosis Hepatitis B Hepatitis A Influenza Pneumococcal disease	PPD Hepatitis B vaccine Hepatitis A vaccine Influenza vaccine Pneumococcal vaccine	Indian Health Service/ Tribal health programs/ Medicare	9, 43 14, 48 49 50
Settings where large numbers of young adults congregate (eg, colleges, military bases, health care settings)	Rubella	Rubella vaccine		51
Recent divorce or separation Unemployment Bereavement	Depression	Mental health counseling Possible referral and hospitalization		5, 26, 33, 55
	Suicide	Question regarding preparatory actions		

Table A.4. Risk Factor Category: Geographic and Ethnic Background - All Ages

Risk Factor	Prevention Target Condition	Preventive Service and/or Referral	Reimbursement Strategy	*Clinician's Handbook* Chapter
African, African-American, Latin American, Caribbean, Southeast Asian, Middle Eastern or Mediterranean ethnicity	Hemoglobinopathy (pregnant women)	Hemoglobin electrophoresis		1, 27
African-American, Mexican-American, American Indian, Alaska Native ethnicity; Immigrants from developing countries	Lead poisoning (children 1–5 years of age)	Blood lead level Residential lead hazard control	EPSDT	7
African-American, Hispanic, Pacific Island ethnicity (also see low-income)	Tuberculosis	PPD		9, 43
American Indian, Hispanic, African-American ethnicity	Diabetes mellitus	Fasting glucose Obesity screening Nutritional counseling Exercise counseling		10, 38 3, 29 20, 56 21, 57
Immigrants from areas with high prevalence of tuberculosis, hepatitis B, or HIV (includes most countries in Africa, Asia, or Latin America)	Tuberculosis Hepatitis B STD/HIV	PPD Hepatitis B vaccine STD/HIV counseling STD/HIV screening	Medicare	9, 43 14, 48 23, 59 40
African-American ethnicity	Glaucoma (≥40 years of age) Prostate cancer	Ophthalmology referral for screening Digital rectal exam* Prostate specific antigen*		45 30 39
Asian Indians who use chewing tobacco or betel nut	Oral cancer	Oral exam Cessation counseling Regular dental exam		30 60 19, 54
Caucasian females	Post-menopausal osteoporosis	Nutritional counseling Exercise counseling Smoking cessation counseling Post-menopausal hormone replacement therapy		56 57 60 47, 62

*Whether these procedures diminish the morbidity and mortality associated with prostate cancer is controversial.

Table A.5. Risk Factor Category: Occupational, Recreational, Residential, and Environmental Exposures - All Ages

Risk Factor	Prevention Target Condition	Preventive Service and/or Referral	Reimbursement Strategy	*Clinician's Handbook* Chapter
Children living with someone whose job or hobby involves lead exposure, living near lead industry, or using lead-based pottery	Lead poisining	Blood lead level Residential lead hazard control	EPSDT	iii, 7
Health care workers	Tuberculosis	PPD		9,43
	Hepatitis B	Hepatitis B vaccine	Medicare	14,48
	Influenza	Influenza vaccine	Medicare	49
Multiple sex partners Commercial sex worker Illicit drug use	Hepatitis B Hepatitis C	Hepatitis B vaccine	Medicare	14, 48
	HIV/STDs Pelvic inflammatory disease Chronic pelvic pain	Gonorrhea and chlamydia screening RPR for syphilis HIV serology HIV/STD counseling		10, 40, 23, 59
	Unintended pregnancy Ectopic pregnancy Infertility	Unintended pregnancy counseling		25, 61
Employed in dye, leather, tire or rubber industry	Bladder cancer	Smoking cessation counseling		60
Exposure to dusts and fumes related to work in welding, construction, shipyards, or foundry	Respiratory problems	Smoking cessation counseling Counsel on use of personal protective equipment		60
Lead exposure related to work or hobby (eg, radiator repair, metal worker, construction, bridge painter, shooting gallery)	Lead poisoning	Blood lead level Occupational/residential lead hazard control		7 iii
Exposure to excessive noise levels related to work or hobby (eg, construction, maintenance, manufacturing, aerospace, musicians)	Hearing impairment	Refer to work site program for audiogram Counsel on use of personal protective equipment		iii, 35

Table A.6. Risk Factor Category: Substance Abuse - Adolescents and Adults

Risk Factor	Prevention Target Condition	Preventive Service and/or Referral	Reimbursement Strategy	*Clinician's Handbook* Chapter
Use of tobacco products	Lung cancer	Smoking cessation counseling		24, 60
	Oral cancer			30
	Chronic obstructive pulmonary disease			
	Asthma			
	Coronary heart disease	Obesity screening		3, 29
	Stroke	Blood pressure screening		2, 28
		Cholesterol screening		4, 31
		Nutritional counseling		20, 56
		Exercise counseling		21, 57
		Aspirin therapy (if indicated)		46
Excessive alcohol use		Alcohol counseling and referrals		18, 53
	Injuries and violence	Injury and violence counseling		22, 26, 55
	STD/HIV	STD/HIV counseling		23, 59
		STD/HIV screening		40
	Tuberculosis	PPD		9, 43
	Liver disease	Hepatitis B vaccine	Medicare	14, 48
	Cardiomyopathy			
	Malnutrition	Nutritional counseling		20, 56
		Consider also:		
		Influenza vaccine	Medicare	49
		Pneumococcal vaccine	Medicare	50
Illicit drug use, especially intravenous		Drug counseling and referrals		18, 53
	Tuberculosis	PPD		9, 43
	STD/HIV	STD/HIV counseling		23, 40, 59
		STD/HIV screening		
	Hepatitis B	Hepatitis B vaccine	Medicare	14, 48
	Hepatitis C			
	Malnutrition	Nutritional counseling		20, 56
	Depression	Assess for depression		5, 26, 33, 55
	Suicide	Question regarding preparatory actions Mental health counseling (possible referral and hospitalization)		

Table A.7. Risk Factor Category: Personal Medical History - All Ages

Risk Factor	Prevention Target Condition	Preventive Service and/or Referral	Reimbursement Strategy	*Clinician's Handbook* Chapter
Perinatal infection with herpes, syphilis, rubella cytomegalovirus or toxoplasmosis Birth weight <1,500 g Severe perinatal asphyxia Malformations involving head or neck Admission to intensive care nursery	Hearing impairment	Refer for auditory brainstem response or oto-acoustic emission testing		6
Recurrent otitis media Use of ototoxic medications Prior bacterial meningitis	Hearing impairment	Refer for hearing evaluation		6
Pre-term and low-birth-weight infants Infants whose primary dietary intake is non-fortified cow's milk	Iron-deficiency anemia	CBC, ferritin Counsel about iron-enriched foods and breast-feeding		1 20
Women in periconception period with prior pregnancy affected by neural tube defect	Neural tube defect	Referral for amniocentesis Alpha-fetoprotein measurement Folic acid supplementation		56
Obesity	Coronary heart disease Hypertension	Obesity screening Blood pressure screening Cholesterol screening Nutritional counseling Exercise counseling Aspirin therapy (if indicated)		3, 29 2, 28 4, 31 20, 56 21, 57 46
	Diabetes mellitus	Fasting glucose		10, 38
Radiation exposure to head and neck during infancy or childhood	Thyroid cancer Hypothyroidism	Palpation of thyroid Thyroid function tests		30 42
History of cryptorchidism or atrophic testes	Testicular cancer	Clinician or self-examination Counsel about increased risk and screening options		30
Down's syndrome	Hypothyroidism	Thyroid function tests		8, 42

continued

Table A.7. Risk Factor Category: Personal Medical History - All Ages—*Continued*

Risk Factor	Prevention Target Condition	Preventive Service and/or Referral	Reimbursement Strategy	*Clinician's Handbook* Chapter
Recurrent and/or unexplained injuries	Child abuse/neglect	Screening questions Documentation Report to local child protective agency		22, 26
History of dysplastic or congenital nevi History of immunosuppression History of severe sunburn in childhood Poor tanning ability; light skin, hair, or eyes; freckles	Skin cancer	Avoid sun exposure between 10:00 a.m. and 3:00 p.m. Protective clothing, sunscreen Consider dermatology referral for those at highest risk		30
Severe myopia	Glaucoma	Ophthalmology referral for screening		11, 45
Depression	Suicidal ideation	Question regarding preparatory actions Mental health counseling (possible referral and hospitalization)		5, 18, 26, 33, 53, 55
Diabetes mellitus	Influenza	Influenza vaccine	Medicare	49
	Penumococcal disease	Pneumococcal vaccine	Medicare	50
	Early retinopathy and glaucoma	Referral for screening		11, 45
	Early nephropathy	Urine screen for microalbuminuria		10, 44
	Coronary heart disease	Obesity screening Blood pressure screening Cholesterol screening Nutritional counseling Exercise counseling Smoking cessation counseling Aspirin therapy (if indicated)		3, 29 2, 28 4, 31 20, 56 21, 57 24, 60 46
Ulcerative colitis, duration >10 years	Colorectal cancer	Referral for colonoscopy (possible surgical consult for prophylactic colectomy)		30, 34, 41

Table A.8. Risk Factor Category: Family Medical History - All Ages

Risk Factor	Prevention Target Condition	Preventive Service and/or Referral	Reimbursement Strategy	*Clinician's Handbook* Chapter
Diabetes mellitus	Diabetes mellitus and subsequent complications	Fasting Glucose Obesity screening Nutritional counseling Exercise counseling		10, 38 3, 29 20, 56 21, 57
Glaucoma	Glaucoma	Referral for screening		11, 45
Hereditary childhood sensorineural hearing loss	Hearing impairment	Refer for auditory brainstem response or oto-acoustic emission testing		6, 35
Breast cancer	Breast cancer	Mammography Clinical breast exam	Medicare	30, 36
Hereditary polyposis or hereditary non-polyposis colerectal cancer	Colorectal cancer	Referral for colonscopy (possible surgical consult for prophylactic colectomy)		30, 34, 41
Colorectal cancer prior to age 50	Colorectal cancer (patients aged 40–60 years)	Fecal occult blood testing Sigmoidoscopy		30, 34, 41
Multiple endocrine neoplasia (MEN) type II	Medullary thyroid cancer	Referral to endocrinology		30
Ovarian cancer especially hereditary ovarian cancer syndrome (HCS)	Ovarian cancer	Ultrasound Pelvic exam CA-125 measurement		30
Prostate cancer	Prostate cancer	Digital rectal exam* Prostate specific antigen*		30 39
Skin cancer (eg, familial atypical moles, melanoma)	Skin cancer	Consider dermatology referral for those at a highest risk		30

*Whether these procedures diminish the morbidity and mortality associated with prostate cancer is controversial.

Table A.9. Risk Factor Category: Sexual History - Adolescent and Adult Males

Risk Factor	Prevention Target Condition	Preventive Service and/or Referral	Reimbursement Strategy	Clinician's Handbook Chapter
Muliple sex partners Sex with other males Sex for money or drugs Prior history of STD Urban adolescent clinic	Hepatitis B STD/HIV	Hepatitis B vaccine STD/HIV counseling STD/HIV screening	Medicare	14, 48 23, 59 40

Table A.10. Risk Factor Category: Sexual History - Adolescent and Adult Females

Risk Factor	Prevention Target Condition	Preventive Service and/or Referral	Reimbursement Strategy	Clinician's Handbook Chapter
Multiple sex partners Sex for money or drugs Prior STD	Hepatitis B	Hepatitis B vaccine	Medicare	14, 48
	STD/HIV Pelvic inflammatory disease Chronic pelvic pain Ectopic pregnancy Infertility Unintended pregnancy	STD/HIV counseling STD/HIV screening		23, 59 40
		Unintended pregnancy counseling		25, 61
		Substance abuse counseling		18, 53
Ever sexually active especially multiple sex partners and early onset of sexual activity	Cervical cancer	Papanicolaou smear	Medicare	30, 37, 40

Table A.11. Risk Factor Category: Reproductive History - Female

Risk Factor	Prevention Target Condition	Preventive Service and/or Referral	Reimbursement Strategy	*Clinician's Handbook* Chapter
All pregnant women	Asymptomatic bacteriuria pyelonephritis/ bacteremia	Urinalysis and culture		44
	Anemia	CBC		27
	D (Rh) incompatibility	D blood typing and antibody testing		
	Preeclampsia	Periodic blood pressure measurement		2, 28
	Neural tube defect	Folic acid supplementation		20, 56
	Domestic violence	Direct questioning about abuse using screening instrument; referral for counseling; referrals to crisis center, shelter, and social services; notify protective authorities		26, 55
	Problems related to substance abuse including alcohol, tobacco and illicit drugs	Screen for use and counsel regarding personal hazards, effects on fetus, and potential to transmit drugs through breast milk		18, 24, 58, 60
	Nutritional and immunological deficiencies	Counsel regarding adequate calcium intake and breast feeding		20, 56
	Vertical transmission of hepatitis B, and HIV	Hepatitis B surface antigen HIV serology		14, 48 23, 40
	Obstetric complications related to STDs	STD/HIV screening STD/HIV counseling		23, 59 40
	Hemoglobinopathy	Hemoglobin electrophoresis and counseling		27

continued

Table A.11. Risk Factor Category: Reproductive History - Female—*Continued*

Risk Factor	Prevention Target Condition	Preventive Service and/or Referral	Reimbursement Strategy	*Clinician's* Handbook Chapter
Periconception period with prior pregnancy affected by neural tube defect	Neural tube defect	Referal for amniocentesis with α-fetoprotein measurement		
		Folic acid supplementation		20, 56
Pregnant women <35 years of age, and no prior pregnancy affected with Down's syndrome	Down's syndrome	Serum multiple-marker screening and counseling		
Pregnant women ≥35 years of age, or prior pregnancy affected with Down's syndrome	Down's syndrome	Refer for amniocentesis or chorionic villus sampling OR multiple-marker screening and counseling		
Pregnant women ≥35 years, with obesity or glucosuria on screening urinalysis	Gestational diabetes mellitus Fetal macrosomia Birth trauma	Glucose tolerance test		38
Post-partum period	Thyroid dysfunction	Thyroid screening		42
Early menopause	Osteoporosis	Hormonal treatment		47, 62
	Coronary heart disease	Obesity screening		29
		Blood pressure screening		28
		Cholesterol screening		31
		Nutritional counseling		56
		Exercise counseling		57
		Smoking cessation counseling		60
		Aspirin therapy (if indicated)		46

B

IMMUNIZATION

Appendix B provides information regarding standards for immunizations, Federal and State programs and resources to help ensure the safe and timely delivery of immunizations, and information about immunization registries.

Appendix B is organized into the following sections:

Childhood Immunizations

- Access: Vaccines for Children Program (VFC)
- True Contraindications for Immunizations
- Recording Procedures
- National Vaccine Injury Compensation Program
- Reporting Of Adverse Events: Vaccine Adverse Event Reporting System (VAERS)
- Patient-Oriented and Community-Based Approaches

Adult Immunizations

Immunization Registries

Childhood Immunizations

A comprehensive list of standards for the delivery of childhood immunizations is in Table B.1. Most of these standards are relevant to the clinical practices of providers.

Immunization Access: The Vaccines for Children Program (VFC)

The Vaccines for Children Program (VFC) was created in 1994 to increase the levels of childhood immunization by providing vaccines at no charge to participating private and public health care providers to administer to eligible children. Recent estimates indicate approximately 60% of US children will benefit from this program. Table B.2 provides information on the program.

True Contraindications for Immunizations

Many opportunities to immunize children are missed because clinicians withhold immunizations for invalid reasons. General guidelines regarding con-

Table B.1. National Vaccine Advisory Committee Standards for Childhood Immunization Practices

1. Immunization services are readily available.
2. There are no barriers or unnecessary prerequisites to the receipt of vaccines.
3. Immunization services are available free or for a minimal fee.
4. Providers utilize all clinical encounters to screen and, when indicated, immunize children.
5. Providers educate parents and guardians about immunization in general terms.
6. Providers question parents or guardians about contraindictions, and before immunizing a child, inform them in specific terms about the risks and benefits of the immunization their child is to receive.
7. Providers follow only true contraindications.
8. Providers administer simultaneously all vaccine doses for which a chld is eligible at the time of each visit.
9. Providers use accurate and complete recording procedures.
10. Providers co-schedule immunization appointments in conjunction with appointments for other child health services.
11. Providers report adverse events following immunization promptly, accurately and completely.
12. Providers operate a tracking system.
13. Providers adhere to appropriate procedures for vaccine management.
14. Providers conduct semi-annual audits to assess immunization coverage levels and to review immunization records in the patient population they serve.
15. Providers maintain up-to-date, easily retrievable medical protocols at all locations where vaccines are administered.
16. Providers operate with patient-oriented and community-based approaches.
17. Vaccines are administered by properly trained individuals.
18. Providers receive ongoing education and training on current immunization recommendations.

From: National Vaccine Advisory Committee. *Standards for Pediatric Immunization Practices.* Atlanta, Ga: Centers for Disease Control and Prevention; 1993.

traindications and precautions for administering childhood immunizations are presented in Table B.3. Precautions and contraindications for specific childhood immunizations are listed in chapters 12 to 17.

Documentation

The National Childhood Vaccine Injury Act (NCVIA) requires that for each of the covered vaccines (DTP/DTaP or component antigens, MMR or component antigens, IPV/OPV, Hep B, Hib and VZV), the vaccine recipient's permanent medical record or a permanent office log contains the following information:

■ date the vaccine was administered

■ vaccine manufacturer and lot number

■ name, address, and title of the person administering the vaccine.

Table B.2. The Vaccines for Children Program

Eligibility
Children (18 years or younger) eligible for free vaccine under the program are:
- Medicaid Insured*
- Uninsured*
- All American Indian or Alaska Native children*
- Children with health insurance that does not cover vaccines as a benefit†

Provider Information
Any health care provider licensed by a state to administer vaccines can participate in the Vaccines for Children Program and receive free vaccines at an estimated savings of $270 per child in out-of-pocket expenses. This program has been designed to provide easy enrollment to providers and has several benefits:
- Ensures that patients get vaccinated on time
- Eliminates the need for private health care providers to refer patients to public clinics
- Does not require new patients to be served based on their eligibility
- Fee caps on vaccinations are adequate for administration; no fee caps are set for the office visit.

More information can be obtained from your State health department's immunization program.

---

*May go to any qualified health care provider who chooses to participate in the program.

†May receive services through such facilities as a Federally Qualified Health Center (FQHC) or a Rural Health Clinic.

From: National Immunization Program. *Vaccines for Children*, Vol 1, No 1. Atlanta, Ga: Centers for Disease Control and Prevention; 1994.

The Advisory Committee on Immunization Practices (ACIP) recommends that the above information be recorded for all vaccines, not only for those covered by the NCVIA.

National Vaccine Injury Compensation Program

The National Vaccine Injury Compensation Program (VICP) is a Federal "no-fault" system designed to compensate individuals injured by specific vaccines. The vaccines currently covered under the VICP include: DTP/ DTaP or component antigens; MMR or component antigens, and OPV/IPV. In addition, HepB, Hib, and VZV vaccines were recently added to the VICP. The effective date of coverage of these new vaccines is August 6, 1997. See Table B.4 for specific information related to reporting and compensation.

Further information about VICP can be obtained by calling (800)338-2382 or visiting the VICP website at http://www.hrsa.dhhs.gov/bhpr/vicp.

Reporting Of Adverse Events: Vaccine Adverse Event Reporting System (VAERS)

To help ensure the safety of vaccines distributed in the US, the Department of Health and Human Services has established the Vaccine Adverse Event Re-

Table B.3. Contraindications and Precautions for Childhood Immunizations*

True Contraindications and Precautions	NOT Contraindications (vaccines may be given)
Anaphylactic reaction to a vaccine contraindicates further doses of that vaccine Anaphylactic reaction to a vaccine constituent contraindicates the use of vaccines containing that substance	Moderate or severe illness with or without fever Mild to moderate local reaction (soreness, redness, swelling) following a dose of an injectable antigen Mild acute illness with or without low-grade fever Current antimicrobial therapy Convalescent phase of illnesses Prematurity (same dosage and indications as for normal, full-term infants) Recent exposure to an infectious disease History of penicillin or other nonspecific allergies or fact that relatives have such allergies

*This information is based on the recommendations of the Advisory Committee on Immunization Practices (ACIP) and those of the Committee on Infectious Diseases (Red Book Committee) of the American Academy of Pediatrics (AAP). These recommendations may vary from those contained in the manufacturers' package inserts.

From: National Vaccine Advisory Committee. *Standards for Pediatric Immunization Practices.* Atlanta, Ga: Centers for Disease Control and Prevention; 1993.

porting System (VAERS). VAERS provides a database management system for the collection and analysis of post-vaccination adverse events.

Mandated reportable events are:

- Adverse events listed in Table B.4 that occur within the time period specified or within 7 days, whichever is longer.

- Any event listed in the manufacturer's vaccine package insert as a contraindication to vaccination

In addition, individuals are encouraged to report any clinically significant or unexpected events (even if they are not certain the vaccine caused the event) for any vaccine, whether or not it is listed in Table B.4. Manufacturers are also required by regulation (21 CFR 600.80) to report to the VAERS program all adverse events made known to them for any vaccine.

To improve the ability to detect new adverse events, clinicians, vaccine manufacturers and parents are encouraged to report to VAERS any clinically significant adverse event following administration of any vaccine licensed in the United States, not just those mandated for reporting.

Table B.4. National Childhood Vaccine Injury Act: Reporting and Compensation Tables[1]

Vaccine	Adverse Event	Interval from Vaccination to Onset of Event	
		For Reporting[2]	**For Compensation**[3,4]
I. Tetanus toxoid-containing vaccines (DTaP, DTP, DT; Td, TT)	A. Anaphylaxis or anaphylactic shock	0-7 days	0-4 hours
	B. Brachial neuritis	0-28 days	2-28 days
	C. Any acute complication or sequela (including death) of above events	No limit	No limit
	D. Events described in manufacturer's package insert as contraindications to additional doses of vaccine	No limit	Not applicable
II. Pertussis antigen-containing vaccines (DTaP, DTP, P, DTP-Hib)	A. Anaphylaxis or anaphylactic shock	0-7 days	0-4 hours
	B. Encephalopathy (or encephalitis)	0-7 days	0-72 hours
	C. Any acute complication or sequela (including death) of above events	No limit	No limit
	D. Events described in manufacturer's package insert as contraindications to additional doses of vaccine	No limit	Not applicable
III. Measles, mumps and rubella virus-containing vaccines in any combination (MMR, MR, M, R)	A. Anaphylaxis or anaphylactic shock	0-7 days	0-4 hours
	B. Encephalopathy (or encephalitis)	0-15 days	5-15 days
	C. Any acute complication or sequela (including death) of above events	No limit	No limit
	D. Events described in manufacturer's package insert as contraindications to additional doses of vaccine	No limit	Not applicable
IV. Rubella virus-containing vaccines (MMR, MR, R)	A. Chronic arthritis	0-42 days	7-42 days
	B. Any acute complication or sequela (including death) of above event	No limit	No limit
	C. Events described in manufacturer's package insert as contraindications to additional doses of vaccine	No limit	Not applicable
V. Measles virus-containing vaccines (MMR, MR, M)	A. Thrombocytopenic purpura	0-30 days	7-30 days
	B. Vaccine-Strain Measles Viral Infection in an immunodeficient recipient	0-6 months	0-6 months
	C. Any acute complication or sequela (including death) of above events	No limit	No limit
	D. Events described in manufacturer's package insert as contraindications to additional doses of vaccine	No limit	Not applicable

VI. Polio live virus-containing vaccines (OPV)	A. Paralytic Polio
	  –in a non-immunodeficient recipient
	  –in an immunodeficient recipient
	  –in a vaccine assoc. community case
		
		0-30 days
		0-6 months
		No limit
			
			0-30 days
			0-6 months
			No limit

	B. Vaccine-Strain Polio Viral Infection
	  –in a non-immunodeficient recipient
	  –in an immunodeficient recipient
	  –in a vaccine assoc. community case
		
		0-30 days
		0-6 months
		No limit
			
			30 days
			0-6 months
			No limit

	C. Any acute complication or sequela (including death) of above events	No limit	No limit
	D. Events described in manufacturer's package insert as contraindications to additional doses of vaccine	No limit	Not applicable

continued

Table B.4. National Childhood Vaccine Injury Act: Reporting and Compensation Tables[1]—*Continued*

Vaccine	Adverse Event	Interval from Vaccination to Onset of Event	
		For Reporting[2]	For Compensation[3,4]
VII. Polio inactivated-virus containing vaccines (IPV)	A. Anaphylaxis or anaphylactic shock	0-7 days	0-4 hours
	B. Any acute complication or sequela (including death) of above event	No limit	No limit
	C. Events described in manufacturer's package insert as contraindications to additional doses of vaccine	No limit	Not applicable
VIII. Hepatitis B antigen-containing vaccines[5]	A. Anaphylaxis or anaphylactic shock	0-7 days	0-4 hours
	B. Any acute complication or sequela (including death) of above event	No limit	No limit
	C. Events described in manufacturer's package insert as contraindications to additional doses of vaccine	No limit	Not applicable
IX. Hemophilus influenzae type b polysaccharide vaccines (unconjugated, PRP vaccines)[5]	A. Early-onset Hib disease	0-7 days	0-7 days
	B. Any acute complication or sequela (including death) of above event	No limit	No limit
	C. Events described in manufacturer's package insert as contraindications to additional doses of vaccine	No limit	Not applicable
X. Hemophilus influenzae type b polysaccharide conjugate vaccines[5]	A. No Condition Specified for Compensation	Not applicable	Not applicable
	B. Events described in manufacturer's package insert as contraindications to additional doses of vaccine	No limit	Not applicable
XI. Varicella virus-containing vaccines[5]	A. No Condition Specified for Compensation	Not applicable	Not applicable
	B. Events described in manufacturer's package insert as contraindications to additional doses of vaccine	No limit	Not applicable
XII. Any new vaccine recommended by the Centers for Disease Control and Prevention for routine administration to children, after publication by the Secretary of a notice of coverage.	A. No Condition Specified for Compensation	Not applicable	Not applicable
	B. Events described in manufacturer's package insert as contraindications to additional doses of vaccine	No limit	Not applicable

1. Effective date: March 24, I997
2. Taken from the Reportable Events Table (RET), which lists conditions reportable by law (42 USC 300aa-25) to the Vaccine Adverse Event Reporting System (VAERS), including conditions found in the manufacturers package insert.
3. Taken from the Vaccine Injury Table (VIT) used in adjudication of claims filed with the National Vaccine Injury Compensation Program.
4. Claims may also be filed for a condition with onset outside the designated time intervals or a condition not included in the Table.
5. The effective date of coverage is August 6, 1997.

Adult Immunizations

The National Coalition for Adult Immunization has published standards for adult immunization practice (Table B.5).

Patient-Oriented And Community-Based Approaches

The use of a patient or parent-held record is an example of a patient-oriented approach to immunization. All States have official immunization cards for childhood immunizations, and immunization record forms are incorporated into several comprehensive health records for children, such as the *Child*

Health Guide of the Put Prevention Into Practice campaign. Use of these records has been shown to be related to increased immunization rates for children in the United States, over a range of socioeconomic groups.

Immunization Registries

In 1996, 23 States were operating immunization registries in the public health sector. Plans are underway to establish basic statewide networks. Local and State immunization registries should become the cornerstone of a future immunization delivery system, assuring that every child is immunized on schedule. When the registries become fully functional, all children will be enrolled from birth. Parents can be reminded automatically when immunizations are

---

Table B.5. National Coalition for Adult Immunization Standards for Adult Immunization Practices, 1990

---

1. Encourages the promotion of appropriate vaccine use through information campaigns for health care practitioners and trainees, employers, and the public about the benefits of immunizations.
2. Encourages physicians and other health care personnel (in practice and in training) to protect themselves and prevent transmission to patients by assuring that they themselves are completely immunized.
3. Recommends that all health care providers routinely determine the immunization status of their adult patients, offer vaccines to those for whom they are indicated, and maintain complete immunization records.
4. Recommends that all health care providers identify high-risk patients in need of influenza vaccine and develop a system to recall them for annual immunization each autumn.
5. Recommends that all health care providers and institutions identify high-risk adult patients in hospitals and other treatment centers and assure that appropriate vaccination is considered either prior to discharge or as part of discharge planning.
6. Recommends that all licensing/accrediting agencies support the development by health care institutions of comprehensive immunization programs for staff, trainees, volunteer workers, inpatients, and outpatients.
7. Encourages States to establish pre-enrollment immunization requirements for colleges and other institutions of higher education.
8. Recommends that institutions that train health care professionals, deliver health care, or provide laboratory or other medical support services require appropriate immunizations for persons at risk of contacting or transmitting vaccine-preventable illnesses.
9. Encourages health care benefit programs, third-party payers, and governmental health care programs to provide coverage for adult immunization services.
10. Encourages the adoption of a standard personal and institutional immunization record as a means of verifying the immunization status of patients and staff.

From: National Coalition for Adult Immunization. *Standards for Adult Immunization Practices.* Bethesda, Md: National Coalition for Adult Immunization; 1992.

due and can be recalled when they are overdue. Providers will easily determine the immunization needs of their patients, old or new, at the time of each visit, wherever a child interacts with the health care system, be it a doctor's office, public health clinic, emergency room or elsewhere.

The immunization registries will enable changes in immunization schedules to be rapidly incorporated into software and disseminated. Public health officials will have a simple, quick and inexpensive method to assess immunization coverage in their communities and to identify groups at risk for under-immunization. Local registries can be interconnected, and information on immunization coverage can be shared with local and State agencies, which should expedite information gathering and lower costs.

Patient and Provider Resources

Centers for Disease Control and Prevention (CDC) Vaccine Hotline: 1-800-232-2522 Provides answers to general vaccine questions including vaccine safety.

Centers for Disease Control and Prevention (CDC) Immunization Information Page **http://www.cdc.gov/diseases/immun.html**

National Immunization Program **http://dynares.com/nip**

Vaccine Adverse Event Reporting System (VAERS)

Pre-addressed, postage-paid VAERS forms and instructions maybe obtained by calling the 24-hour VAERS information recording at (800)822-7967. A sample form can be copied from the *Physician's Drug Reference*. Copies of the Reportable Events Table are available through State health departments and can be obtained by calling the 24-hour VAERS recording.

The VAERS form and additional information can be obtained from: http://www.fda.gov/cber/vaers.html

To request for specific information on reports submitted to VAERS contact:
US Food and Drug Administration
Freedom of Information Staff (HFI-35)
5600 Fishers Lane
Rockville, MD 20857, Fax # 301-443-1726

To obtain VAERS data (available to the public for a fee) contact:
National Technical Information Service 5285 Port Royal Road
Springfield, VA 22161
703-487-4650
order #SUB5228

http://www.ntis.gov/health/3he61942.htm

Vaccine Injury Compensation Program (VICP)

Further information can be obtained by calling: (800) 338-2382

VICP Internet address: http://www.hrsa.dhhs.gov/bhpr/vicp

Selected References

Chen RT, Rastogi SC, Mullen JR, et al. The Vaccine Adverse Event Reporting System (VAERS). *Vaccine.* 1994;12:541-550.

Cordero J, Orenstein W. The future of immunization registries. Developing immunization registries. *A J Prev Med.* Supplement. 1997;13:122-124.

Ellenberg SS, Chen RT. The complicated task of monitoring vaccine safety. *Public Health Reports.* 1997;112:10-20.

Robinson CA, Evans WB, Mahanes JA, Sepe SJ. Progress on the child immunization initiative. *Public Health Reports.* 1994;109(5):594-600.

Stratton KR, Howe CJ, Johnston RB Jr, ed. *Adverse Events Associated with Childhood Vaccines. Evidence Bearing on Causality.* Washington, DC: National Academy Press; 1994.

Wood D, Halfon N. The impact of the Vaccine for Children's Program on child immunization delivery. A policy analysis. *Arch Pediatric Adolescent Med.* 1996;150:577-581.

C

REPORTING OF NOTIFIABLE DISEASES

Clinicians are responsible for alerting their local or State health department when a case of a notifiable disease is detected, an important contribution to community and public health. The Centers for Disease Control and Prevention (CDC) of the US Public Health Service USPHS) defines a notifiable disease as "one for which regular, frequent, and timely information on individual cases is considered necessary for the prevention and control of the disease." Reporting furnishes feedback on the effectiveness of preventive measures such as immunizations, aids in tracing sources of infection and routes of spread, describes foci of infections and geographic clustering, and helps determine trends. Nevertheless, clinician reporting in the United States is grossly incomplete, partly because clinicians may be unaware of the usefulness of this information.

In the United States, reporting is regulated at the level of the State and territorial governments. Currently, all States require clinician reporting of certain infectious diseases. Generally, continued failure to report cases of notifiable diseases can result in punitive measures against the responsible party (eg, fines.) Although the majority of States have also instituted requirements for laboratory reporting of certain diseases, clinicians are still obligated to report cases. Not all notifiable diseases are confirmed solely through laboratory testing, and clinician reports often contain important demographic data crucial to investigatory and control procedures that are not available in laboratory reports.

At the national level, reporting is voluntary. The CDC depends on reports from State epidemiologists and lab directors in order to create their national summary statistics. The current list of nationally notifiable diseases, which is updated periodically by the Council of State and Territorial Epidemiologists (CSTE) with input from the CDC, is presented in Table C.1.

All clinicians should be aware that the list of notifiable diseases, case definitions for each disease, particular requirements and protocols for reporting, and the penalties for failing to do so vary from state to state. The CSTE is creating an Internet address that will list and summarize the requirements for each State.

Table C.1. Infectious Diseases Designated as Notifiable at the National Level - United States, 1997

Acquired immunodeficiency syndrome (AIDS)	Measles
Anthrax	Meningococcal disease
Botulism	Mumps
Brucellosis	Pertussis
Chancroid	Plague
Chlamydia trachomatis, genital infections	Poliomyelitis, paralytic
Cholera	Psittacosis
Coccidioidomycosis	Rabies, animal
Cryptosporidiosis	Rabies, human
Diphtheria	Rocky Mountain spotted fever
Encephalitis, California serogroup	Rubella
Encephalitis, eastern equine	Rubella, congenital syndrome
Encephalitis, St. Louis	Salmonellosis
Encephalitis, western equine	Shigellosis
Escherichia coli O157:H7	Streptococcal disease (invasive Group A)
Gonorrhea	*Streptococcus pneumoniae,* drug-resistant
Haemophilus influenzae, invasive disease	invasive disease
Hansen disease (leprosy)	Streptococcal toxic-shock syndrome
Hantavirus pulmonary syndrome	Syphilis
Hemolytic uremic syndrome, post-diarrheal	Syphilis, congenital
Hepatitis A	Tetanus
Hepatitis B	Toxic-shock syndrome
Hepatitis C/non-A, non-B	Trichinosis
HIV infection, pediatric	Tuberculosis
Legionellosis	Typhoid fever
Lyme Disease	Yellow fever
Malaria	

Source: Centers for Disease Control and Prevention. Case definitions for infectious conditions under public health surveillance. *MMWR.* 1997;46(No. RR-10).

Currently, no centralized data base of State reporting requirements exists. Clinicians are urged to contact their State epidemiologist's office at their State Department of Health for a current list of notifiable diseases and procedures for reporting. The clinician's local county department of health is also a valuable source of information regarding reporting requirements for the State.

Provider Resources

Centers for Disease Control and Prevention. Summary of Notifiable Diseases, United States. Published annually in *Morbidity and Mortality Weekly Report.* The CDC, in its annual summary of notifiable diseases, provides a complete listing of State and territorial epidemiologists and lab directors.

Selected References

Centers for Disease Control and Prevention. Summary of notifiable diseases, United States, 1994. *MMWR.* 1994;43(53).

Centers for Disease Control and Prevention. Case definitions for infectious conditions under public health surveillance. *MMWR.* 1997;46(No. RR-10).

Last, JM. *Public Health and Preventive Medicine.* 11th ed. New York, NY: Appleton-Century-Crofts; 1980.

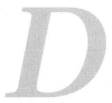

MAJOR AUTHORITIES CITED

(In Alphabetical Order)

American Academy of Dermatology
930 N. Meacham Road
Schaumberg, IL 60173
Tel: (847)330-0230
Fax: (847)330-0050

American Academy of Family
  Physicians
8880 Ward Parkway
Kansas City, MO 64114-2797
Tel: (800)274-2237
Fax: (816)822-0580

American Academy of
  Ophthalmology
P.O. Box 7424
San Francisco, CA 94109
Tel: (415)561-8500
Fax: (415)561-8533

American Academy of Pediatric
  Dentistry
211 E. Chicago Avenue
Suite 700
Chicago, IL 60611
Tel: (312)337-2169
Fax: (312)337-6329

American Association of Pediatric
  Ophthalmology and Strabismus
P.O. Box 193832
San Francisco, CA 94119
Tel: (415)561-8505
Fax: (415)561-8575

American Academy of Pediatrics
141 Northwest Point Boulevard
P.O. Box 6007
Elk Grove Village, IL 60009-0927
Tel: (847)228-5005
Fax: (847)228-5097

American Cancer Society
1559 Clifton Road NE.
Atlanta, GA 30329-4251
Tel: (404)320-3333
(800)ACS-2345

American College of Obstetricians
  and Gynecologists
409 12th Street SW.
Washington, DC 20024
Tel: (202)863-2502
Fax: (202)484-5107

American College of Physicians
Independence Mall West
Sixth Street at Race
Philadelphia, PA 19106
Tel: (215)351-2400
Fax: (215)351-2829

American College of Preventive
  Medicine
1660 L Street, NW
Suite 206
Washington, DC 20036-5603
Tel: (202)466-2044
Fax: (202)466-2662

American College of Radiology
1891 Preston White Drive
Reston, VA 22091
Tel: (703)648-8900

American College of Sports Medicine
P.O. Box 1440
Indianapolis, IN 46202-1440
Tel: (317)637-9200
Fax: (317)634-7817

American Dental Association
211 E. Chicago Avenue
Chicago, IL 60611
Tel: (800)621-8099
Fax: (312)440-7494

American Diabetes Association
1660 Duke Street
Alexandria, VA 22314
Tel: (703)549-1500
(800)ADA-DISC

American Dietetic Association
216 W. Jackson Boulevard
Suite 800
Chicago, IL 60606-6995
Tel: (312)899-0040
Fax: (312)899-1979

American Gastroenterological
  Association
6900 Grove Road
Thoroughfare, NJ 08086
Tel: (609)848-1000
Fax: (609)853-5991

American Geriatrics Society
770 Lexington Avenue
Suite 300
New York, NY 10021
Tel: (212)308-1414
Fax: (212)832-8646

American Heart Association
7320 Greenville Avenue
Dallas, TX 75231
Tel: (800)242-1793
Fax: (214)987-4334

American Medical Association
515 N. State Street
Chicago, IL 60610
Tel: (312)464-4804
Fax: (312)464-4184

American Nurses Association
600 Maryland Avenue SW. #100W
Washington, DC 20024-2571
Tel: (202)554-4444
Fax: (202)651-7004

American Optometric Association
243 N. Lindbergh Boulevard
St. Louis, MO 63141
Tel: (314)991-4100
Fax: (314)991-4101

American Society of Colon and
  Rectal Surgeons
85 W. Algonquin Road
Suite 550
Arlington Heights, IL 60005
Tel: (847)290-9184
Fax: (847)290-9203

American Society of Dentistry for
  Children
875 N. Michigan Ave #440
Chicago, IL 60611-1901
Tel: (312)943-1244
Fax: (312)943-5341

American Speech-Language-Hearing
  Association
10801 Rockville Pike
Rockville, MD 20852
Tel: (301)897-5700
(800)638-8255
Fax: (301)571-0457

American Thoracic Society
1740 Broadway
14th Floor
New York, NY 10019
Tel: (212)315-8700
Fax: (212)315-8872

American Thyroid Association
Montefiore Medical Center
111 E. 210th Street
Bronx, NY 10467
Tel: (718)882-6047
Fax: (718)882-6085

American Urological Association
1120 N. Charles Street
Baltimore, MD 21201-5559
Tel: (410)727-1100
Fax: (410)223-4370

Bright Futures
Guidelines for Health Supervision
   of Infants, Children, and
   Adolescents
2000 15th St. North
Suite 701
Arlington, VA 22201-2617
Tel: (703)524-7802
Fax: (703)524-9335

Canadian Task Force on Periodic
   Health Examination
Parkwood Hospital—Room A-240
801 Commissioners Road East
London, Ontario, Canada
N6C 5J1
Tel: (519)685-4292 ext. 2327
Fax: (519)685-4016

Joint Commission on Accreditation
   of Health Care Organizations
1 Renaissance Blvd
Oakbrook Terrace, IL 60180
Tel: (708)916-5600
Fax: (708)916-5644

Joint Committee on Infant Hearing
Allan O. Diefendorf PhD., Chair
Indiana University School of
   Medicine
Riley Hospital for Children
Suite 0860
720 Barn Hill Dr.
Indianapolis, IN 46202
Tel: (317)630-8980
Fax: (317)630-8958

National Medical Association
1012 10th Street NW.
Washington, DC 20001
Tel: (202)347-1895
Fax: (202)842-3293

National Osteoporosis Foundation
1150 17th St NW
Suite 500
Washington, DC 20036-4603
Tel: (800)624 BONE
Fax: (202)223-2237

Skin Cancer Foundation
245 5th Ave.
Suite 1403
New York, NY 10016
Tel: (212) 725-5176
Fax: (212) 725-5751

World Health Organization
525 23rd St NW
Washington, DC 20037
Tel: (202) 974-3000
Fax: (202) 974-3663

U.S. Federal Agencies

Agency for Health Care Policy and Research

The Alzheimer's Disease and Related
Dementias Panel of the Agency for
Health Care Policy and Research
6000 Executive Blvd.
Suite 310
Rockville, MD 20852
Tel: (301) 594-4015
Fax: (301) 594-4027

The Sickle Cell Disease Guideline
Panel of the Agency for Health
Care Policy and Research
Suite 310
Rockville, MD 20852
Tel: (301) 594-4015
Fax: (301) 594-4027

The Smoking Cessation Guideline
Panel of the Agency for Health
Care Policy and Research
Suite 310
Rockville, MD 20852
Tel: (301) 594-4015
Fax: (301) 594-4027

U.S. Preventive Services Task Force
Agency for Health Care and Policy
Research
Office for the Forum for Quality and
Effectiveness in Health Care
6000 Executive Blvd.
Suite 310
Rockville, MD 20852
Tel: (301) 584-4015
Fax:(301) 594-4027

Centers for Disease Control and Prevention

Advisory Committee on
Immunization Practices
Centers for Disease Control and
Prevention
Mailstop A-20
Atlanta, GA 30333
Tel: (404) 639-3851

Advisory Council for the Elimination
of Tuberculosis
Center for Disease Control and
Prevention
1600 Clifton Rd.. NE
Mailstop EO7
Atlanta, GA 30333
Tel: (404)639-8000
Fax: (404)639-8600

Lead Poisoning Prevention Branch
Division of Environmental Hazards
and Health Effects
National Center for Environmental
Health
Center for Disease Control and
Prevention
4770 Buford Highway, NE
Mailstop F42
Atlanta, GA 30341-3724
Tel: (770)488-7330
Fax: (770)488-7335

National Institutes of Health

National Cancer Institute
Building 31, Room 10A24
Bethesda, MD 20892
Tel: (800)4-CANCER
National Eye Institute
Box 20/20
Bethesda, MD 20892
Tel: (301)496-5248

National Cholesterol Education
Program
NHLBI Information Center
P.O. Box 30105
Bethesda, MD 20824-0105
Tel: (301)251-1222
Fax: (301)251-1223

National Cholesterol Education
Program Expert Panel on Blood
Cholesterol Levels in Children and
Adolescents
NHLBI Information Center
P.O. Box 30105
Bethesda, MD 20824-0105
Tel: (301)251-1222
Fax: (301)251-1223

National Cholesterol Education
Program
Expert Panel on Detection,
Evaluation, and Treatment of High
Blood Cholesterol in Adults
NHLBI Information Center
P.O. Box 30105
Bethesda, MD 20824-0105
Tel: (301)251-1222
Fax: (301)251-1223

National High Blood Pressure
Education Program
NHLBI Information Center
P.O. Box 30105
Bethesda, MD 20824-0105
Tel: (301)251-1222
Fax: (301)251-1223

National Heart, Lung, and Blood
Institute Task Force on Blood
Pressure Control in Children
NHLBI Information Center
P.O. Box 30105
Bethesda, MD 20824-0105
Tel: (301)251-1222
Fax: (301)251-1223

National Institute of Dental Research
9000 Rockville Pike
Bethesda, MD 20892
Tel: (301)496-4261
Fax: (301 496-9988

National Institutes of Health
Consensus Development Panel on
Breast Cancer in Women Ages 40-49
NIH Consensus Program Information
Center
P.O. Box 2577
Kensington, MD 20891
Tel: (888)NIH-CONSENSUS
Fax: (301)816-2494

National Institutes of Health
Consensus Panel on Physical
Activity and Cardiovascular Health
NIH Consensus Program Information
Center
P.O. Box 2577
Kensington, MD 20891
Tel: (888)NIH-CONSENSUS
Fax: (301)816-2494

National Transportation Safety Board
490 L' Enfant Plaza East, SW
Washington, DC 20594
Tel: (202)314-6000
U.S. Department of Agriculture

Center for Nutrition Policy &
Promotion
1120 20th St., NW
Suite 200 North Tower
Washington, DC 20036
Tel: (202)418-2312
Fax: (202)208-2322

E

COPYRIGHT CONSIDERATIONS

The *Clinician's Handbook of Preventive Services* contains information that is subject to copyright; that information has been included in this publication subject to the specific terms of permission received from the copyright holders, who reserve all other rights. All such information is clearly marked in the text of the *Handbook*. It is a violation of copyright law to reproduce any copyrighted information from this publication without first obtaining separate permission from the copyright holder or holders, except as detailed herein.

That portion of the content of the *Handbook* produced by the Federal Government is in the public domain, although it is subject to certain legal restrictions: any portion reproduced must be clearly identified as Federal information produced by the U.S. Department of Health and Human Services; and the following disclaimer must appear on any information product that is linked in a substantive way with the Put Prevention Into Practice campaign or the *Handbook*— "The U.S. Department of Health and Human Services does not endorse any particular organization or its activities, products, or services." If supplemental information, such as a preface or appendix, is incorporated in a reprint, all supplemental pages must be clearly labeled as such.

The *Handbook* has been published by the U.S. Department of Health and Human Services (DHHS) through the U.S. Government Printing Office (GPO) and is available to the public through the GPO Sales Program, which markets Federal publications on a revolving-fund basis, and Federal Depository Libraries, which provide access to collections of Federal documents.

DHHS received permission to reproduce the copyrighted information in this publication subject to the following conditions:

1. Permission was granted for publication of a single edition of the *Handbook* for distribution by DHHS and GPO.

2. This edition of the *Handbook* may be reprinted by the Government or other parties (with separate permissions) only in its entirety.

3. DHHS's formal partners among voluntary and professional organizations in the Put Prevention Into Practice campaign may reprint this edition of the *Handbook*—again, only in its entirety—to promote its use in medical

and educational settings, including sale to their individual members at a price not exceeding the price set by GPO for sale to the general public.

4. Reprints of this book by other parties shall not include the use of the DHHS or PHS seals.

Any organization or individual intending to make commercial use of any of the copyrighted information in the *Handbook* must obtain separate permission from all copyright holders. ("Commercial use" is defined as incorporation of any portion of the *Handbook* that is subject to copyright in another publication or sale of reprints of the *Handbook* at a price higher than that set by GPO for sale to the general public.)

Index

CLINICIAN'S HANDBOOK
OF PREVENTIVE SERVICES

Note that page numbers followed by "f" designate figures; those followed by "t" designate tables.

☆ U. S. GOVERNMENT PRINTING OFFICE: 1998-434-007